Disclaimer of Liability

The Essential Brain Injury Guide has been prepared under the auspices of the Brain Injury Association of America. The information in this guide reflects the current state of knowledge at the time of its revision in November 2006. It is designed to provide useful information with the recognition that there will be future developments in scientific information and technology. The Essential Brain Injury Guide will be periodically reviewed and updated.

The Essential Brain Injury Guide is distributed with the understanding that the Brain Injury Association of America and the Academy of Certified Brain Injury Specialists are not engaged in rendering professional rehabilitation services. If rehabilitation or medical advice or assistance is required, the services of a competent rehabilitation professional or physician should be sought.

The recommendations contained in the Essential Brain Injury Guide may not be appropriate for use in all circumstances. The decision to adopt any particular recommendation or procedure contained in the Essential Brain Injury Guide is the sole responsibility of the individual using the Essential Brain Injury Guide and is not the responsibility of any individual associated with the Brain Injury Association of America, the Academy of Certified Brain Injury Specialists, or the publisher of the Essential Brain Injury Guide. Any and all use of any recommendations or procedures in the Essential Brain Injury Guide should be based upon the facts and circumstances in each particular case and on the basis of all available resources.

This manual provides a body of knowledge that can be utilized in preparation for brain injury specialist certification. Purchase or use of this manual does not represent a guarantee of certification.

Copyright 2009 © Academy of Certified Brain Injury Specialists,
Brain Injury Association of America.

All rights reserved. No part of the publication may be reproduced in whole or in part without prior written permission.

Design and layout, Heidi Reyst, PhD, CBIST
Rainbow Rehabilitation Centers, Inc., Livonia, MI

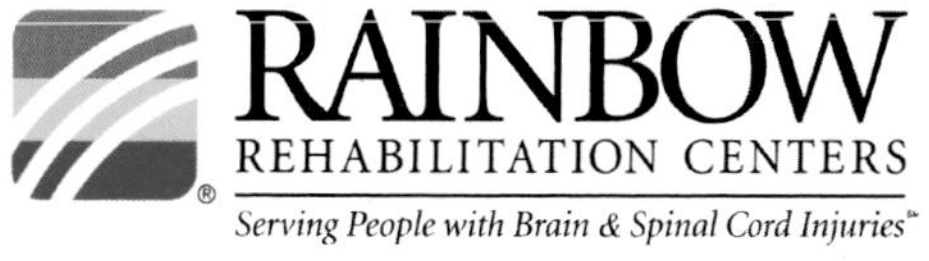

The Academy of Certified Brain Injury Specialists and the Brain Injury Association of America would like to thank the following companies who contributed to the inaugural printing of the Essential Brain Injury Guide:

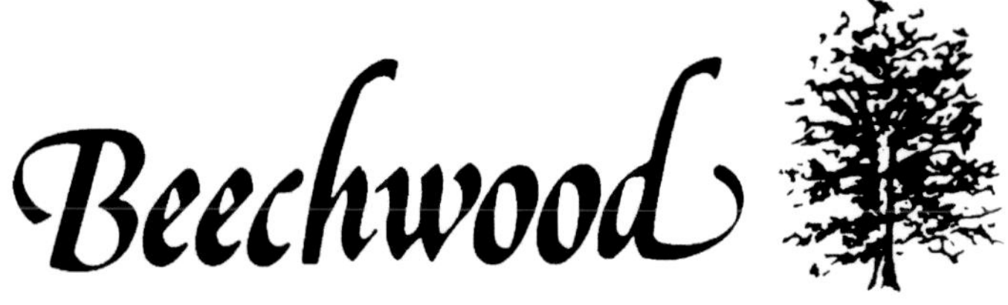

Beechwood Rehabilitation Services
A Program of Woods Services
469 East Maple Avenue
Langhorne, PA 19047
(800) 782-3299
www.beechwoodrehab.org
Inaugural and second printing sponsor

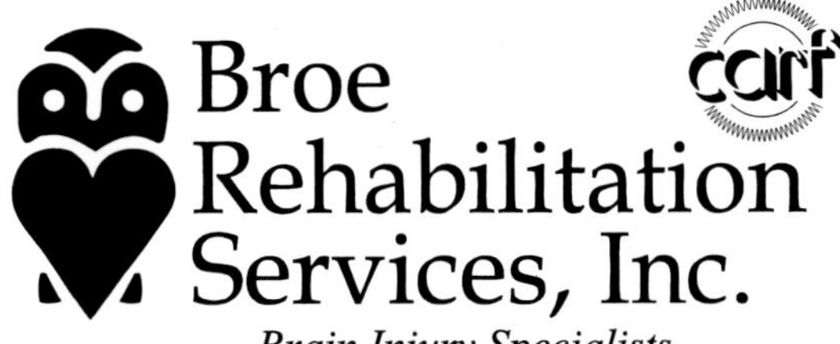

Broe Rehabilitation
Services, Inc.
33634 W. 8 Mile Road
Farmington Hills, MI 48335
(248) 476-4990
www.broerehab.com
Inaugural printing sponsor

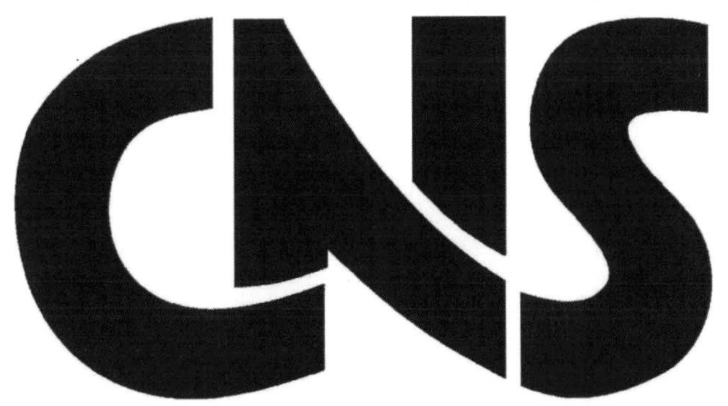

3650 Mt Vernon Avenue, Bakersfield, CA 93306
1320 West Walnut Hill Lane, Irving, Texas 75038
16542 Ventura Blvd., Suite 500, Encino, CA 91436
800-922-4994
www.neuroskills.com
Inaugural printing sponsor

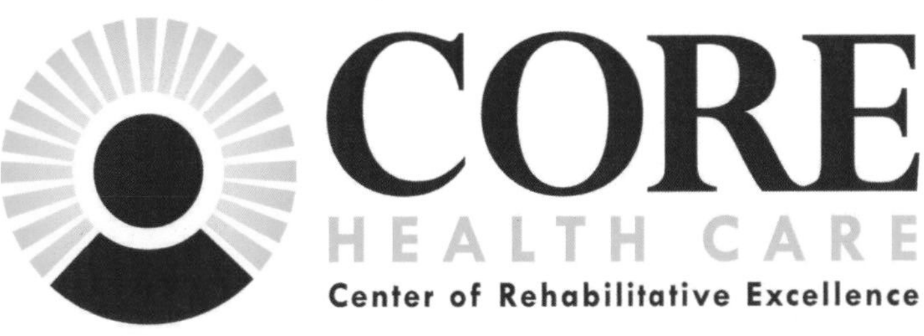

CORE Health Care
P.O. Box 419
Dripping Springs, TX 78620
(866) 683-1007
www.corehealth.com
Inaugural and second printing sponsor

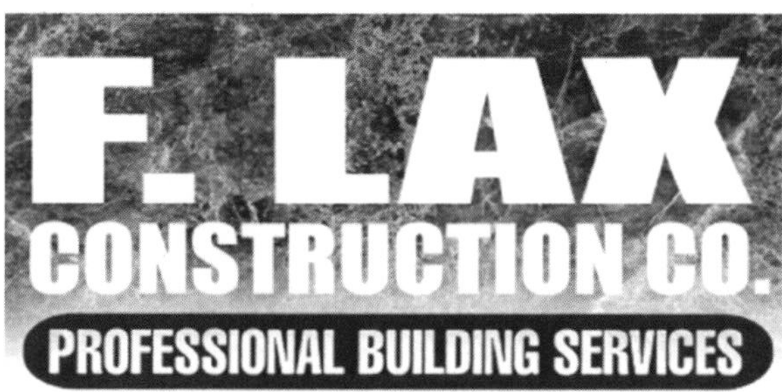

Barrier Free Modifications

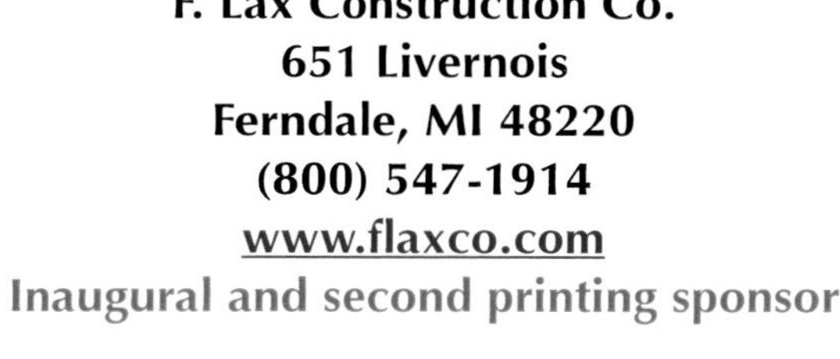

F. Lax Construction Co.
651 Livernois
Ferndale, MI 48220
(800) 547-1914
www.flaxco.com
Inaugural and second printing sponsor

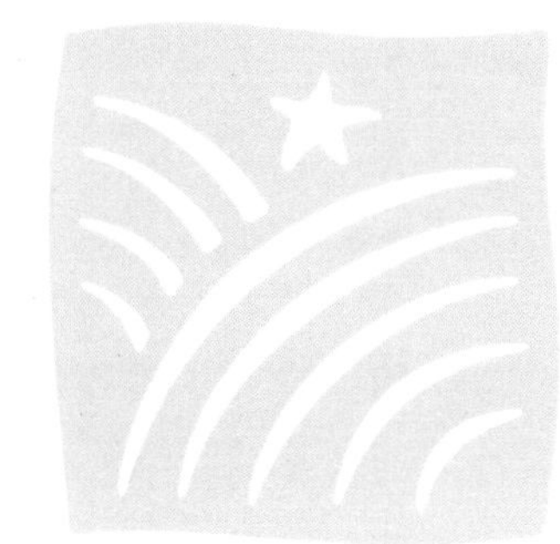

Healthcare Associates:
Northeast Center for Special Care
300 Grant Avenue
Lake Katrine, NY 12449
(854) 336-7899
Fax (845) 336-7899
www.northeastcenter.com
Inaugural printing sponsor

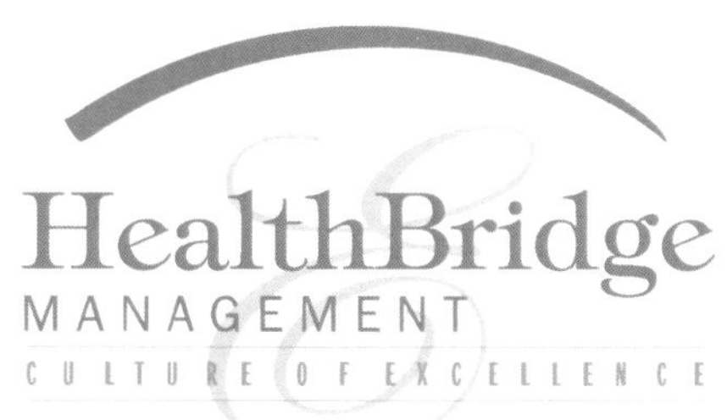

Healthbridge
57 Old Road to Nine Acre Corner
Concord, MA 01742
978-318-9425
866-999-9498
Fax (978) 318-0462
www.healthbridgecareers.com
Inaugural and second printing sponsor

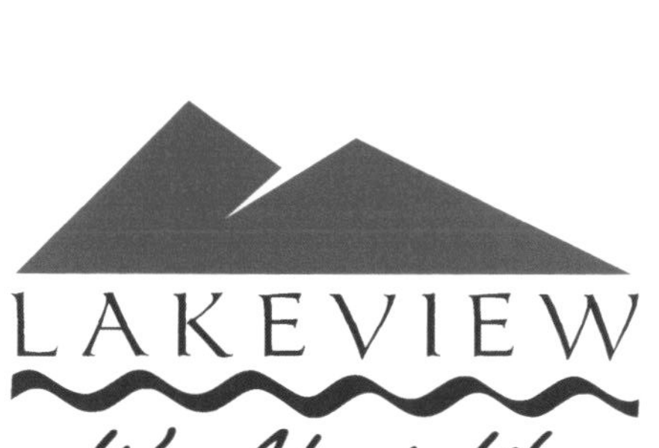

Lakeview NeuroRehabilitation Center
244 Highwatch Road
Effingham, NH 03882
(800) 473-4221
www.lakeviewsystem.com
Inaugural and second printing sponsor

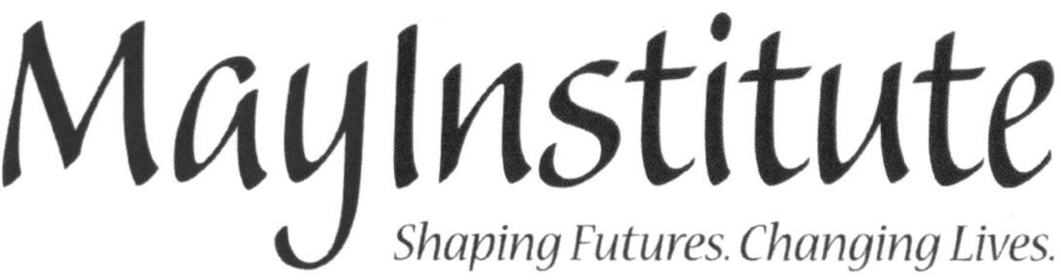

May Center for Education & Neurorehabilitation
(May Institute)
596 Summer Street, Brockton MA 02302
508-588-8800, 800-778-7601
www.mayinstitute.org
Inaugural printing sponsor

The Academy of Certified Brain Injury Specialists and the Brain Injury Association of America would like to thank the following companies who contributed to the inaugural printing of the Essential Brain Injury Guide:

MENTOR ABI

MENTOR ABI
www.mentorabi.com
800-203-5394
abiinfo@thementornetwork.com
Inaugural printing sponsor

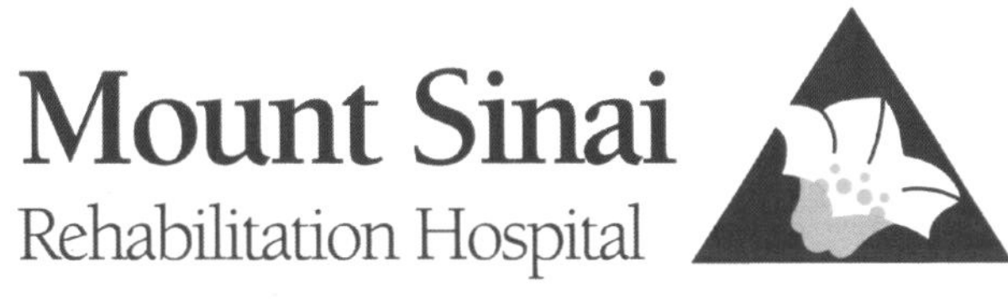

a SAINT FRANCIS *Care* Provider

Mount Sinai Rehabilitation Hospital
490 Bluehills Avenue
Hartford, CT 06112
(860) 714-3500
(800) 789-7709
www.rehabct.com
Inaugural and second printing sponsor

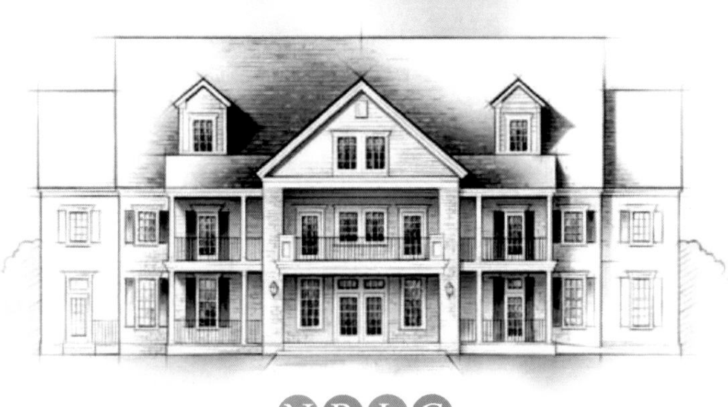

NRLC
Neurological Rehabilitation Living Centers

Neurological Rehabilitation Living Centers
Robert Voogt & Associates, Inc.
1851 Old Donation Parkway
Virginia Beach, VA 23454
(757) 481-5772 Voice
(757) 481-12147 Fax
rva@rvarehab.com
Inaugural printing sponsor

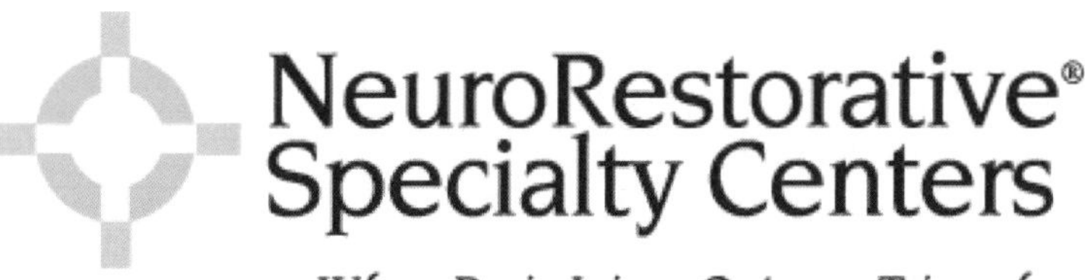

... Where Brain Injury Outcome Triumphs

Neurorestorative Specialty Centers
4500 West Commercial Drive
North Little Rock, AR 72116
(501) 758-8799
(800) 743-6802 Referral
www.neurorestorative.com
Inaugural and second printing sponsor

NRC
NEURO-REHABILITATION
CENTERS AT
MIDDLEBORO & WORCESTER

A WINGATE HEALTHCARE COMMUNITY
www.neurorehabcenters.com

Wingate Healthcare
1 Charles River Place
63 Kendrick St
Needham, MA 02494
www.neurorehabcenters.com
Inaugural and second printing sponsor

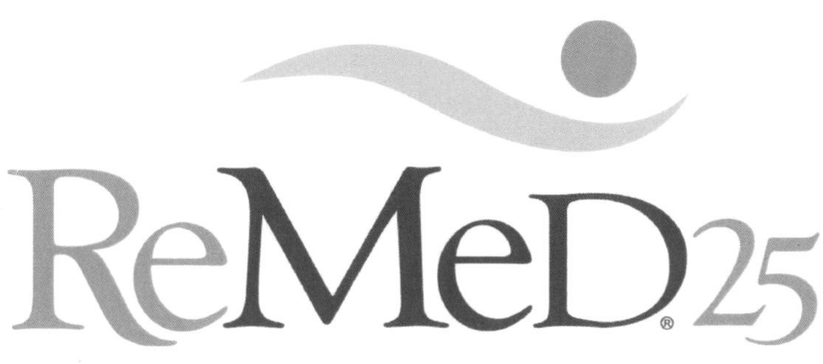

ReMed
16 Industrial Boulevard
Suite 201
Paoli, PA 19301
(800) 84ReMed
(484) 595-9300
www.remed.com
Inaugural and second printing sponsor

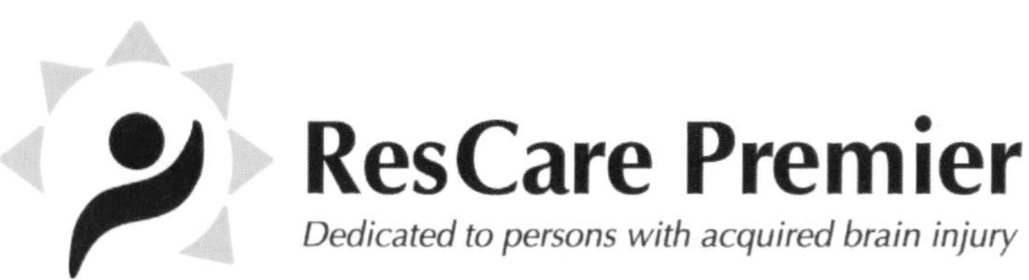

ResCare Premier
220 W. Hutchison St.
San Marcos, TX 78666
800.28.brain
(800) 282-7246
www.rescarepremiertexas.com
Inaugural printing sponsor

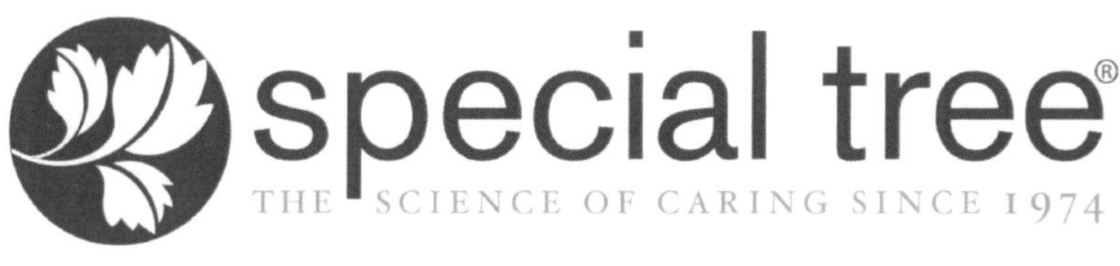

Special Tree
Rehabilitation System
39000 Chase Rd.
Romulus, MI 48174
(800) 648-6885
www.specialtree.com
Inaugural and second printing sponsor

Western Michigan Brain Injury Network

Hope Network Rehabilitation Services

Mary Free Bed Rehabilitation Hospital

Spectrum Health Continuing Care Neurorehabilitation Services

Inaugural and second printing sponsor

Table of Contents

Chapters

The Brain Injury Associaton of America & the Academy of Certified Brain Injury Specialists gratefully acknowledge the contributions of the chapter authors:

Chapter 1: Overview of Brain Injury

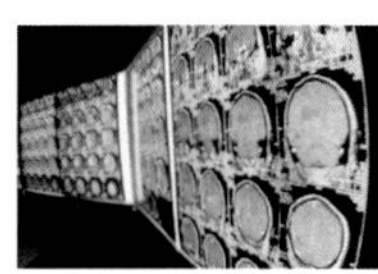

Cathy Ficker-Terrill, MS
Karen Flippo, MRA
Terri Antoinette, MHSA, RNC
Debra Braunling McMorrow, PhD

Chapter 2: Philosophy of Rehabilitation

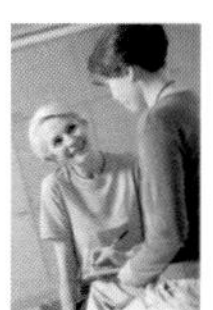

Al Condeluci, PhD
Marty McMorrow, MS

Chapter 3: Understanding the Brain & Brain Injury

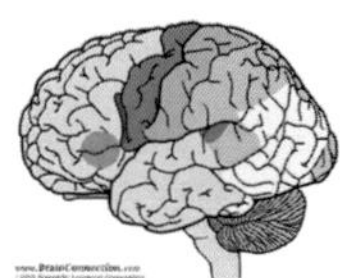

Ron Savage, EdD

Chapter 4: Health, Medications and Medical Management

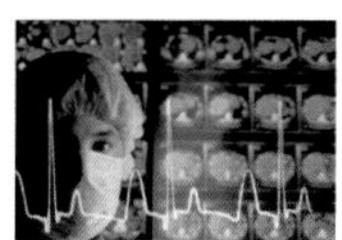

Terry Page, PhD

Chapter 5: Understanding & Treating Functional Impacts of Brain Injury

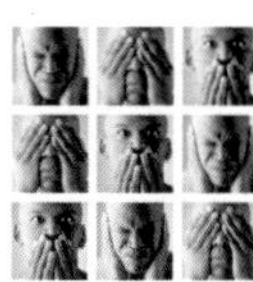

Terri Antoinette, MHSA, RNC
David Strauss, PhD
Tina Trudel, PhD

Chapter 6: Children and Adolescents with Brain Injuries

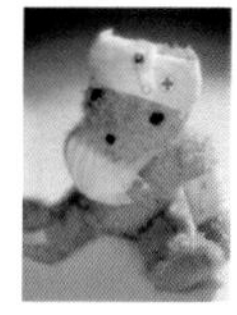

Ron Savage, EdD
Janet Tyler, PhD

Chapter 7: Family

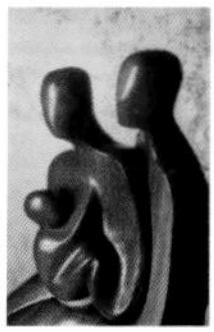

Debra Russell, PhD

Chapter 8: Legal and Ethical Issues

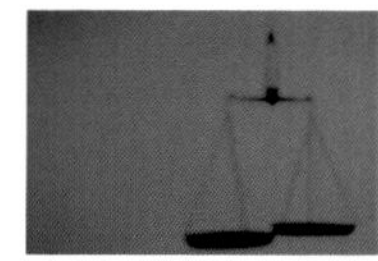

Harvey Jacobs, PhD
Kevin Ann Huckshorn, RN, MSN, CAP
Allan Bergman
Anne Parrette Rohall, Esq

The Essential Brain Injury Guide is a revised version of the previously published ACBIS Training Manual (versions I, II and III). This fourth printing incorporates the work of many dedicated professionals during the publication's history. BIAA and ACBIS gratefully acknowledge the work of Marilyn Lash, MSW as editor and Heidi Reyst, PhD, CBIST as graphic designer. We would also like to thank the following individuals whose contributions made this guide such a valuable resource.

Terri Antoinette, MHSA, RNC
Andrea Beaudry
Debra Braunling McMorrow, PhD
Lynley Ebeling
Elie Elovic, MD
Harvey Jacobs, PhD

Linda Mackay, MA, CCC-SLP, BRS-S, CBIST
George Mendez, RN
Ann Pereira-Ogan, BA
Linda Robinson, RN, MAMS
Janet Tyler, PhD
Jeff Victoroff, MD

Acknowledgment

The Academy of Certified Brain Injury Specialists (ACBIS), a program administered under the auspices of the Brain Injury Association of America, was created in 1996 to address a growing need to provide a standard of training for persons working with those with brain injury. The second edition of the manual was published in 1998 and reprinted in 1999.

During the last decade, ACBIS has grown into a nationally recognized certification body with a mission to improve the quality of care by establishing accepted competency standards for the education and training of individuals working in brain injury rehabilitation. Current certifications include Certified Brain Injury Specialists (CBIS) and Certified Brain Injury Specialist Trainers (CBIST).

In the process of establishing ACBIS and the training curriculum and certifications, a great deal of collaboration was sought from experts in the field, family members and brain injury survivors. It is due to this tremendous support and participation that we have been able to provide these updated and enhanced materials to better train those working with persons with brain injury and their families, and thereby provide a higher quality of support for individuals with brain injury.

We thank all who have generously contributed to this process. We commend each of you for participating in this training and certification program and we are confident that your certification will serve you well in your career in the field of brain injury. Thank you for helping us to create a better future.

Jim Misko, PsyD
Chair - Board of Governors
Academy of Certified Brain Injury Specialists

Susan H. Connors
President and CEO
Brain Injury Association of America

ACBIS Board of Governors

Chairperson

James Misko, Psy.D., CBIST
Brown-Karhan Healthcare

Immediate Past Chair

Linda Mackay, MA, CCC-SLP, BRS-S, CBIST
St. Francis Hospital & Medical Center/
The Mount Sinai Rehabilitation Hospital

Chairperson Elect

Erika Mountz, MBA, OTR/L, CBIST
Children's Hospital of Philadelphia

Vice Chairperson for Finances

Michael P. Mozzoni, Ph.D., BCBA, CBIST
Timber Ridge Ranch

Vice Chairperson for Information Management

Heidi Reyst, Ph.D., CBIST
Rainbow Rehabilitation Centers, Inc.

Vice Chairperson for Governance

Thomas Hall, MA, CBIST
Wingate Healthcare -
Post Acute Neurobehavioral Care

Committee Members

Cynthia Boyer, Ph.D.
Bancroft Neurohealth

Julie Buxton, OTR/L, CBIST
Children's Hospital of Philadelphia

Ellen Deibert, MD, CBIST, CIC
Berkshire Medical Center

Brant A. (Bud) Elkind, MS, CBIST
Robin Hill Farm, Inc.

Caroline Feller, MS, OTR, CCM, CBIST
Mentor ABI

Marianne Fenoglietto, CCM, CBIST
UPMC IRR at UPMC South Side

Mary Ferraro, Ph.D., OTRL
Drucker Brain Injury Center

Sharon Grandinette, MS, CBIST
ABI Educational Consultant and Trainer

Ken Handwerger, MA
Special Tree Rehabilitation System

Angie Jackson, MS-CCC/SLP, CBIST
Pate Rehab

Michael Mason, CBIS
Neurological Rehabilitation Institute
at Brookhaven Hospital

Lucille Raia, RN, MS, ARNP, GNP, NEA-BC, CBIST
James A. Haley VAMC

Eric Spier, MD
Mentis Neuro

Beth Spriegel, MS
Remed

ACBIS board members are accomplished professionals in brain injury rehabilitation.
They have varied educational backgrounds, and professional expertise.

To Obtain More Information about the Academy of Certified Brain Injury Specialists, to apply to become ACBIS certified, or to order additional manuals, please contact:

Brain Injury Association of America
1608 Spring Hill Road, Suite 110
Vienna, VA 22182
Tel 703.761.0750 Fax 703.761.0755
www.biausa.org

email: acbis@biausa.org
www.acbis.pro

To speak with the ACBIS program coordinator,
call 703.761.0750

Foreword

The ACBIS program is predicated on the value that individuals sustaining a brain injury shall receive superior service leading to outcomes that enhance their quality of life. Skill, sensitivity, and competence are necessary attributes of a brain injury specialist. To deliver services and supports to persons with brain injuries, the specialist is required to understand the causes, incidences, epidemiology, treatment modalities, community services, and funding sources and requirements. Familiarity with laws and regulations that guarantee rights and fund treatment, from the onset of an injury through community reentry or long-term care, is paramount. Knowledge and skills are essential, but equally important are the embracing principles and values that guide practice. In the United States, there are at least 3.17 to 5.3 million individuals living with traumatic brain injuries – each of them has a story. Each story is different, and each requires a professional approach that is respectful, person-centered, and outcome focused. This manual begins with the story of two individuals who have sustained traumatic brain injuries. Their words express what they expect from service providers.

Dear Caregivers:

Hello, we are two young men, roommates, people who have survived brain injury, living in the community in our own apartment. We primarily depend on people outside of our families for support. However, we have both had the experience of living in institutions also - a nursing home and a group home. Even though we are both survivors of brain injury, we are each very different - unique, if you will. If you get nothing else from this introduction, we hope you will understand and remember that.

When we sustained our brain injuries, we were instantly different. If you have not lived through such an experience, it is impossible for you to understand all the feelings and emotions. Please don't tell us you do understand unless you are another survivor of brain injury!! Because you can't possibly. However, you can ask us how we feel - give us a chance to work through all of the emotions we are experiencing, especially those of loss - loss of the person we were.

Our bodies changed, our personalities changed. We may never be who we were before, but with your help we can be 100% of who we are now. Please allow us to ask for that help - don't just assume you know what we need. We need to be allowed to try to succeed on our own, and even permitted to fail - just like the rest of the world. Allow us to take responsibility for ourselves - even encourage us to do this. Help us find our strengths, but not by pointing out our weaknesses. Help us learn strategies that compensate for our weaknesses. Help us learn to ask for accommodations that we need, how to advocate for ourselves.

Put yourself in our shoes for a moment. You're in a wheelchair. You are capable of speaking for yourself but can't, because your brain injury left you without speech for the most part. We both use augmentative communication devices. We will depend on you to help us with them. Please be patient - give us time to get our points across. Don't assume you know what we're going to say. We beg you to try and see the world through our eyes, with our perspective. Don't force your perspective on us. Challenge us, but accept us. Take the time to really get to know us, even though we aren't easy to understand.

Neither of us is paralyzed, but both of us are restricted in our movements - both in different ways. Remember we will depend on you to even help us shift our positions - a normal person wouldn't sit long periods in the same position, neither should we. Even though we both use wheelchairs, we both enjoy getting out of them and sitting on our "regular" furniture - sofa and recliners. You would get tired of sitting in just one chair all day, day after day - so do we. Help make everything in our world accessible to us. We want to be as independent as possible, so allow us to try to do things on our own. Help when we ask - not before. It is so easy to just do something for us, but please don't get in that habit. It diminishes us and you.

We need friends just like anyone else. Just because you are our caregiver doesn't mean you can't be our friend. We would much prefer you be our friend and companion, not just "caregiver" in the strictest sense of the word. Relationships are just as important to us as they are to you. We like to kid around and joke just like you do. We like to go shopping, see movies, and just "hang out" in the community. Isolation is a terrible thing. It makes us question whether we have any worth. Please don't allow anyone to isolate us - it diminishes our value. All we want is to live, love, laugh and pray - just like everyone else. Above all, please recognize that we still have dreams – just like everyone else. Help us find our inner worth and live each day to its fullest, always remembering the sky's the limit!!

Please let us choose who we want as caregivers. For instance, we're both more comfortable with male caregivers for our personal needs, but we enjoy the company of females out in the community. Talk to us - ask us what our preferences are. We understand that sometimes we may have to use someone we aren't really fond of because of scheduling problems. But for the most part, please try to give us a choice. Think of having your most personal needs taken care of by someone you are totally uncomfortable with. You wouldn't like it - neither do we.

Please let us know what we can do to make your job easier and better, what we can do for you. We want this to be a career for you - not just a job!! It is important to us that we have a stable surrounding, yes, a home - not just lots of people coming and going.

As we said in the beginning, remember first and foremost that we are individuals - your help needs to be specific to our individual needs. This isn't a "one size fits all" kind of job. Above all, remember, we have brain injuries, but we are persons first - just like you. We want and need dignity and respect - just like you.

Thank you for letting us introduce you to our world - living with a brain injury!

Robert "Bear" Packwood
Jamie (J.J.) Rose
January 1, 1998

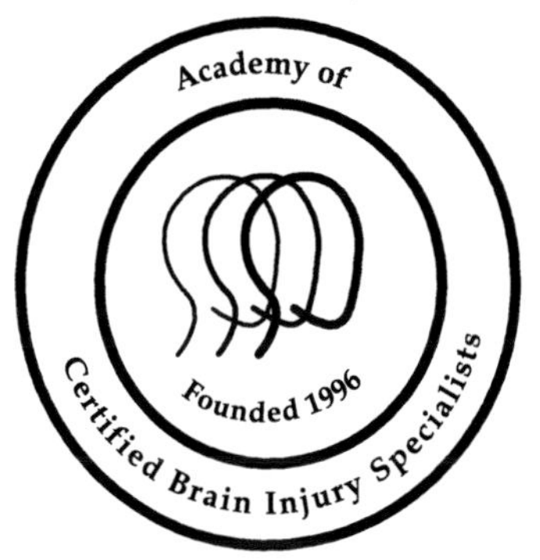
Academy of
Founded 1996
Certified Brain Injury Specialists

Chapter 1

Overview of Brain Injury

Learning Objectives

By the end of this chapter, you will be able to:

- Describe the incidence, prevalence and epidemiology of brain injury.
- Distinguish between traumatic brain injury and acquired brain injury.
- Describe systems of care available in the rehabilitation continuum.
- Demonstrate several of the funding issues for the support of persons with brain injury.
- Explain the Traumatic Brain Injury Act of 1996 and its impact on services and funding for persons with brain injury.

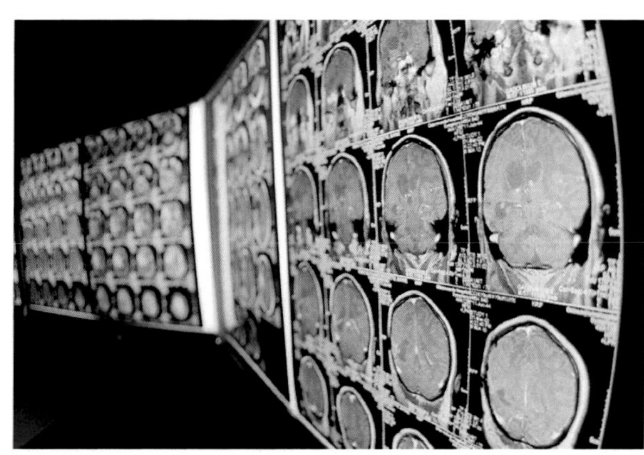

Introduction

"Traumatic brain injury (TBI) is an important public health problem in the United States. Because the problems that result from TBI, such as those of thinking and memory, are often not visible, and because awareness about TBI among the general public is limited, it is frequently referred to as the "silent epidemic."

The preceding quote is from the Centers for Disease Control (CDC) report on Traumatic Brain Injury in the United States: Emergency Department Visits, Hospitalizations, and Deaths (Langlois, Rutland-Brown & Thomas 2006, p. 3). It highlights the relative lack of awareness about brain injury that continues to exist. Brain injury is indeed a public health problem, and understanding the incidence and prevalence of brain injury is one way for brain injury specialists to help spread awareness about this epidemic. But before brain injury epidemiology is addressed, it is important to clearly understand the definitions of brain injury.

Definitions

Establishing a uniform working definition has been difficult and controversial. No universal definition can be all inclusive and uniform for surveillance and research, yet simple and understandable enough to facilitate public response to education and prevention efforts. In 1986, the National Head Injury Foundation (NHIF), now known as the Brain Injury Association of America (BIAA), adopted a definition of traumatic brain injury. This definition is used in data registries and serves as a standard definition for use by lay and professional advocates in the development of services.

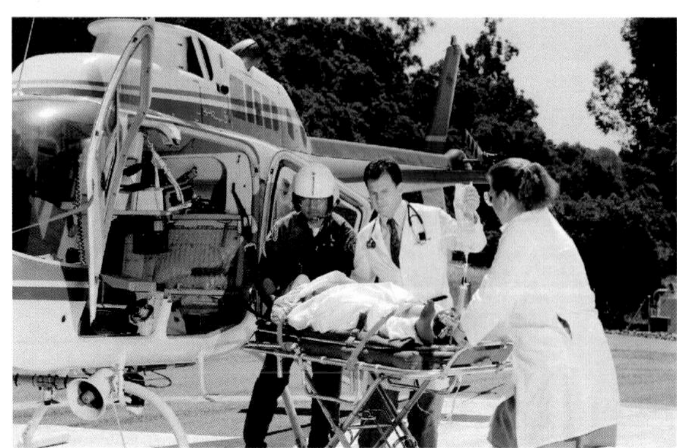

Traumatic Brain Injury

Traumatic brain injury (TBI) is an insult to the brain, not of a degenerative or congenital nature but caused by an external physical force, that may produce a diminished or altered state of consciousness, which results in an impairment of cognitive abilities and/or physical functioning. It can also result in the disturbance of behavioral or emotional functioning. These impairments may be either temporary or permanent and cause partial or total functional disability or psychosocial maladjustment.

In 1997, the Brain Injury Association of America adopted a definition of acquired brain injury (ABI) to broaden the definition of brain injury beyond that only produced by trauma.

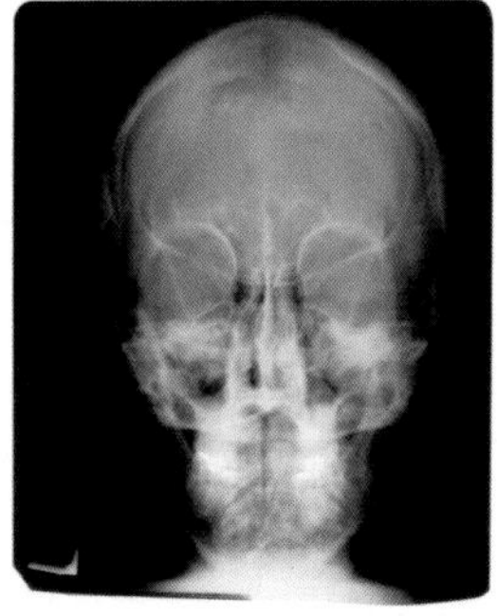

Acquired Brain Injury

An acquired brain injury (ABI) is an injury to the brain that has occurred after birth and is not hereditary, congenital or degenerative. The injury commonly results in a change in neuronal activity, which affects the physical integrity, the metabolic activity, or the functional ability of the cell. The term does not refer to brain injuries induced by birth trauma.

The definition of an acquired brain injury is more comprehensive and includes not only injuries caused by the trauma of external physical force applied to the head and/or neck (TBI), but also internal insults to the brain.

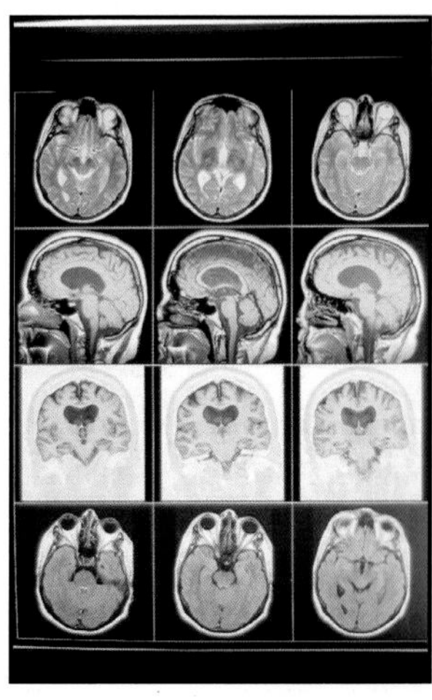

An acquired brain injury may result in mild, moderate, or severe impairments in one or more areas including:

- **Cognition**
  (e.g., speech & language communication; memory, attention and concentration, reasoning, and abstract thinking).

- **Physical functions**
  (e.g., ambulating, seeing, hearing, balancing).

Causes of Acquired Brain Injury

- TBI.
- Tumors.
- Blood Clots.
- Strokes.
- Seizures.
- Toxic Exposures (e.g., substance abuse, ingestion of lead, inhalation of volatile agents).
- Infections (encephalitis, meningitis).
- Metabolic Disorders (insulin shock, diabetic coma, liver and kidney disease).
- Neurotoxic Poisoning (airway obstruction, strangulation, cardiopulmonary arrest, carbon monoxide poisoning, drowning).
- Lack of oxygen to the brain.

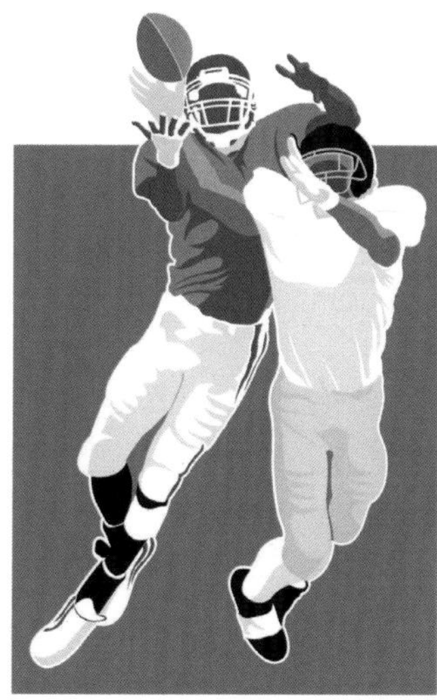

- **Psychosocial behavior**
  (e.g., social skills, anger management, impulsivity).

Any of these impairments often are the cause of major stresses in peer and family relationships as well as educational and employment settings.

While it is important to understand the different definitions of brain injury, the term brain injury is used throughout this manual to refer to acquired brain injury. When reference is specifically made to injury caused by trauma due to external physical force, the term traumatic brain injury (TBI) is used.

Causes of Traumatic Brain Injury

- Motor Vehicle Crashes.
- Falls.
- Gunshot Wounds.
- Sports Injuries.
- Workplace Injuries.
- Shaken Baby Syndrome.
- Child Abuse.
- Domestic Violence.
- Military Actions.
- Other injuries caused by trauma.

Another distinction is open versus closed head injuries. An open head injury occurs when the skull has been penetrated and the brain is exposed. A closed head injury occurs when the skull is intact but the brain has been impacted.

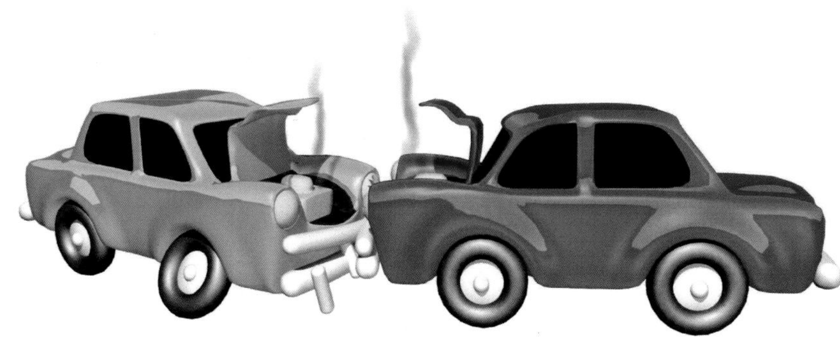

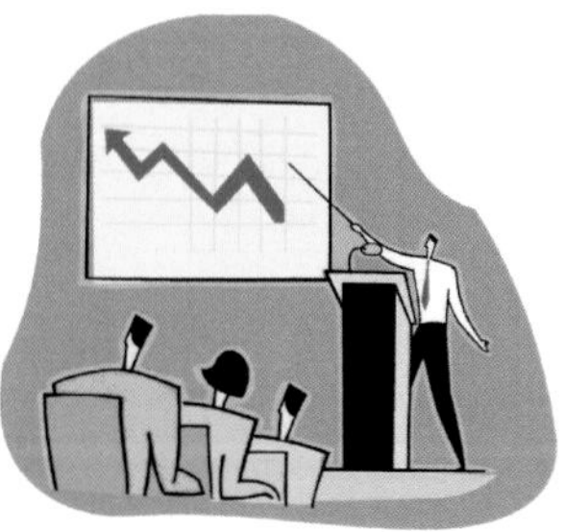

Epidemiology of Traumatic Brain Injury

A traumatic brain injury can happen to a child or adult of any age, race, gender, religion or socioeconomic status. In other words, it does not discriminate. But it may disproportionately affect some groups of people more than others. For that reason, it is important to quantify how, and to whom, brain injury happens. This is done by conducting surveillance.

Through the process of surveillance, an objective determination can be made regarding the number of traumatic brain injuries that occur, where and how they occur and which population groups are at highest risk. Specifically, it provides incidence and prevalence rates (see the sidebar below for definitions). This information helps program planners effectively allocate resources for prevention and improve the quality and delivery of care.

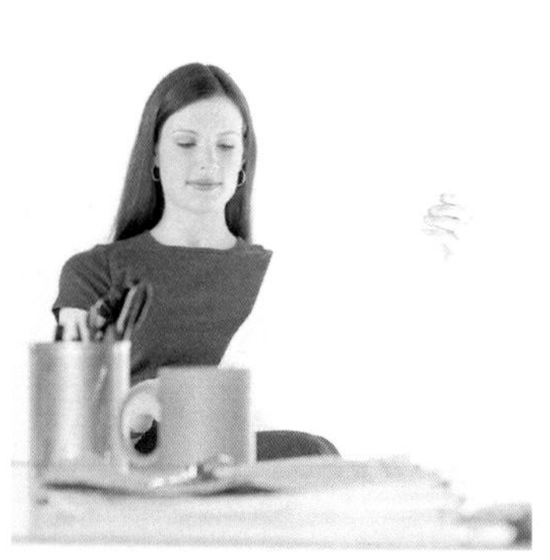

Surveillance

Surveillance is the ongoing and systematic collection, analysis and interpretation of data used to describe and monitor a health event.

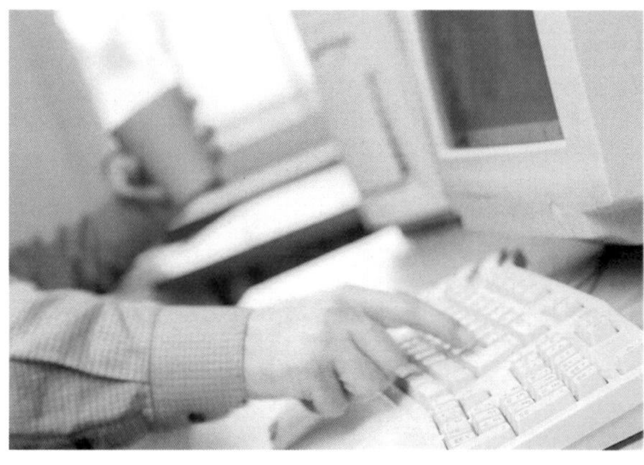

Epidemiology

Epidemiology is a branch of medical science that deals with the incidence, distribution, and control of disease in a population.

Incidence

Incidence is the number of cases of disease having their **onset** during a prescribed period of time. the It is a measure of morbidity or other events that occur within a specified period of time, and is often expressed as a rate.

Example:

- In 2005, 1.5 million new case of diabetes were diagnosed in people aged 20 or older.

Prevalence

Prevalence is the number of cases of a disease **present** during a particular interval of time. It is often expressed as a rate.

Examples:

- In 2005, 20.8 million people were living with diabetes.
- In 2005, about 1 in every 400-600 children had Type I diabetes.
- In 2005, 12.8% of American Indians / Alaska Natives over age 20 had diagnosed diabetes.

All definitions and data from www.cdc.gov.

Prevalence

Earlier in the chapter it was noted that TBI is called the "Silent Epidemic." When looking at prevalence data for rates of disability due to various types of ailments, it is clear that brain injury is prevalent, and it is less clear why so few know about it's public health impact. In comparison with other persons with disabilities, traumatic brain injury ranks third in prevalence. Yet, it remains a largely unrecognized major public health problem.

Figure 1 presents rates of disability in the general population of Americans. The numbers show that there are approximately:

- 18.8 million: depressive disorders (National Institute of Mental Health).
- 6.2. - 7.5 million: mental retardation (Association for Retarded Citizens).
- 3.17 - 5.3 million: TBI CDC.
- 4.7 million: stroke (Stroke Association).
- 4 million: Alzheimer's disease (Alzheimer's Association).
- 2.3 million: epilepsy (CDC).
- 500,000: cerebral palsy (United Cerebral Palsy).
- 200,000: spinal cord injuries (CDC).

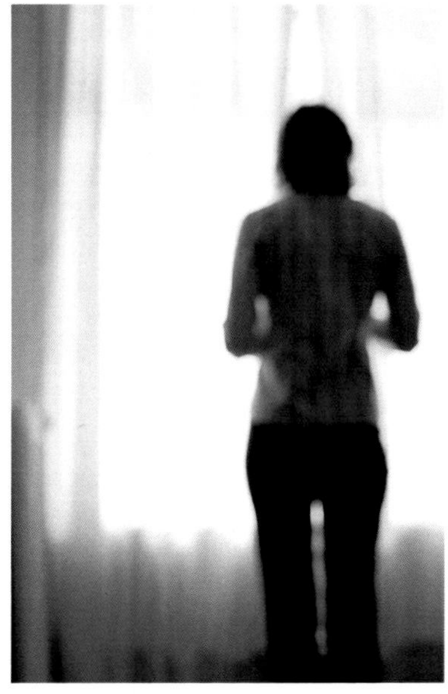

An estimated 10 million Americans are affected if the rates for disability due to Stroke (4.7 million) and TBI (5.3 million) are combined. This makes brain injury the second most prevalent injury and disability in the United States (National Institutes of Health). Overall, the number of individuals currently living with disability due to stroke and TBI combined represents 3.8 percent of the U.S. population.

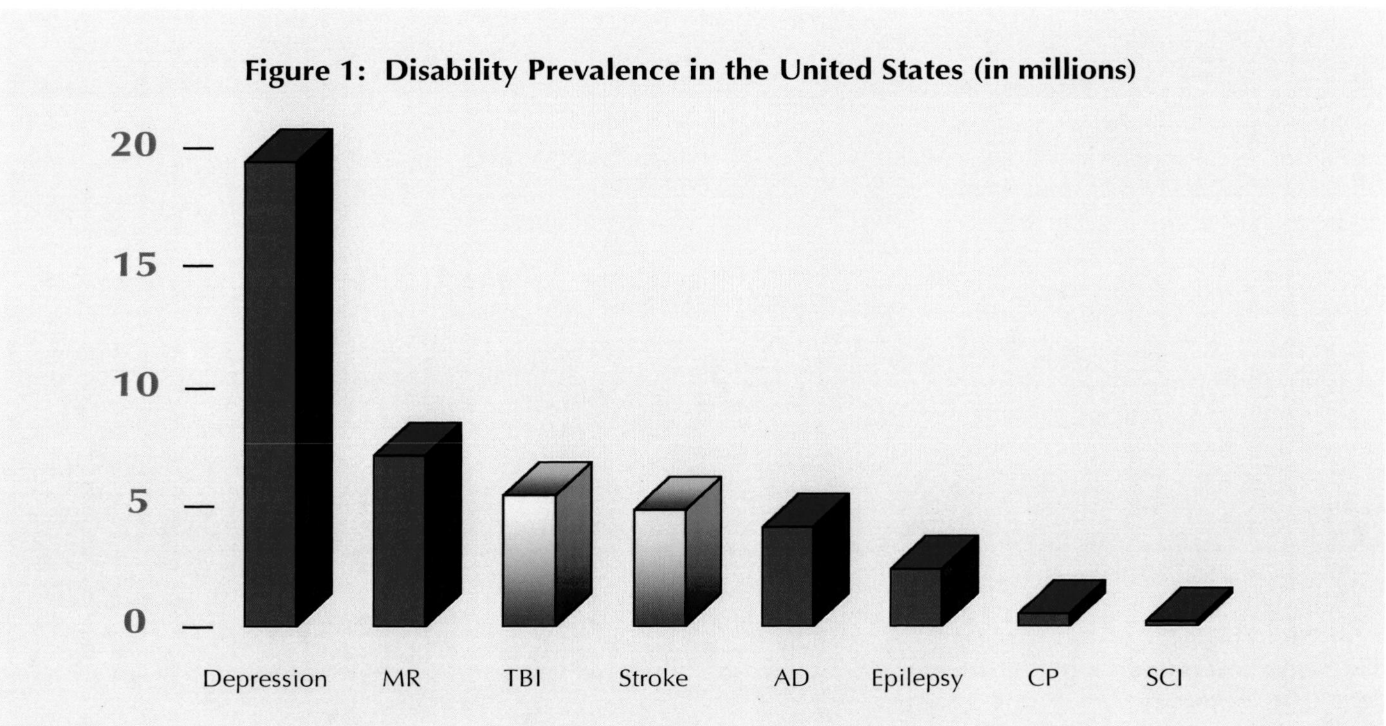

Incidence

In January of 2006, the CDC published Traumatic Brain Injury in the United States: Emergency Department Visits, Hospitalizations, and Deaths.* This publication included data from the years 1995 to 2001 for the United States population. It included hospitalization data, death data, and for the first time, emergency department (ED) visits of people treated and released.

Annual Rates of TBI

Overall, annually in the U.S., 1.4 million people sustain a traumatic brain injury. Of these 1.4 million, there are:

- 50,000 Deaths
- 235,000 Hospitalizations
- 1,100,000 ED Visits

Figure 2 highlights the overall percentages by category. Based on these numbers, if 1.4 million people sustain a TBI every year, it follows that a TBI occurs every 23 seconds in the United States. According to the CDC (2001), 80,000-90,000 Americans experience the onset of a long-term disability following traumatic brain injury each year.

Previous data from 15 state trauma registries reported an annual estimated incidence of TBI at a rate of 91 per 100,000 (Thurman, Alverson, & Dunn et al., 1999). However, it is important to note that certain variables can influence data reporting. If emergency room visits or outpatient visits without hospitalization are included, the numbers can rise dramatically. Data from the CDC report (2006), which includes ER visit numbers, show an annual incidence rate of 506 per every 100,000 persons.

**** For the remainder of this manual, this report will be referred to as the 2006 CDC Report.***

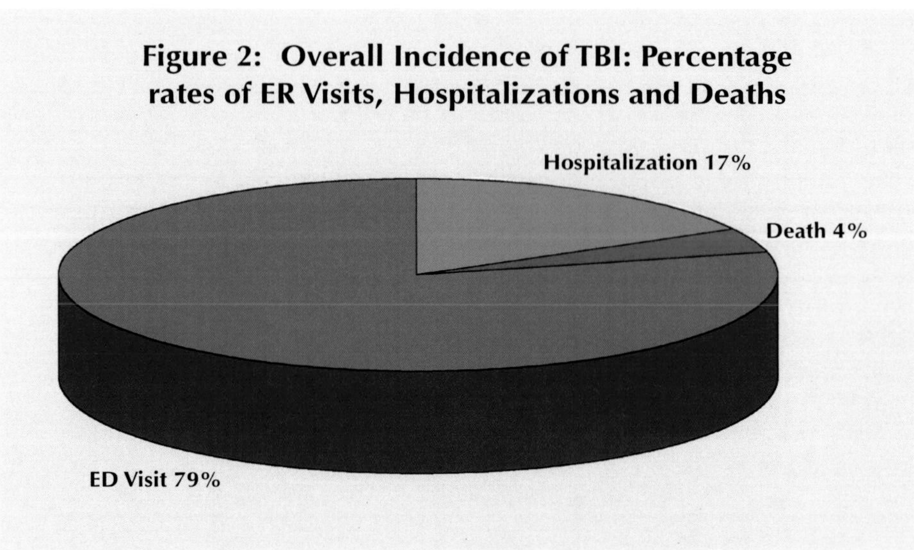

If TBI incidence data is compared against other disease data, the term silent epidemic is further reinforced. As can be seen in Figure 3, compared to some other well known health problems, TBI incidence is quite high.

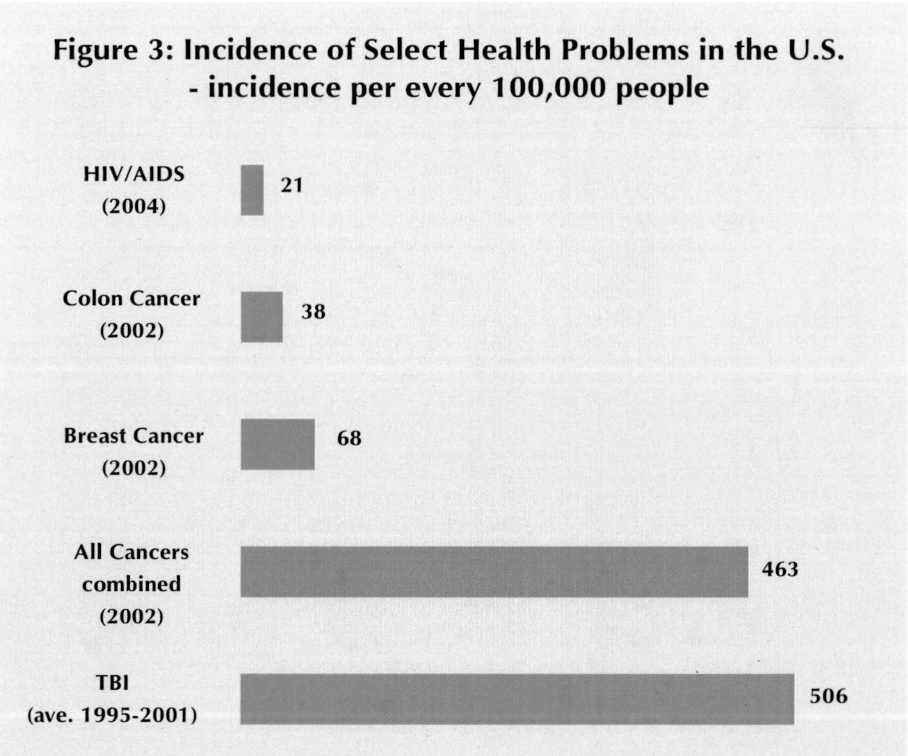

Risk Factors

The overall incidence and prevalence rates are only part of the story. What is not addressed in this data is whether these rates include individuals who have sustained multiple TBIs. This is an important issue, as it has been estimated that after incurring 1 TBI, the risk for a 2nd is 3 times greater, and when an individual sustains a 2nd TBI, the risk for another is 8 times higher. While there is not definitive information available as to how many individuals within the prevalence data have multiple TBI's, the CDC report has provided interesting data along many demographic lines. This data is presented below.

The increased morbidity and mortality among males may be related to the following factors: fire-arm use, alcohol use, work related incidents (particularly in the farming and construction fields), and/or participation in contact sports (Kraus & McArthur, 1999).

> **Risk Factors**
>
> After one TBI, the risk for a 2nd is 3 times greater.
>
> After two TBI's, the risk is 8 times greater.

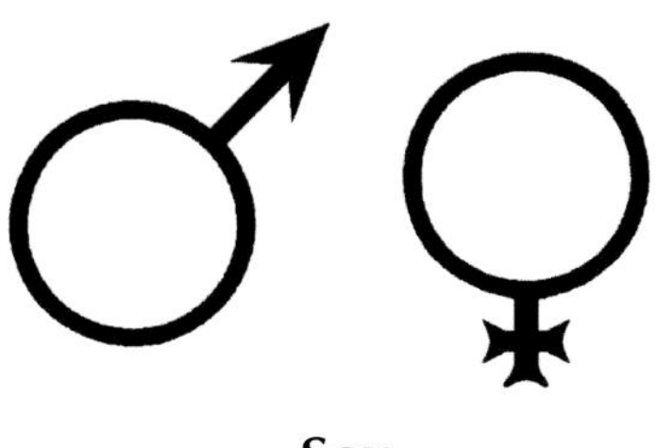

Sex

Traumatic brain injury is more common in males than females in nearly every category and for the entire spectrum of injury severity. When the 2006 CDC Report data are examined by sex, rates differed considerably. Males accounted for 59 percent of TBIs, while females account for 41 percent (Figure 4). Overall, males had 1.5 times the number of TBI's than did females.

Relative to females, males also had higher rates of hospitalization (62 % males; 38 % females), ER visits (59% males; 41 % females) and deaths due to TBI (74 % males; 26 % females). As can be seen in Figure 5, male rates of TBI exceed that of females in ER visits, hospitalizations and deaths.

Figure 4: Annual Incidence of TBI - Overall percentage rates by Sex

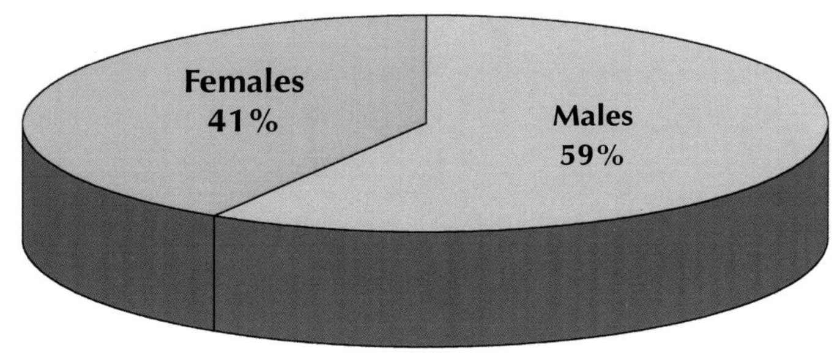

Figure 5: Annual Incidence of TBI: ER Visit, Hospitalization and Death Percentage Rates by Sex

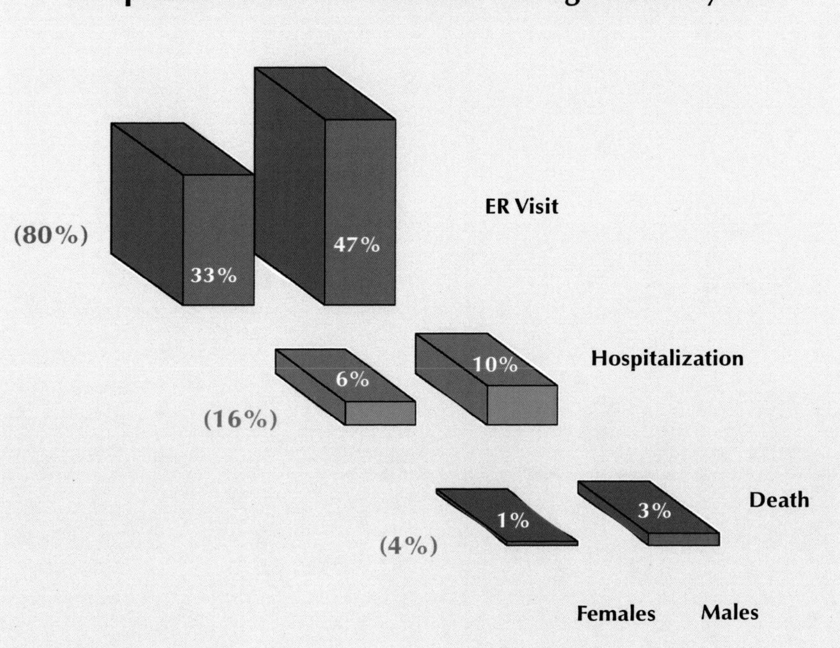

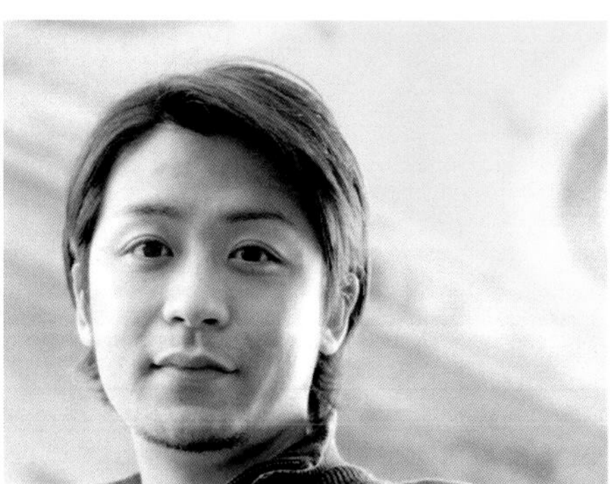

Race

Past studies have reported conflicting findings regarding the relationship between race and the incidence of traumatic brain injury. Some studies suggested that black and other non-white races have higher rates of injuries, while others suggested little difference.

In looking at the the data from the 2006 CDC Report, it is not readily apparent whether there are differences across race just by examining overall percentages as show in Figure 6. However, when examining the incidence rates per every 100,000 people by race, the numbers show that blacks have a higher incidence rate than both whites and American Indian/Alaska Native/Asian & Pacific Islander (AI/AN & API). Blacks sustain 486 TBI's per 100,000, which is 85 more than whites, and over 200 more than individuals in the category of AI/AN&API (Figure 7).

Figure 6: Overall Incidence of TBI - Percentage Rates by Race

White 81%

Black 16%

American Indian/ Alaska Native & Asian/Pacific Islander 3%

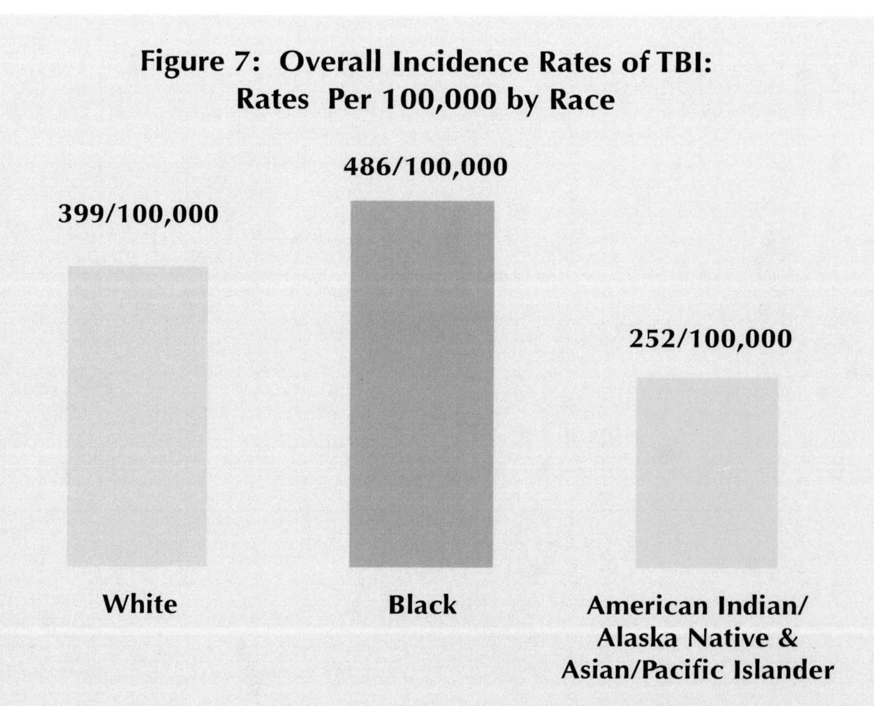

Figure 7: Overall Incidence Rates of TBI: Rates Per 100,000 by Race

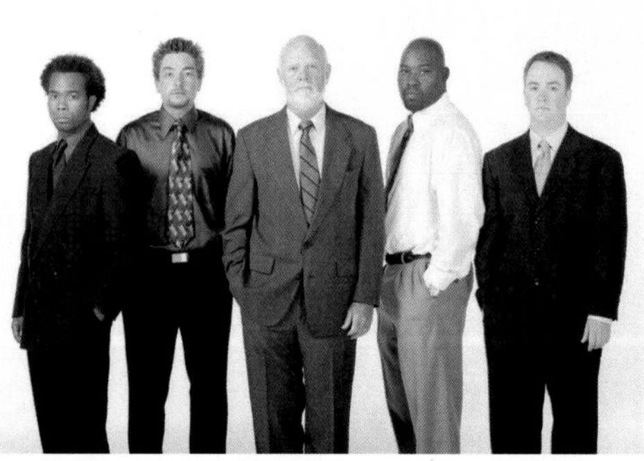

Age

Historically, the incidence of TBI has been highest in the 15-24 age group (Kraus, Black & Hessol et al., 1984; Kraus, Rock & Hemyari, 1990; Elovic & Antoinette, 1996). Recent data from the 2006 CDC report show the highest rates in the age groups of **0-4** (1121 per 100,000), **15-19** (814 per 100,000), **5-9** (659 per 100,000), and **75 or older** (659 per 100,000). Figure 8 presents incidence per 100,000 data by age.

Figure 8: Annual Incidence of TBI - Rates per 100,000 by Age

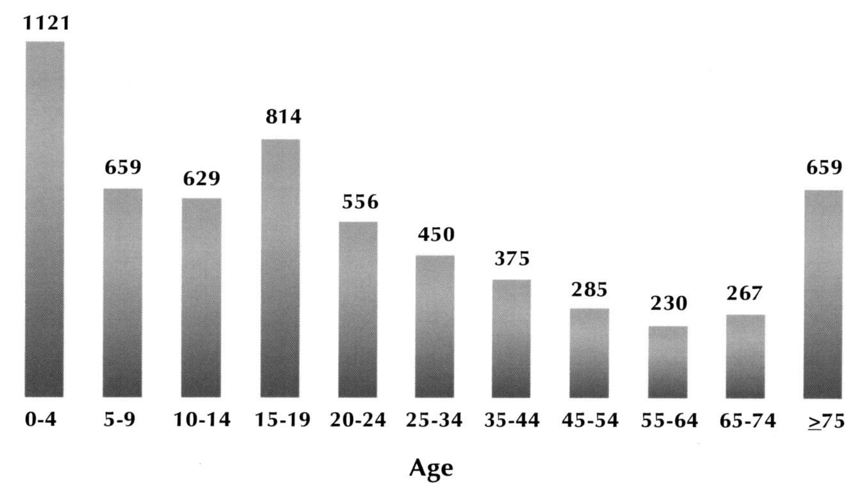

When looking at ER visits, hospitalizations and deaths due to TBI, rates vary across the age span. The highest rates of **death** occurred in the **75 and older** group (51 per 100,000) followed by ages **20-24** (28 per 100,000), and **15-19** (24 per 100,000).

The highest rate of **hospitalization** was also in the **75 and older** group (272 per 100,000). Adolescents aged **15-19** had a rate of hospitalization of 129 per 100,000, followed by young adults aged **20-24** (99 per 100,000).

When it came to **emergency department visits**, the age group of **0 to 4** had significantly higher rates than any other age group at 1,035 per every 100,000 people. The next closest rates were **15-19** years (661 per 100,000), **5-9** years (603 per 100,000) and **10-14** years (567 per 100,000).

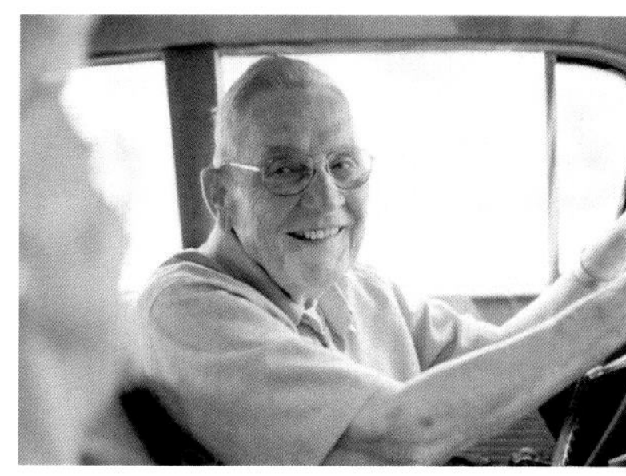

Figure 9: Annual Incidence of TBI Rates per every 100,000 people - ER Visits, Hospitalizations and Deaths by Age

Age	0-4	5-9	10-14	15-19	20-24	25-34	35-44	45-54	55-64	65-74	≥75
Death Rate	6	3	5	24	28	20	17	16	17	23	51
Hospitalization Rate	80	53	57	129	99	74	67	58	62	87	272
ER Visit Rate	1035	603	567	661	429	358	291	211	151	158	336

When examining TBI incidence by age and race, it is the pattern of incidence across the age range that is of interest. Figure 10 illustrates the patterns of TBI per 100,000 people. For Males, Females, Whites and Blacks, the data on ED Visits (blue), Hospitalizations (green) and Deaths (red), generally shows the highest rates in the range of **0-4** years, with a spike in the **15-19** age range, and a spike in the **over 75** age range.

In looking at the highest rate of incidence per 100,000 people across Age by Sex and Age by Race, the similarities across categories are remarkabley consistent. The table below presents the highest rate of ED Visits by Race and Age. For all categories with large enough sample sizes, the highest rate per 100,000 was the age group of **0-4**. For Hospitalizations, the age group of **75 years or older**, had the highest rate of incidence. In the category of deaths due to TBI, Males, Females, Whites, and AA/AI & API, the **75 and older** age group had the highest rate of incidence. Blacks were the exception, where the highest rate of death due to TBI occurred in the age range of **20-24**.

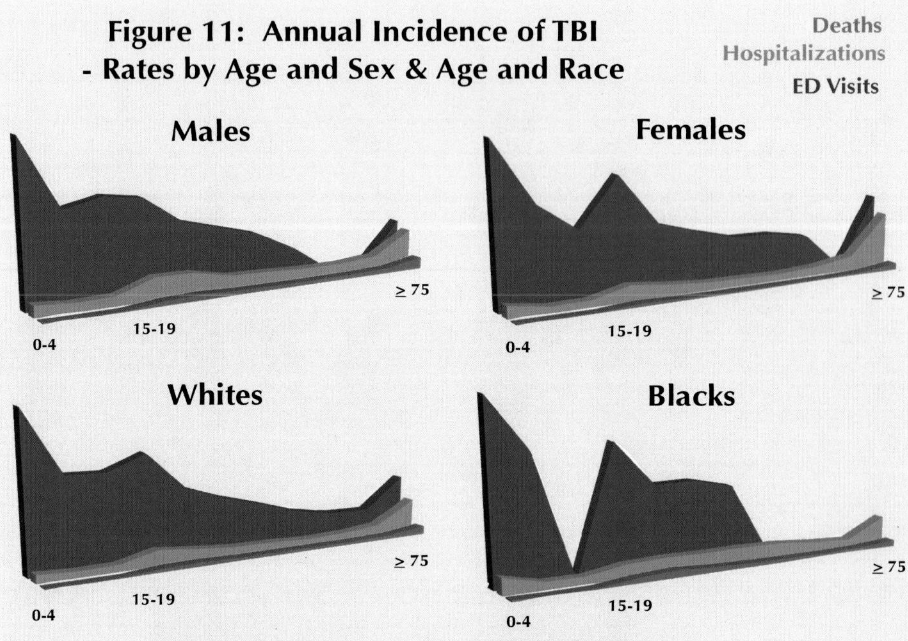

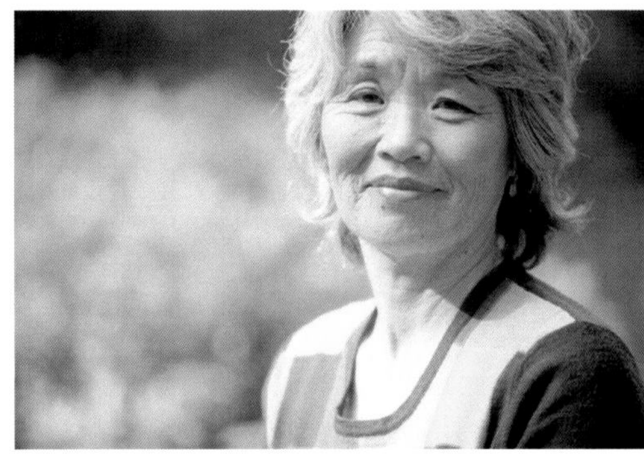

Table 1: Rates /100,000 of ED Visits, Hospitalizations and Deaths by Sex and Race

	ED Visits		Hospitalizations		Deaths	
	Age Group	Per 100,000	Age Group	Per 100,000	Age Group	Per 100,000
Males	0-4	1254	≥ 75	275	≥ 75	84
Females	0-4	806	≥ 75	270	≥ 75	40
White	0-4	1046	≥ 75	210	≥ 75	52
Black	0-4	991	≥ 75	144	20-24	40
AA/AI & A/PI	Sample size too small		≥ 75	272	≥ 75	44

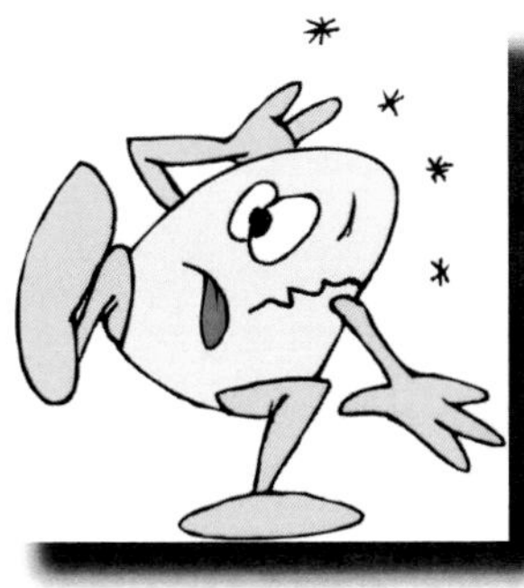

As the preceding page illustrates, incidence rates for children are some of the highest across the lifespan. Because of special circumstances related to brain injury in children - particularly because young brains are not fully developed and because many of these injuries and deaths are potentially preventable, special attention to TBI incidence in children is warranted.

Data from the 2006 CDC report show that over 450,000 children, aged **0-19**, sustain a TBI annually. These injuries are the result of motor vehicle/traffic accidents, falls, sport related injuries and abuse. Of these 450,000 TBIs, there were:

- 7,400 Deaths
- 62,000 Hospitalizations
- 384,000 ED Visits

These numbers represent 30 percent of all TBI's annually. Incidence rates per 100,000 relative to overall rates show differences for children aged **0-19**. Figure 12 shows incidence rates for ED visits, Hospitalizations and Deaths for children. The overall incidence rate for all age groups per 100,000 for Deaths (red) is 18. In the **15-19** age group, this rate was exceeded.

In the category of Hospitalizations (green), the overall incidence rate is 85 per 100,000. Again, the **15-19** age group had a higher incidence rate. For ED Visits (blue), all 4 age groups greatly exceeded the overall incidence rate of 403 per 100,000. In the **0-4** age group, the rate exceeds the overall rate by more than double.

In addition to the numbers of traumatic brain injuries, countless other children are hospitalized with other acquired brain injuries resulting from:

- Anoxic injuries (choking, strangulation, etc.)
- Infections (encephalitis, meningitis)

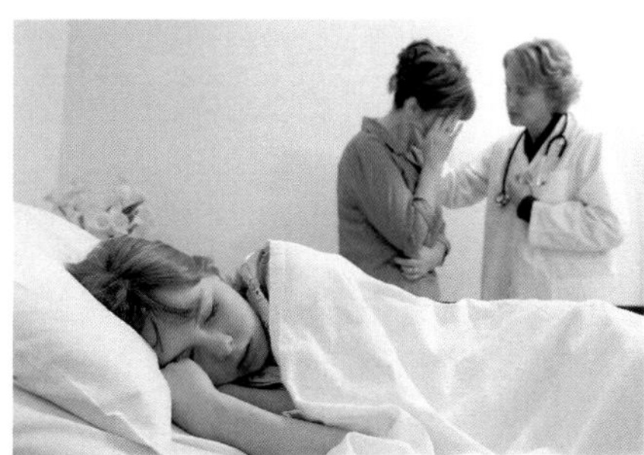

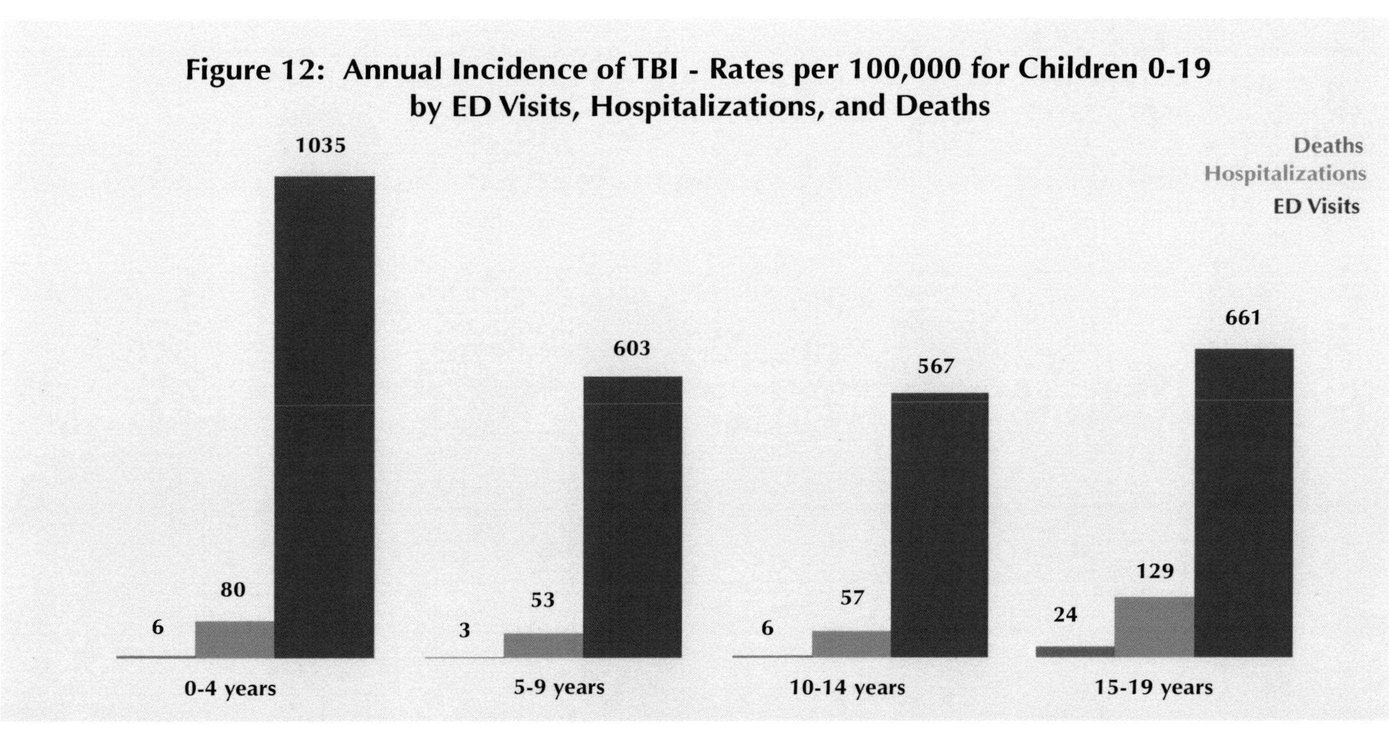

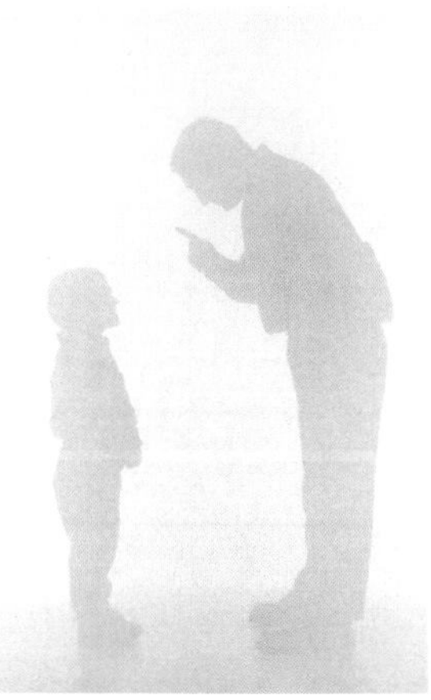

- Tumors
- Strokes and other vascular accidents
- Neurotoxic poisonings, and
- Metabolic disorders (insulin shock, liver and kidney disease).

Research has determined that age is a strong predictor of the cause of brain injury in children: For example:

- Non-accidental trauma is the cause of at least 80% of deaths from head trauma in children, under two years old.
- Two-thirds of the children under three years old, who are physically abused, have traumatic brain injuries.

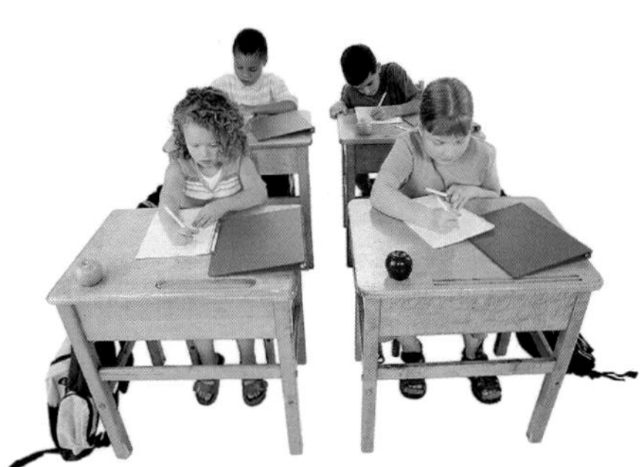

Cause of Injury

Determining the cause of injury is critically important, particularly because traumatic brain injury is often the result of preventable incidents and/or intentionally inflicted injuries. Accurate epidemiological information can provide the basis for implementing preventive strategies. These can target the prevention of the event itself that leads to an injury, as well as the prevention of sustaining a traumatic brain injury when these events do occur. For example, prevention of car crashes can occur by reducing speed limits, but seat/lap belts and air bags help to prevent a traumatic brain injury when the collision occurs.

A review of the data on this important epidemiological information, again, is variable depending on which population group is being studied. It is also important to differentiate incidence rates of injury versus incident rates of death due to the injury (Elovic and Antoinette, 1996).

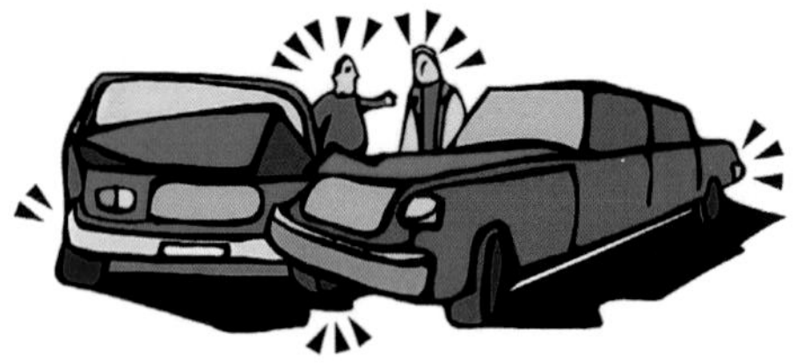

Historically, the majority of studies have reported transportation related incidents as the number one cause of traumatic brain injury.

Prevention efforts have been successful in reducing transportation related traumatic brain injuries from 11.1 per 100,000 in 1980 to 6.9 per 100,000 in 1994 (Division of Acute Care, 1999).

Recent data shows that this trend of falling motor vehicle rates has resulted in Falls surpassing Motor Vehicle /Traffic as the number one cause of TBI. Figure 13 presents this data. Falls acount for 29 percent of TBIs, followed by Motor Vehicle/Traffic at 20 percent, and Struck by/Against at 19 percent.

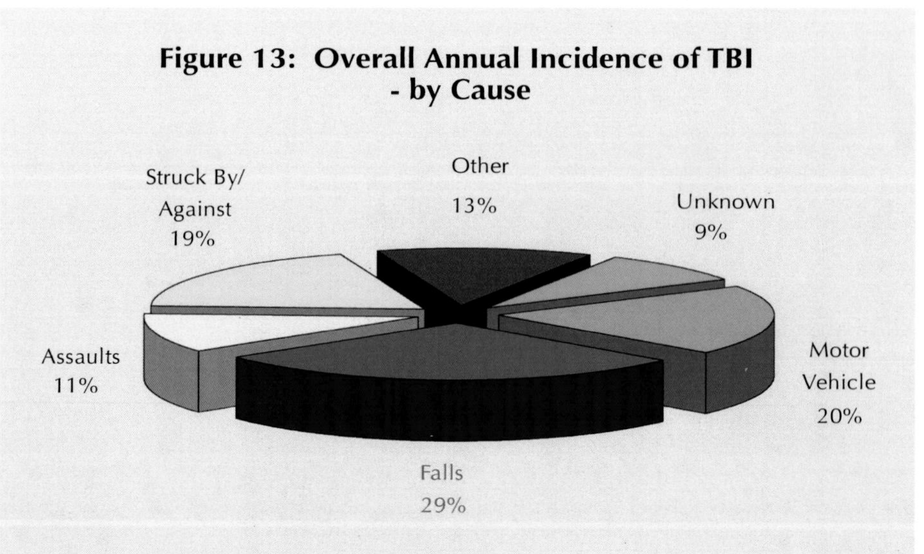

Figure 14: Annual Incidence of TBI - ED Visits

Struck By/ Against 24%
Other 11%
Unknown 4%
Motor Vehicle 18%
Falls 31%
Assaults 12%

Figure 15: Annual Incidence of TBI - Hospitalizations

Unknown 36%
Motor Vehicle 25%
Falls 21%
Assaults 6%
Struck By/ Against 3%
Other 9%

Figure 16: Annual Incidence of TBI - Deaths

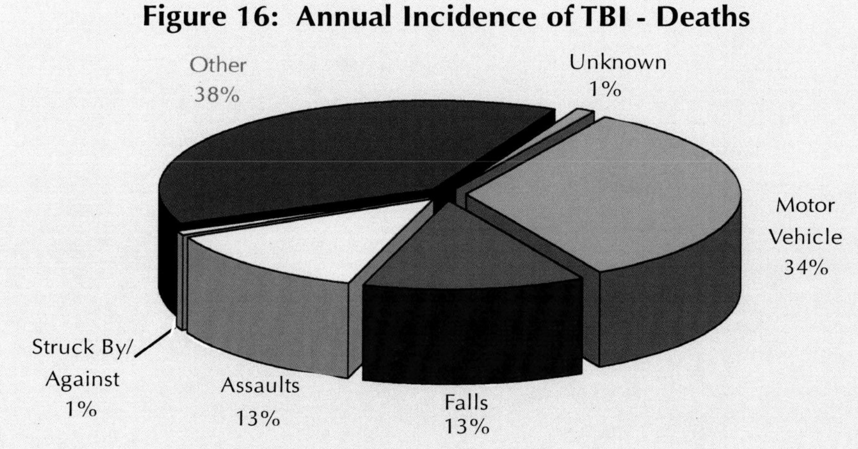

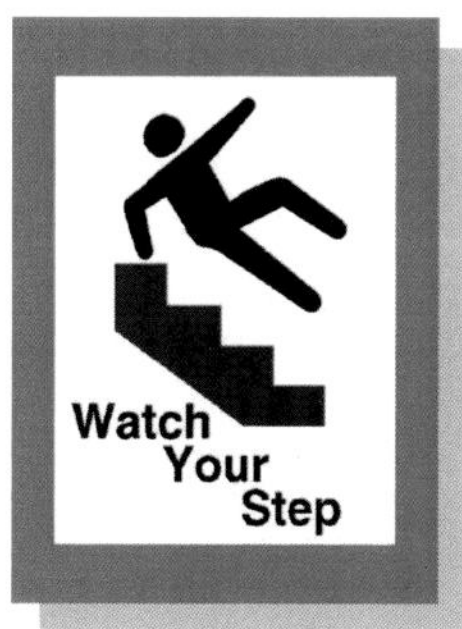

For individuals age 65 and older, falls are the leading cause of traumatic brain injury at 52 percent. For children aged 0-14, falls account for 39 percent of TBIs.

The leading cause of TBI resulting in ED Visits, was falls at 31 percent, followed by Struck by/Against at 24 percent (Figure 14). The leading cause of Hospitalizations due to TBI was in the category of Unknown (36%) followed by Motor Vehicle/Traffic at 25 percent (Figure 15). The leading cause of Death due to TBI was in the category of Other at 36 percent followed by Motor Vehicle/Traffic at 34 percent (Figure 16).

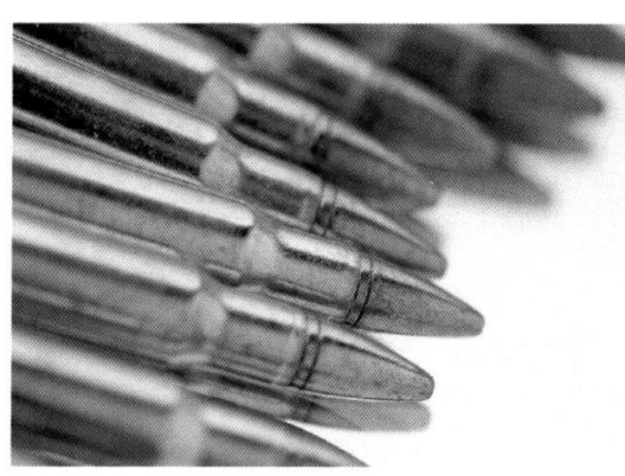

Previous data has shown that firearms are a significant cause of traumatic brain injury fatalities (Sosin, Sniezek, Waxweiler, 1995). This is not surprising if one considers that the mortality rate of firearm related TBI is greater than 90% (Gennarelli, Champion, Sacco et al, 1989). In addition, 2/3^{rds} of firearm-related traumatic brain injuries are classified as suicidal in intent.

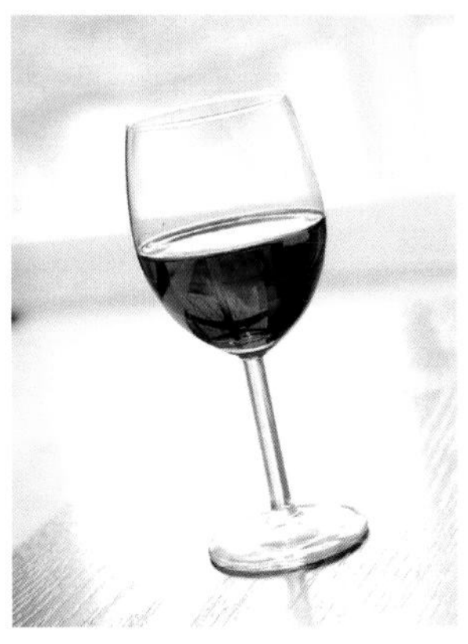

Alcohol is also a significant factor in injury etiology. The correlation between alcohol and injury is well established. In a systematic review of publications examining alcohol intoxication at the time of injury, Parry-Jones, Vaughan and Miles Cox (2006), found rates ranging from 37 to 51%.

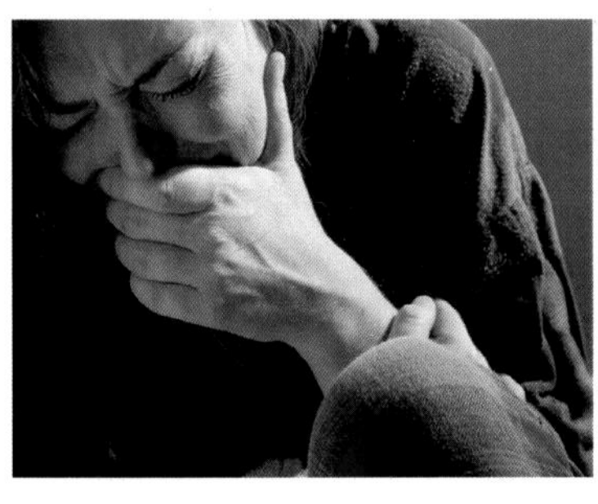

Another factor in injury etiology is domestic violence. Intimate violence is the leading cause of serious injury to American women between the ages of 15 and 44. It is estimated that a woman is beaten every 12 seconds in the United States. Each year, two to four million women are physically abused by someone with whom they are intimate. The head, face and neck are the most frequent sites of injury, with TBI a result of this violence far too often.

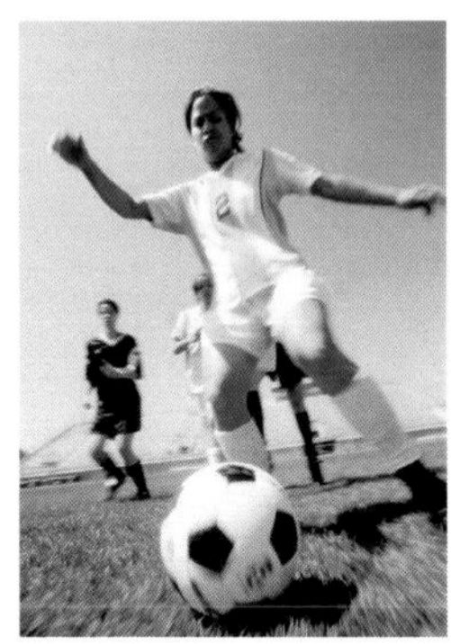

It is estimated that sports/recreational injuries account for approximately 750 fatalities annually. Nearly 50% were related to playground equipment, 10% horseback riding with skateboarding, skiing, sledding and children's toys accounting for many of the remainder of the injuries (Krauss, McArthur, 1999).

Injury Severity

Individuals with traumatic brain injury are typically identified as having a mild, moderate or severe injury. Mild traumatic brain injury is a common injury resulting in an estimated 290,000 hospital admissions each year (Whyte, 1998; Marshal and Marshal, 1985).

Recent studies suggest that up to 80% of all individuals with traumatic brain injuries are diagnosed as having a mild injury. The number of persons who sustain mild traumatic brain injuries would be much higher, however, if the data included persons who do not require hospitalization. This data, however, is hard to collect. Mild traumatic brain injuries are often called concussions and there is still a lack of education among the general public that a concussion is a brain injury.

- Between 10 and 30% of traumatic brain injuries are considered moderate (Kraus and McArthur 1996).
- Between 5% and 25% of traumatic brain injuries are considered severe (Kraus and McArthur, 1996).
- Between 50,000 and 75,000 persons sustain a severe traumatic brain injury each year, and between one-third and one-half of them die (Whyte, 1998).

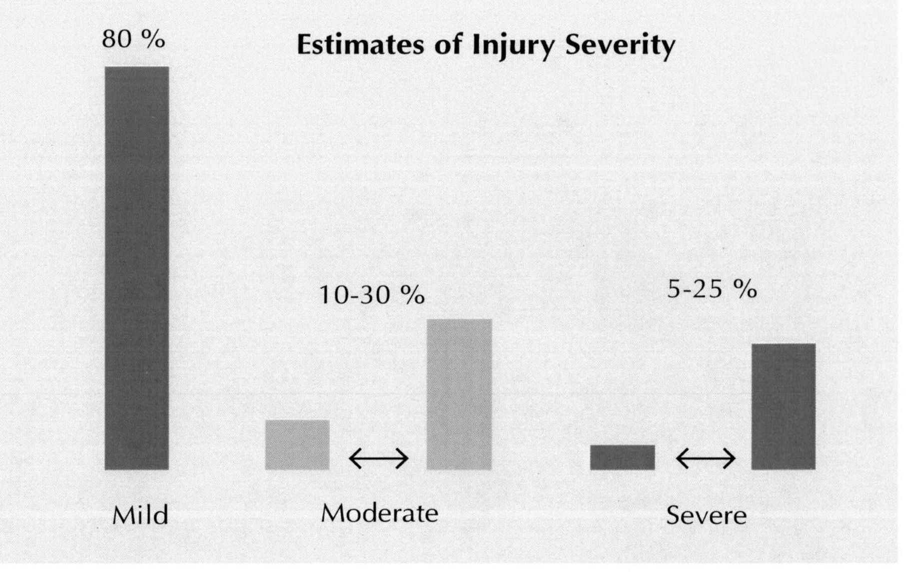

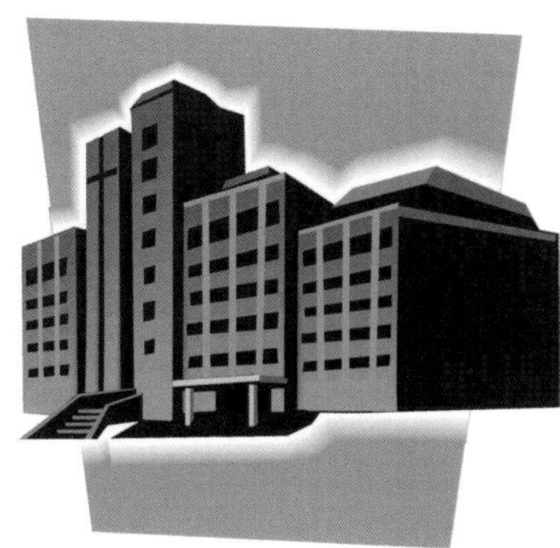

Systems of Care

Brain injury rehabilitation can encompass services from the onset of injury throughout the person's life. By necessity, options must be available to accommodate the diverse needs of individuals with brain injuries. However, not everyone has access or chooses to access these services. Nor are all systems appropriate for every individual. The following are examples of services available in the continuum of care:

Hospital-Based Services

Acute Hospital Care

Physicians, nurses and other medical staff are primarily focused on saving the individual's life and preventing further injury. A person may be in a coma during this phase of support. Surgery may be necessary to repair internal injuries, broken bones and other complications secondary to the brain injury. The individual may participate in acute hospitalization and acute rehabilitation in the same hospital. Studies have demonstrated that the earlier and more aggressive rehabilitation is in the acute hospital, the better the outcomes (Mackay et al., 1992).

Acute Rehabilitation

This phase provides a high intensity of skilled service delivery (e.g., physical therapy, occupational therapy, speech therapy, recreational therapy, neuropsychological and physical medicine and rehabilitation services) while optimizing the person's medical condition and improving basic functioning. Depending upon medical stability, the focus is on developing basic skills such as bowel and bladder control, communication, mobility, basic hygiene, orientation and learning.

Post-Hospital Services

Skilled Nursing Facility (Sub-acute)

This level of care is appropriate for persons at continued medical risk with complex nursing needs. Participation in rehabilitation in this setting is affected by medical stability. The rehabilitative goals and therapies may be similar to those offered in a rehabilitation setting.

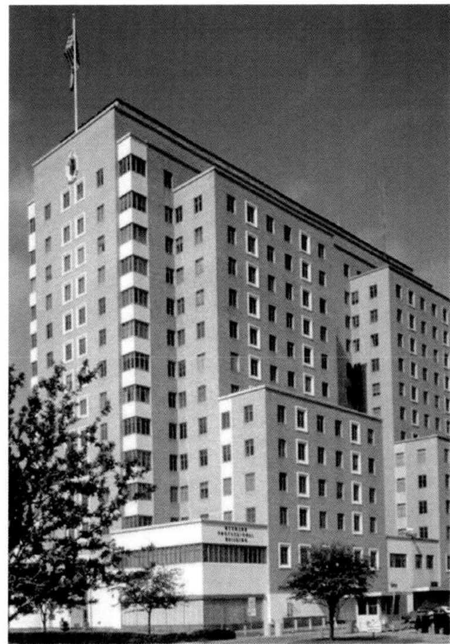

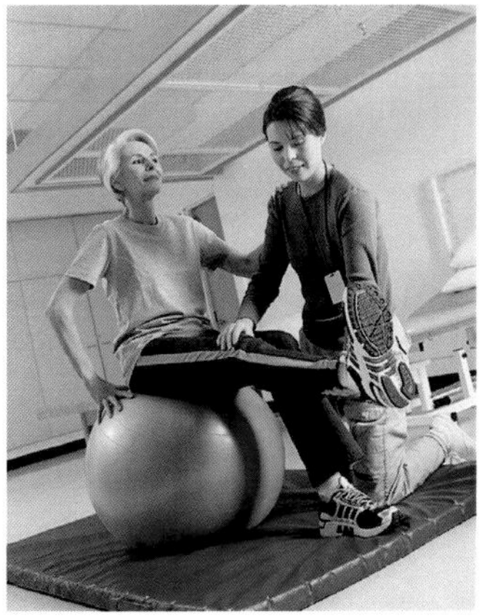

Post-Acute Rehabilitation

Individuals at the post acute stage of recovery are not typically at high medical risk and can participate more fully in rehabilitation. The focus of rehabilitation is on functional, physical, cognitive, behavioral and emotional skills. Community-based activities are used to help the individual return to and ease reintegration into home and community. Typically, this may include activities of daily living, meal preparation, community errands and leisure or pre-vocational or vocational activities.

Outpatient Services

Outpatient rehabilitation services are for persons not residing in a rehabilitation facility, but accessing them from home. They may be provided hourly or for a partial or full day.

Supported Living

Supported living is designed to support an individual's preferred lifestyle as integration occurs into the community. Options include residential, community and group living settings with varying levels of support based on the individual's needs.

Accreditation & Licensure

National accreditation agencies such as the Joint Commission on the Accreditation of Health-care Organizations (JCAHO) and the Commission for the Accreditation of Rehabilitation Facilities (CARF) have established set standards for rehabilitation programs. In addition a number of states have required licenses for programs serving persons with brain injury.

Accredited programs and services have demonstrated that they are in compliance with quality and performance standards as outline and promulgated by the accrediting agency. The goal of accreditation standards is to ensure that the organization has the capacity to meet the needs of individuals with disabilities. Skilled and knowledgeable professionals who practice in the field conduct an on-site survey. These surveyors not only hold the organization accountable for compliance with standards, but also offer consultation to enhance the ongoing delivery of services.

Accreditation reinforces trust and confidence that an organization has made a commitment to the enhancement of quality through a voluntary, independent process of accountability.

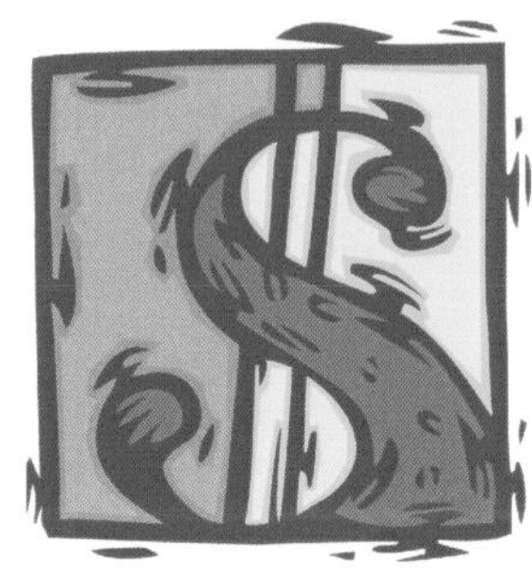

Costs of Traumatic Brain Injury

The costs of TBI can be staggering and are often due to the resultant life-long disability. According to Finkelstein, Corso and Miller (2006) in their book The Incidence and Economic Burden of Injuries in the United States, they estimated that:

- Traumatic brain injuries cost more than $60 billion in the year 2000.
- For all of the traumatic brain injuries incurred in 2000, the estimated lifetime costs are $406 billion.
    - $80 billion is in direct costs.
    - $326 billion is in lost productivity costs
- Males account for $283 billion.
- Injuries in the age group 25-44 account for 40% of costs, while they account for only 30% of the population.
- Motor vehicle accidents account for $89 billion (22%).
- Falls account for $68 billion (20%) of costs.

It is clear from these numbers that the costs of TBI are staggering. What is not so clear is if and where the funding will come from to cover these enormous costs.

Funding

While services for persons with brain injury have unquestionably improved the quality of life of individuals, these advancements have far outdistanced society's ability to pay for such services. And based on the above numbers, the costs are staggering.

Whatever the funding source, it is essential that:

- Advocacy for necessary support is provided and,
- Available funding is appropriately and cost effectively managed.

These two elements are essential to maximize outcomes and the supports needed for the individual, whether on a short-term or life-long basis. The Brain Injury Association of America estimates that only 5% of individuals with severe brain injuries have adequate funding for long-term treatment.

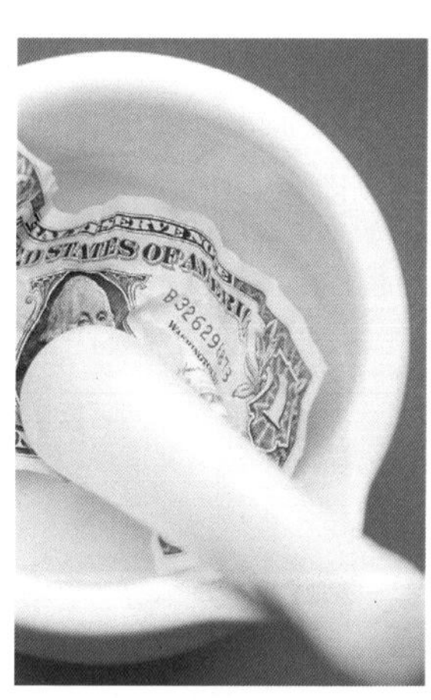

Private Funding

Indemnity Insurance

In the past several years, funding has moved from indemnity insurance to managed care. Prior to managed care, most insurance policies were indemnity policies in which the insurer assumed the responsibility of paying medical benefits for services performed and covered under the policy in return for premium payments. The employee typically pays a deductible. An enrollee can use any doctor or hospital and simply files a claim for reimbursement. In the past several years, enrollment in this kind of plan has declined.

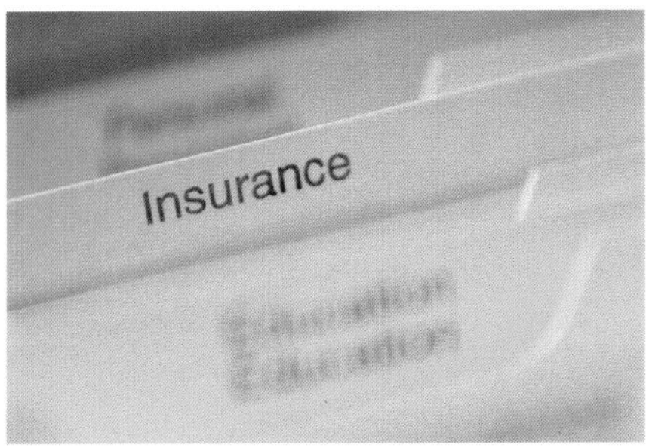

Managed Care

This consists of programs known as health maintenance organizations (HMOs) and preferred provider organizations (PPOs). The main characteristics of managed care include:

- An organizational structure that oversees the care of the individual, with a gate-keeping mechanism that can include incentives for enrollees to use network providers.
- Elective contracting with providers such as hospitals, physicians, etc., to obtain the best price available for health-related services.
- Quality controls to ensure that services provided are necessary and appropriate.
- Risk-sharing arrangements in which fiscal responsibility is shared by the managed care organization, the provider of services and the consumer.

These programs were developed to offer health care choices to employees, yet still allow a mechanism for controlling health care expenses to employers. Employees typically have lower health care costs but must use designated providers.

Public Funding

Medicaid provides health care for more than 40 million people throughout the US, including low-income families and people who are blind, aged 65 and older or who have disabilities. Most services provided under the standard Medicaid program are medically oriented (in-patient, hospital, skilled nursing facility, etc.). Basic Medicaid programs generally do not provide many of the after-hospital or long-term community-based support services needed by many persons with traumatic brain injury. Medicaid can fund some of these services through the use of waivers.

Funding

The BIAA estimates that only 5% of individuals with severe brain injuries have adequate funding for long term treatment.

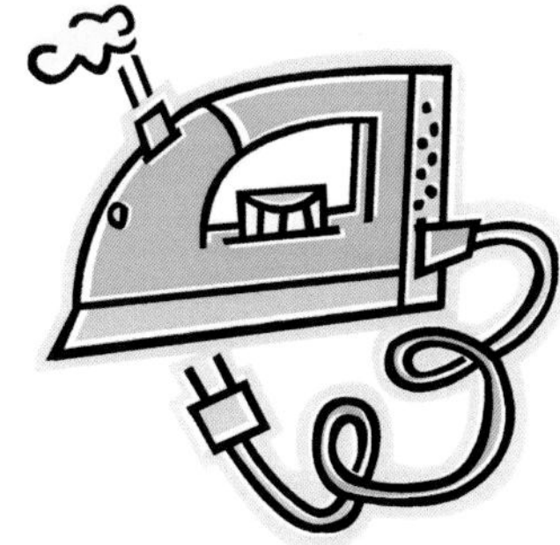

Home and Community-Based Services Waivers

Under a Medicaid Home and Community-Based Services (HCBS) waiver, a state with Centers for Medicare and Medicaid approval, can waive one or more of the requirements of eligibility for funding and provision of services. However, the average per capita cost of providing these services cannot exceed the cost of institutional care. States may select the services, the service definition, target population, and number of individuals included under each Central Management Services (CMS) approved Home and Community-Based Services waiver.

Waivers are intended to give states flexibility to try new approaches to delivering health care services or to adapt existing programs to the special needs of particular areas or groups of people. In 2002, 24 states and the District of Columbia had state waiver services for adults with brain injury. Home and community based services may include:

- Case management
- Homemaker service
- Home health aide services
- Personal care

- Adult day health
- Habilitation services
- Respite care
- Day treatment or other partial hospitalization services, psychosocial rehabilitation services and clinic services for individuals with chronic mental illness
- Other services requested by the state and approved by CMS as cost effective and necessary to avoid institutionalization (such as emergency response systems, assistive technology, etc) and;
- Expanded habilitation services to recipients who have been discharged from a Medicaid-certified nursing facility or intermediate care facility for persons with mental retardation, regardless of when the discharge occurred. Expanded habilitation services may include prevocational services to prepare an individual for paid or unpaid employment.

Public Spending on *Traumatic Brain Injury*

The first attempt to compile data on public resources and services provided for persons with traumatic brain injury was a study that Congress requested of the Government Accounting Office (GAO). Published in 1998, the GAO noted that:

"Despite strategies implemented, service gaps are likely - the number of adults with TBI who are provided services remains small relative to

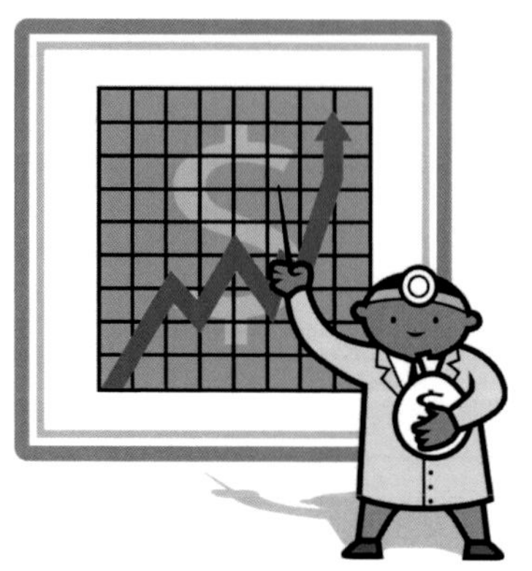

estimates of the total number. According to program representatives and experts, those most likely to have difficulty accessing services are:

- Individuals with cognitive impairment but who lack physical disabilities;
- Individuals without an effective advocate to negotiate the social service system or without a social support system; and
- Individuals with problematic or unmanageable behaviors, such as aggression, destructiveness, or participation in illegal behaviors.

Without treatment, individuals with problematic or unmanageable behaviors are the most likely to become homeless, institutionalized in a mental facility, or imprisoned."

The GAO also reported that:

"While both the private and public sectors finance acute care services to adults with TBI, federal and state governments pay for a large part of post-acute services received by adults with TBI. This is primarily because private insurance generally limits post-acute services and does not pay for long-term care. Individuals may quickly exhaust personal resources. In addition, individuals' longevity may be unaffected by the injury, and adults with TBI may require post-acute services for an extended period of time - some for the remainder of their lives."

The report concluded that:

"Despite state efforts to provide services, some adults with TBI encounter substantial barriers in accessing services that will support their reintegration into the community" (GAO 1998).

The 1997 GAO report on Traumatic Brain Injury determined that Medicaid and Home and Community Based Waiver programs covered an estimated 2,478 individuals and

Public Spending on Brain Injury

1997 HCB Waivers

	# People Helped	Dollars Spent
TBI:	**2,478**	**$118 Million**
MR:	**236,000**	**$ 5.8 Billion**

spent $118 million. By comparison in the same year, waivers covered an estimated 236,000 individuals with mental retardation/ developmental disabilities and spent approximately $5.8 billion!

"The Olmstead Decision"

Lois Curtis and Elaine Wilson, two women with disabilities who lived in Georgia nursing homes, asked state officials to allow them to move into their own homes in the community. After the state's refusal, a lawsuit was filed generating appeals. The case was finally heard by the US Supreme Court and in July 1999, it issued the Olmstead v. L.C. decision and ruled that the two women receive community options.

The Olmstead decision challenges federal, state, and local governments to develop more opportunities for individuals with disabilities through accessible systems of cost-effective community-based services. The Olmstead decision interpreted Title II of the Americans with Disabilities Act (ADA) and its implementing regulations and requires states to administer their services, programs, and activities "in the most integrated setting appropriate to the needs of qualified individuals with disabilities." The ADA and the Olmstead decision apply to all qualified individuals with disabilities regardless of age.

The decision has resulted in several federal and state initiatives that will make living in the community a reality for more people with disabilities. For example, CMS adopted a number of Medicaid policy reforms and issued grants to facilitate state efforts to improve their community services systems. Also, Congress appropriated funds for "Systems Change" Grants specifically to improve community-integrated services. In February 2001, President George W. Bush announced a broad New Freedom Initiative to "tear down barriers to equality" and grant a "New Freedom" to children and adults of any age who have a disability or long-term illness so that they may live and prosper in their communities (ILRU, 2002).

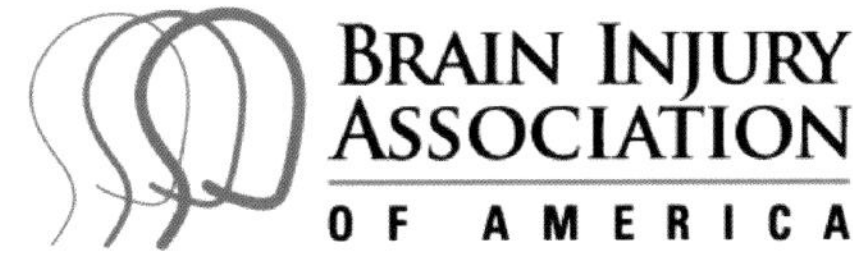

Advocacy & the Brain Injury Association of America

Traumatic brain injury represents a public health problem of great magnitude with profound consequences for persons who have sustained brain injuries, their families and society at large. During the 1970s, improvements occurred in emergency medical services and acute care and specialized models of brain injury rehabilitation were first initiated. In 1980, a group of family members of persons with traumatic brain injuries founded the National Head Injury Foundation. The organization has grown into a national organization including 42 chartered state affiliates.

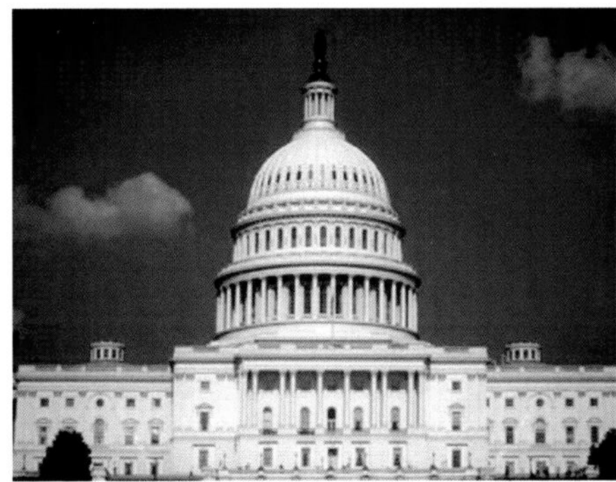

Traumatic Brain Injury Act of 1996

Passed July 29, 1996, this is the single most important piece of legislation because it acknowledged the incidence and prevalence of brain injury nationally and paved the way for surveillance, rehabilitation, and funding.

The Act was passed by Congress "to expand efforts to identify methods of preventing traumatic brain injury; expand biomedical research efforts or minimize the severity of dysfunction as a result of such an injury; and to improve the delivery and quality of services through State Demonstration Projects."

Specifically, the TBI Act of 1996 authorized:

- The Centers for Disease Control and Prevention (CDC) to establish projects to prevent and reduce the incidence of traumatic brain injury.
- The National Institutes of Health to award grants to conduct basic and applied research on developing new methods for more effective diagnosis, therapies and a continuum of care.

The TBI ACT of 1996

Key Points:

- Prevention
- Research
- Improve service delivery

- The Health Resources and Services Administration (HRSA) to make grants to states, to carry out demonstration programs to implement systems that ensure statewide access to comprehensive and coordinated TBI services. States that receive Planning Grants are required to establish "infrastructure core capacity components" prior to developing an implementation plan. These components are:

1. Statewide TBI advisory board.

2. Designated state agency and staff position responsible for TBI activities.

3. Statewide needs assessment to address the full spectrum of services from initial acute treatment through community reintegration for people with traumatic brain injury.

4. Statewide action plan to develop a comprehensive, community-based system of care, encompassing physical, psychological, educational, vocational and social aspects of traumatic brain injury services while addressing the needs of people with traumatic brain injury and their families (HRSA, 1999).

The 2000 reauthorization of the TBI Act extended the appropriation of funds through 2005. On October 17, 2000, President Bill Clinton signed the TBI Act Amendments of 2000, as Title XIII of H.R.4365, the Children's Health Act of 2000, which extended the Act from three to five years. Continued support was given to the CDC to expand state surveillance, education and prevention programs for TBI. The National Institutes of Health were given additional authorization to carry out applied research related to cognitive disorders and neurobehavioral consequences, including the development, modification, and evaluation of therapies and programs of rehabilitation.

State "Demonstration" Projects

The TBI State Grant Program, administered by the HRSA, equips states with seed money to begin work on the integration of services, the establishment of policy, and the procurement of financial support to bring about systems change. This change is achieved by expanding and improving state and local capacity to care for individuals with TBI and their families. To this end, states work to:

- Strengthen the state infrastructure
- Improve community supports and services
- Develop and evaluate model approaches to the myriad challenges in integrating TBI services into the broader service delivery system
- Generate support from local and private sources for sustaining their efforts after the grant's completion.

As of 2003, 49 states and the District of Columbia have received funding from this program out of a total number of 56 (50 states, the District of Columbia and 5 Territories).

Centers for Disease Control and Prevention (*CDC*)

The CDC carries out projects to reduce the incidence of TBI. As one of its activities, the CDC published TBI surveillance methods and guidelines for public health purposes and funded 15 states, which resulted in the creation of a multi-state, uniform reporting system to provide nationally representative data to define groups at higher risk, causes and circumstances of injury and outcomes of injury.

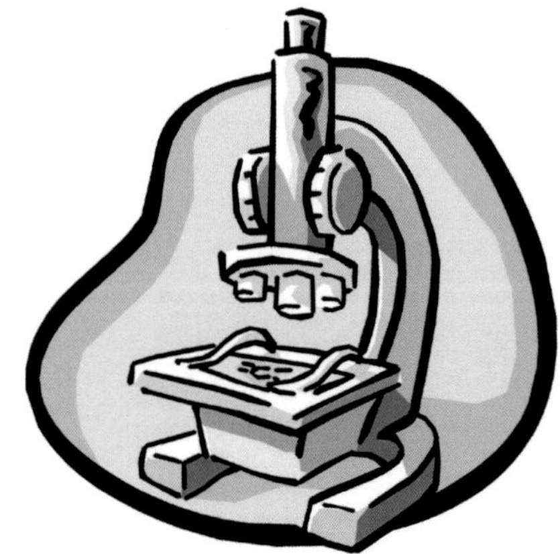

TBI Research

In 1987, The US Department of Education's National Institute on Disability and Rehabilitation Research

(NIDRR) provided funding to establish the Traumatic brain injury (TBI) Model Systems of Care. These research and demonstration grants focus primarily on:

- Developing and demonstrating a model system of care for persons with traumatic brain injury, emphasizing continuity and comprehensiveness of care.
- Maintaining a standardized national database for innovative analyses of TBI treatment and outcomes.

The TBI Model Systems (TBIMS) are involved in prospective, longitudinal multi-center efforts to examine the course of recovery and outcomes following TBI. Each center provides a coordinated system of emergency care, acute neurotrauma management, comprehensive inpatient rehabilitation and long-term interdisciplinary follow-up services. As of 2003, sixteen centers were funded.

NIDRR also maintains the TBI Model Systems National Data Base, which contains hundreds of publications and abstracts of research projects generated from the work of model systems.

Another project is the NIDRR web site (www.ed.gov/about/offices/list/osers/nidrr/index.html), which contains the Center on Outcome Measurement in Brain Injury (COMBI). The COMBI is an online resource for detailed information and support on outcome measures for persons with brain injuries. See www.tbims.org/combi for more information.

The National Institutes of Health conducted research on the development of new methods and modalities for more effective diagnosis, measurement of degree of injury, post-injury monitoring and assessment of care models for brain injury recovery and long term care.

Conclusion

As stated in the House Committee on Commerce report, 104-652, of June 27,1996,

"Because of the serious consequences of TBI and the failure of human services systems and educational programs to meet their needs properly, people with TBI want to be identified as people with brain injuries, not be labeled as having some other disability. This is extremely important if appropriate services are to be developed and targeted and prevention efforts are to be conducted. TBI is different from other disabilities due to the severity of cognitive loss. Most rehabilitation programs are designed for people with physical disabilities, not cognitive disabilities which require special accommodations."

Brain injury is the silent epidemic and continues to be a largely unrecognized major public health problem. While progress has been made in epidemiological data collection and government attention and funding has increased, it remains a challenge to ensure that persons with brain injury have access to much needed ongoing support and services.

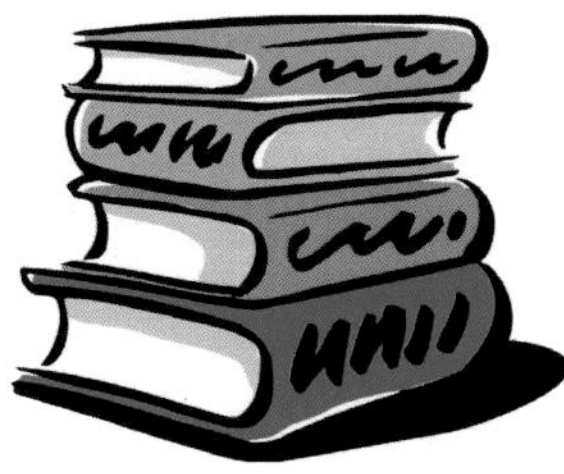

References

Analysis by the CDC National Center for Injury Prevention and Control, using data obtained from state health departments in AK, AZ, CA, CO, LA, MD, MO, NY, OK, RI, SC and UT, 1999.

Annegers JF, Garbow JD& Kurtland LT et al. (1980). The Incidence, Causes and Secular Trends of Head Trauma in Olmstead County, Minnesota 1935-1974. Neurology 30:912-919.

Batshaw, M. (1997). Children With Disabilities. Baltimore: Paul H. Brookes Publishing Co.

Cancer Registry Public Information Data: 1999-2002, WONDER On-line database. United States Department of Health and Human Services, National Program of Cancer Registries, Centers for Disease Control and Prevention. November 2005.

Centers for Disease Control (1999). "Traumatic brain injury in the United States: A Report to Congress."

Centers for Disease Control (2006). "Traumatic Brain Injury in the United States: Emergency Department Visits, Hospitalizations, and Deaths."

Centers for Disease Control. "Cases of HIV Infection and AIDS in the United States, by Race/Ethnicity, 2000-2004.

Division of Acute Care, Rehabilitation Research, and Disability Prevention - National Center for Injury Prevention and Control- CDC - U.S. DHHS. TBI in the United States: A report to Congress, 1999.

Elovic & Antoinette T. (1996). Epidemiology and Primary Prevention of Traumatic brain injury. In: Horn LJ, Zasler ND (Eds.) Medical Rehabilitation of Traumatic brain injury. Philadelphia: Hanley & Belfus.

Elovic E & Kirshbaum S. (1999). Epidemiology of Spinal Cord Injury and TBI: The scope of the problem. Topics in Spinal Cord Medicine 52:1-20.

Finkelstein E.A., Corso, P.S. & Miller, T.R. (2006). Incidence and Economic Burden of Injuries in the United States. Oxford Press.

Gennarelli TA, Champion HR & Sacco WJ et al. (1989). Mortality of Patients with Head Injury and Extracranial Injury Treated in Trauma Centers. J Trauma 29 (9):1193-1201.

HRSA/MCHB, TBI State Demonstration Grant Program, Long-Range Plan February 1999.

Kraus JF, Black MA, Hessol N et al. (1984). The Incidence of Acute Brain Injury and Serious Impairment in a Defined Population. Am J Epidemiology 119 (2) 186-201.

Kraus JF, McArthur DL. (1996). Epidemiologic Aspects of Brain Injury. Neurologic Clinics 14:435-448.

Kibby MY, Long CJ (1996). Minor Head Injury: Attempts at clarifying the confusion. Brain Injury 10:159-186.

Lewin –ICF (1992). The Cost of Disorders of the Brain. Washington, DC: The National Foundation for the Brain.

Mackay, LM, Bernstein, BA, Chapman, PE, Morgan, AS, & Milazzo, LS (1992). Early Intervention in Severe Head Injury: Long Term Benefits of a Formalized Program. Archives of Physical Medicine, 73: 635-641.

Marshall L, Marshall S. Current clinical head injury research in the U.S. In: Becker DP, Povlishock JT (eds) Central Nervous System Research in Status Report. Bethesda, MD: NINCDS, 1985.

Narrow, WE. One-year Prevalance of Depressive Disorders among Adults 18 and Over in the U.S.: NIMH ECA prospective data. Population estimates based on U.S. Census estimated residential population age 18 and over on July 1, 1998. Unpublished.

National Health and Nutrition Examination Survey III (NHANES, III, 1988-14), CDC/NCHS.

NIH Consensus Conference, October 1998 Centers for Disease Control and Prevention National Incidence Data for 1995-1996 and Preliminary Data from the Colorado Traumatic brain injury Registry from 1996-1997.

Parry-Jones BL, Vaughan FL, and Miles Cox W (2006). Traumatic brain injury and substance misuse: a systematic review of prevalence and outcomes research (1994-2004). Neuropsychol Rehabil. 2006 Oct;16(5):537-560.

Schootman M & Fuortes LJ (2000). Ambulatory Care for Traumatic Brain Injuries in the US, 1995-1997. Brain Injury 14 (4):373-381.

Sosin DM, Sniezek JE, & Waswei-ler RJ (1995). Trends in Death Associated with Traumatic brain injury. JAMA 273: 1778-1780.

Terrill, KF, (2001). A Guide for State Associations and State Collaborators on Home and Community-Based Waivers (unpublished manuscript).

Thurman D & Guerrero J (1999). Trends in hospitalization associated with traumatic brain injury. JAMA 282 (10):954-957.

"Traumatic Brain Injury – Programs Supporting Long-term Services in Selected States: Report to Congressional Requesters," Government Accounting Office, February 1998; GAO/HEHS-98-55.

Whyte J, Hart T, & Laborde A et al (1998). Rehabilitation of the patient with traumatic brain injury. In J. Delisa, et al. (Eds), Rehabilitation Medicine: Principles and Practice. (3rd ed.) Philadelphia: Lippincott.

www.cdc.gov/ncipc/pub-res/tbi-congress.htm 4/2000

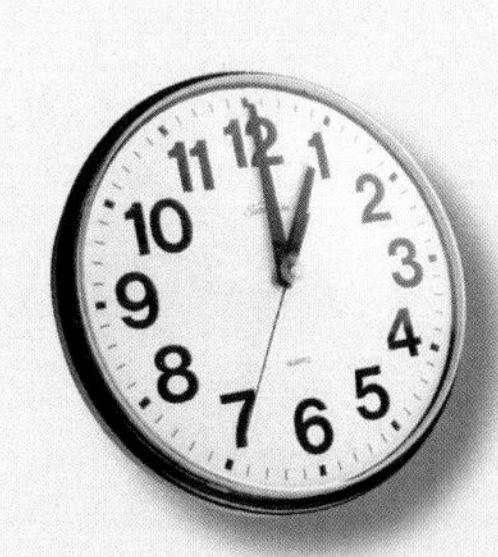

Every 23 seconds, one person in the U.S. will sustain a TBI.

Statistics Summary

Prevalence

3.17 to 5.3 million people are disabled secondary to TBI.

Incidence

1.4 million TBI's occur every year:

- 4% - Death.
- 17% - Hospitalization.
- 79% - Treatment & release from an Emergency Department.

Overall Incidence of TBI: Percentage rates of ER Visits, Hospitalizations and Deaths

Hospitalization 17%

Death 4%

ED Visit 79%

80,000-90,000 people are disabled every year in the U.S. due to TBI.

Sex

Males sustain more TBIs than Females (more than 1.5 times more).

- Males sustain 59% of TBIs.
- Females sustain 41% of TBIs.
- Males have higher rates of Hospitalization, ED Visits and Deaths due to TBI.

Annual Incidence of TBI - Overall percentage rates by Sex

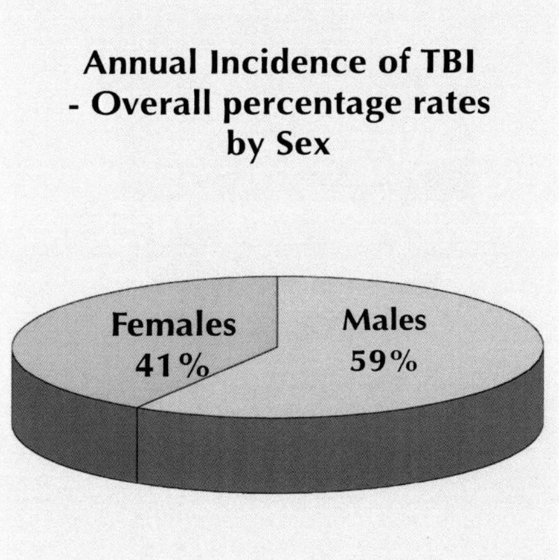

Race

Rates of TBI differ across race.

- Blacks have a highest overall incidence rate (486 per 100,000).
- AI/AN &API have the lowest overall incidence rate (252 per 100,000).
- Overall, Whites account for 81% of TBIs.

Age

Different age groups are disproportionately affected by TBI.

- Highest rate of overall incidence is in the age group of 0-4 (1121 per 100,000).
- The highest Death rate is in the $\geq$ 75 age group (51 per 100,000).
- The highest Hospitalization rate is in the $\geq$ 75 age group (272 per 100,000).
- The highest ED Visit rate is in the 0-4 age group. (1035 per 100,000)

Overall Incidence of TBI - Percentage Rates by Race

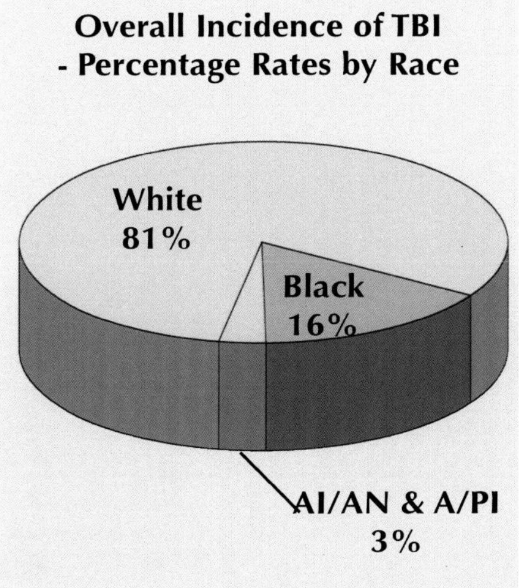

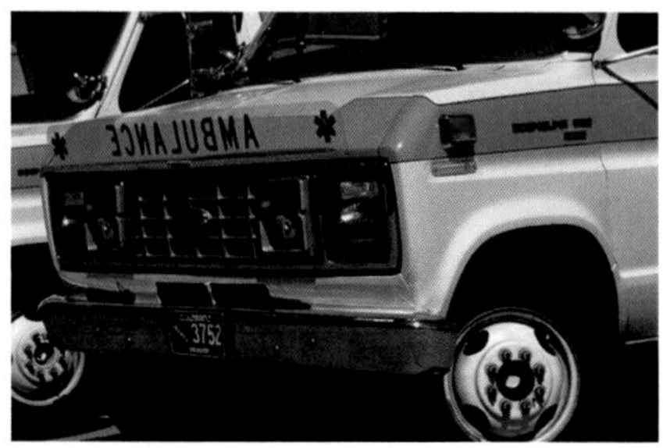

Emergency Department Visits

The highest rates by demographics:

- Males aged 0-4
- Females aged 0-4
- Blacks aged 0-4
- Whites aged 0-4

Falls are the #1 cause of ED Visits at 31%

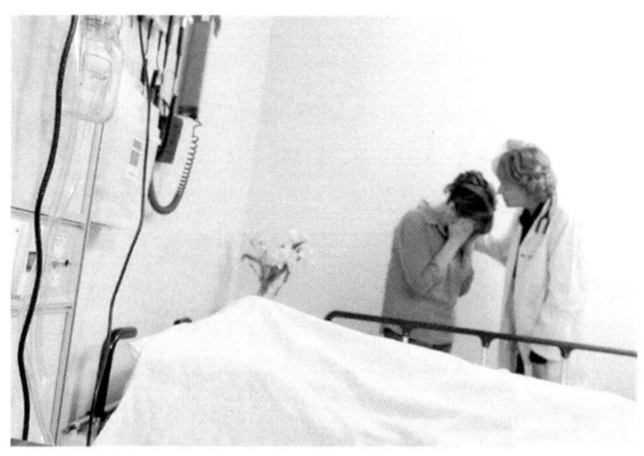

Hospitalizations

The highest rates by demographics:

- Males aged ≥ 75 years
- Females aged ≥ 75 years
- Blacks aged ≥ 75 years
- Whites aged ≥ 75 years

The #1 cause of Hospitalization - Unknown Category (36%)

Deaths

The highest rates by demographics:

- Males aged ≥ 75 years
- Females aged ≥ 75 years
- Blacks aged 20-24
- Whites aged ≥ 75 years

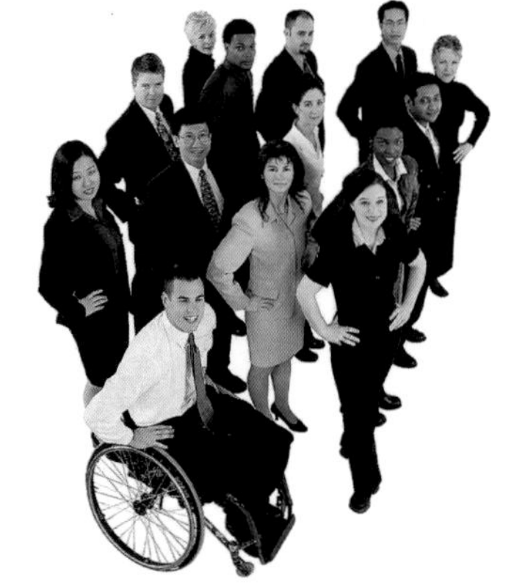

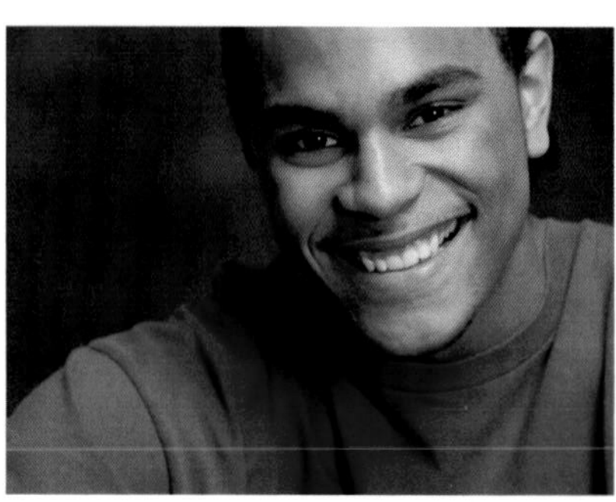

Cause of Injury

The highest rates by demographics:

- Falls are the #1 cause of TBI overall at 29%.
- Falls are the #1 cause of ED Visits (31%)
- The #1 cause of Hospitalization - Unknown Category (36 %)
- The #1 cause of Death - Other Category (38 %)

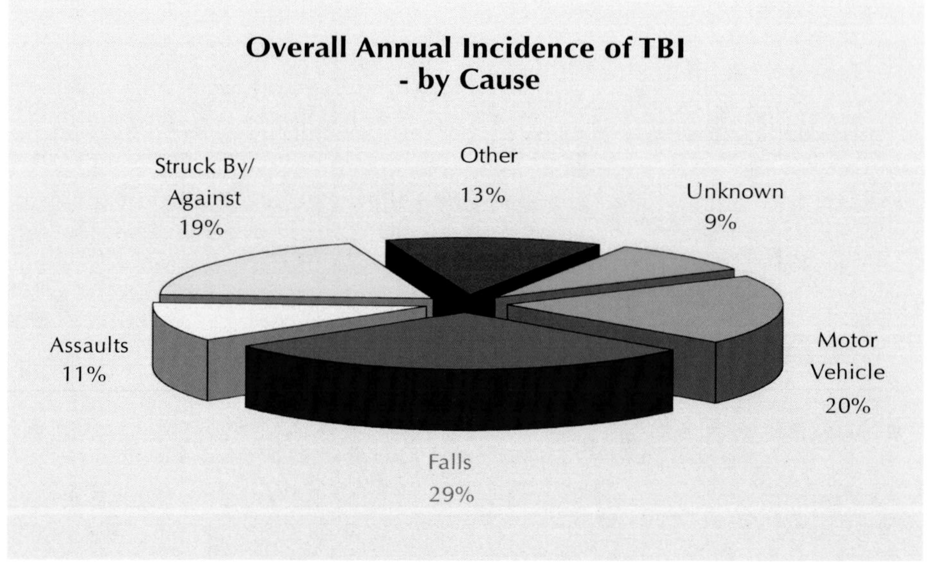

Chapter 2

Philosophy of Rehabilitation

Learning Objectives

By the end of this chapter, you will be able to:

- Distinguish between historical and contemporary rehabilitation philosophies.
- Describe the philosophical basis of the helping role in rehabilitation.
- Identify styles of interacting between those giving and receiving assistance that put contemporary rehabilitation philosophies into practice.

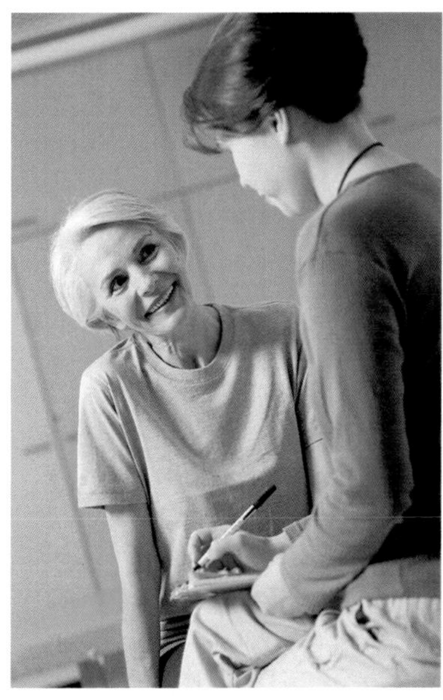

Introduction

It is too simple to view rehabilitation after brain injury as a process of facilitating medical recovery and then providing various therapies to hasten an individual's return to family, school, or work. Yet we often do. Rehabilitation professionals and others refer to remarkable personal outcomes. These occur as a result of a relatively standard set of rehabilitation practices, "natural healing," the individual's progression through "phases of recovery," or some treatment pathway. Considering such optimism, it is no surprise that family members, other loved ones, and staff often have the impression that a person can sustain an intense neurological trauma, learn a few compensatory strategies, and live happily ever after. It is also no surprise that while teaching persons how to assist those with brain injuries, the process may inadvertently be implied to be straightforward and well operationalized. While remarkable personal outcomes do occur, this is not always the case. Many of those involved in the process often wind up disappointed.

The orientation of the person assisting someone with a brain injury can have a dramatic impact on the role that person plays and how that person interacts with others. It also ultimately affects how the person providing care or treatment feels about the impact of those services. How a person interacts may be critical to the outcome. An example is presented below.

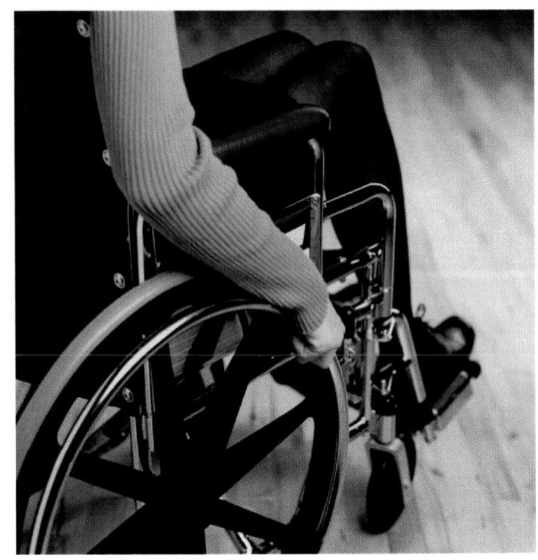

In one way or another, persons involved in providing assistance to others see this sort of phenomenon all the time. Some caregivers char-

Example

Lee was a 32 year old man, who was 4 months post severe frontal-temporal brain injury as a result of a motorcycle accident. Much of the time that he was in the hospital, he was in various sorts of mechanical restraint. This was due to his extreme resistance to support and extreme aggression. When he arrived at a community-based rehabilitation program, Lee was fully verbal and ambulatory. He believed that he lived on a submarine. He often destroyed large plants, because they failed to provide drinks that he requested from them.

Many professionals concluded that Lee was "psychotic and noncompliant" - partially due to these behaviors. Consequently, he was given large doses of psychotropic medications. Staff used a consequence-based behavioral program (i.e., verbal correction after unwanted behavior) when he failed to respond to their requests. It was evident that staff orientation to Lee's difficulty was impacting the way they were interacting with him. Nothing was changing.

One morning, Lee told staff in unusually clear language that he was having "a little difficulty" with his left eye. While nothing was obviously the matter with his eye, staff took the comment seriously because this remark was so clear compared to his other comments. Some felt he might be able to accurately report what he was experiencing in a formal exam. As it turned out, the exam revealed that not only was Lee blind in his left eye, but he had been blind in that eye since his injury.

While the test result had little impact on Lee (e.g., he continued to interpret his blindness as "a little difficulty"), it had an immediate and dramatic impact on how staff perceived him. Suddenly, "living on a submarine" sounded more confused than psychotic from an ex-Navy man. Suddenly, his "failure to respond to requests" was something completely different from noncompliance.

Medications were discontinued. Staff went out of their way to help Lee interpret his environment and organize himself to get through his day. Interactions took on a drastically different look and sound. People worked together. Everything changed.

acteristically view persons they are assisting through some sort of negative, broken, "needs to be corrected," or even "pain in the neck" looking glass. These people act as though the individual they are helping does not perceive that this is their style. More importantly, they do not understand that their style affects the individual's response to them.

Other caregivers have a style where their interactions are delightful to observe. They are unconditionally positive, remarkably effective in eliciting favorable responses, and strangely, at times, subject to criticism. Persons needing assistance avoid negative caregivers and seek out interactions with positive caregivers. Some individuals shift back and forth between these styles, but are unclear on why and when they do this.

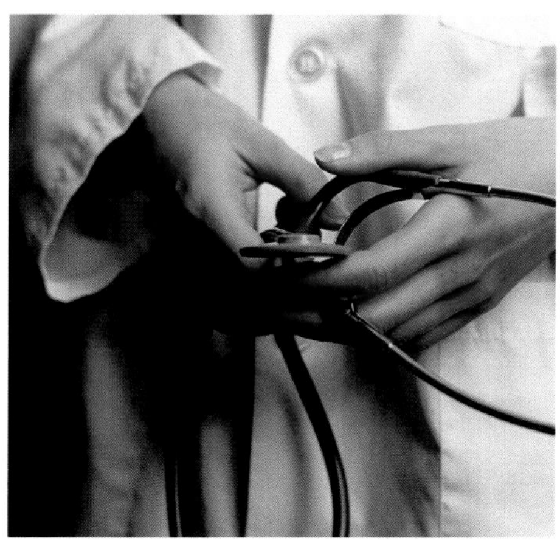

Cultures and the Medical Model

Historic Devaluation

History is riddled with examples of how groups of people have been oppressed and shunned by different societies. From religious persecutions in earliest times to ethnic devaluation and cleansing, particular people have been stigmatized and devalued. More recently, genocide in Germany, apartheid in South Africa, aboriginal separation in Australia, ethnic cleansing in Bosnia and racial discrimination in the United States are vivid examples of how people can be treated in hostile ways because they are devalued. All of these forms of cultural devaluation include some common features (Wolfensberger, 1987).

People are devalued when they are identified by their differences.

Looking at society today, perhaps the most discriminated block of people in the world are people who have been labeled as disabled. Every society has had difficulty, including and welcoming people with disabilities. Certainly in the United States, the climate for inclusion and full community participation for people with disabilities is still remarkably inconsistent.

People with disabilities are caught in this web of cultural devaluation. In spite of rehabilitation services, treatment, legal rights (Americans with Disabilities Act), and charitable approaches, public perceptions of people with disabilities are troubling. Consider that people with disabilities:

- Continue to be labeled at the drop of a hat.

  Usually these labels are medical in nature and create huge cultural stereotypes.

- Are still readily institutionalized.

  Although many institutions have shifted from large, gothic settings to smaller, group facilities, they are still institutions in format. For example, public funding for community supports for people with disabilities is still only offered as a "waiver" to the institutional bias of Medicaid.

- Continue to be viewed as a problem for society.

  Federal and state governments offer funds to address the "disability

Devalued people are:

- Labeled and stereotyped.
- Often congregated in a noticeable way into their own space.
- Thought to be a problem or to pose some kind of threat to those in authority.
- Identified by their label or their difference from those in authority.
- Perceived to be a cost to society, in material or economic ways.

problem," citizens are cautious of having people with disabilities move into neighborhood group homes, some communities actually have ordinances that specify how much distance must be allowed between homes or places where people with disabilities live.

- Are stuck with labels in the community.

  For example, "Jerry's kids," the mentally ill, TBIs, CPs, and MR/DDs are labels used to identify classes of people.

- Are seen as an economic burden.

  For any given classification of disability there are efforts to generate funding to address the specific problems posed by the disability, creating an economic cost to the community.

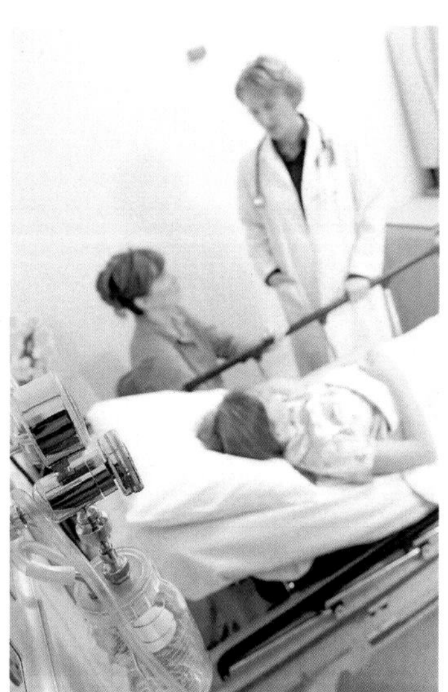

The Medical Model

Medical professionals are often the first "non-family" to become involved when a "disability problem" arises. This may be why the lens generally used by society to view disabilities is still colored by the Medical Model. As a result, members of the community often view a disability as a form of illness or sickness. The Medical Model is prominent and influential in brain injury rehabilitation.

Many theorists have looked at the Medical model as a framework for delivering services. This framework has been summarized in the caption below (Condeluci, 1991):

Since the Medical Paradigm is so pervasive in human services, a deeper examination is warranted. Consider these general characteristics of the paradigm (Zolla, 1986):

- The professional is expert and in charge of the care/treatment.
- Care and treatment is administered through a chain of authority.
- The person who receives treatment is labeled and expected to cooperate.

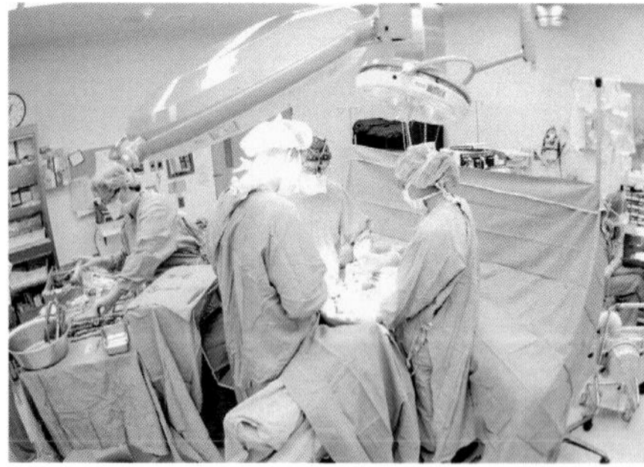

- Main purpose of entry to the paradigm is to restore or fix the person.
- The ailment that brings the person to the paradigm is labeled via a diagnosis.
- Literature and research is used to understand specific features of the ailment.
- The patient is usually offset and congregated with others in like situations.
- Most options for control are held by the expert or other representatives of the paradigm.
- The ailment is usually overshadowed within some therapeutic approach.

Medical Paradigm

- The problem .... The condition
- Core of the problem............... Rests in or with the person
- Actions of the paradigm .... Classify/congregate/treat the problem
- Power person .... The expert (doctor or therapist)
- Goal of the paradigm .... Fix/heal/change the condition/person

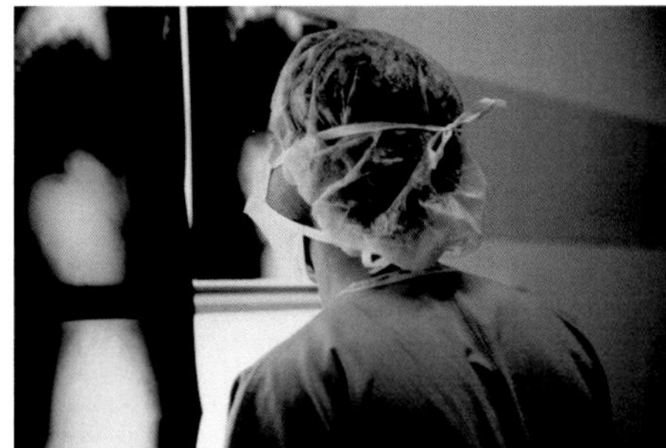

- The ailment can only be treated by the expert or an agent.
- The expert has some credentials or license to treat the ailment.
- The patient is exempt from any real responsibility, except to cooperate.
- Most aspects of the ailment are treated in separate and distinct facilities designed for the ailment.

Exploring the Medical Model reveals other troublesome aspects. These include its emphasis on areas of deficiency, accuracy of predictions of outcome, and its need to validate its own practices. No one is suggesting that these results occur by design. Rather these results are often inadvertent effects of contact with the paradigm. Each of these aspects has internal and external ramifications or unintended consequences. Internally, they begin to shape how the "patient" sees himself and often creates a "sickness identity."

In and of itself, the Medical Model is not bad. Indeed, it does work – when the goal is to address sickness or establish medical stability. However, serious problems arise when its components continue to be used after sickness or medical stability has been addressed. While the Medical Model is relevant during medical instability, a remarkably different model is needed after medical stability has been accomplished.

The ultimate goal of brain injury rehabilitation is not to eliminate sickness (some would argue this!), but to return people who have been injured as fully as possible to their communities. By using this orientation to rehabilitation, our real effort is to help:

- Establish medical stability.
- The individual adapt to the expectations of the community.
- The community accept and respect the differences that people with disabilities may have.

Interdependence, Inclusion and Self-Determination

Interdependence

Finding a philosophy for encouraging community diversity requires a plan that extends the Medical Model. The Interdependent Paradigm has been suggested (Condeluci, 1991). The term Interdependence is not new. However, although it has been used sometimes in human services, it is more often applied to cultural or political issues. Put simply, Interdependence implies a connection or a relationship between two or more entities. It suggests a partnership between parties that maximizes potential for both.

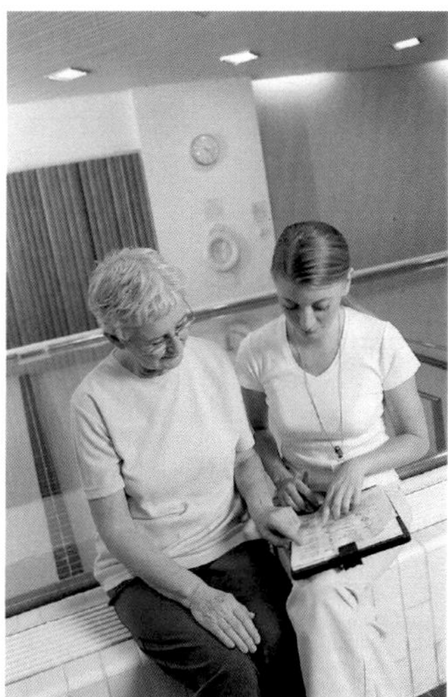

Interdependence Paradigm

- The problem .... Limited or non-existent supports for difference
- Core of the problem............... The system or community
- Actions of the paradigm .... To create supports and empower
- Power person .... The person with the disability
- Goal of the paradigm .... Develop mutually desired relationships

Comparison of Paradigms

Interdependence	Medical
Focuses on capacities	Focuses on deficiencies
Stresses relationships	Stresses congregation
Driven by the person/disability	Driven by the expert/professional
Promotes micro/macro change	Promotes that the person be fixed

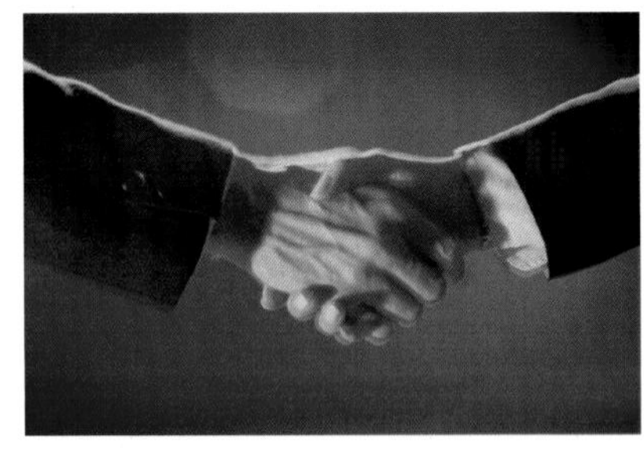

Interdependence is about relating in ways that promote mutual acceptance and respect. Although it recognizes that all people have differences, as a paradigm it encourages acceptance and empowerment for all. Imagine a world in which diverse people learn to interact in a way that improves conditions for everyone.

The best way to appreciate an Interdependent Paradigm is to compare it to the Medical Model. See the box above for this comparison.

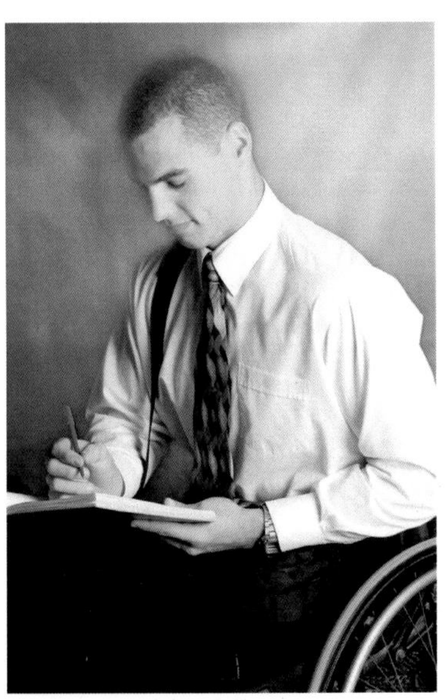

The Interdependent Paradigm offers a fundamentally different perspective on interacting with persons with disabilities. In many ways, the approach is a radical shift from the past. Most of what happens in the early stages of brain injury rehabilitation is offered in the context of the Medical Model. However, as persons prepare to return to the community and receive services, the Interdependent model is a more appropriate framework.

Inclusion

If there were one word that fully captures the ultimate goal of rehabilitation for people with brain injuries, "Inclusion" is that word. Inclusion means that the individual is incorporated and welcomed into the community, regardless of their disability.

Integration is very different from Inclusion. To a large extent, integration expects that people fit in, be alike and reach for similar standards. Although this might fit within the civil rights movement, the notion of having to fit in or be like the "majority" is not realistic in the disability rights movement. To expect people who might not be able to achieve a sense of similarity to be like the majority can be insensitive and inappropriate.

Inclusion brings people to the community regardless of their differences. It does not try to change or alter differences against the person's will or capacity. It does not try to create forced similarity. Inclusion suggests that people join in as they are. Inclusion respects differences, honors diversity, and invites full community participation. It is a term that implies a welcome to all.

Traditional efforts for Inclusion of people with brain injuries have typically focused on changing the

Inclusion

Inclusion brings people to the community regardless of their differences. It does not try to change or alter differences against the person's will or capacity. It does not try to create forced similarity. Inclusion suggests that people join in as they are. Inclusion respects differences, honors diversity, *and invites full community participation. It is a term that implies a welcome to all.*

most obvious behaviors that are presumed related to success in the community (e.g., walking, talking, thinking). Consequently, the majority of rehabilitation programs focus on delivering services to treat problems that accentuate differences between the individual and people in the community. Yet, many people do not and need not accomplish these things to be welcomed in certain communities. It has become clear that rehabilitation must expand its traditional focus.

The Interdependent Paradigm and the concept of Inclusion begin to provide ways to go beyond the traditional focus of brain injury rehabilitation. More contemporary rehabilitation organizations address problems that people with brain injuries can (and have a desire to) address and find ways to include them in their communities as they are. Fostering inclusion represents a change in the very foundation of one's perspective on people.

The concept of Self-Determination revolves around four critical components:

Freedom

Ability to plan a life with supports rather than purchase or be referred to a particular program

Authority

Ability to control a certain sum of dollars to purchase preferred supports

Support

Use of resources to arrange formal and informal supports to live within the community

Responsibility

Role within the community through competitive employment, organizational affiliations, general caring for others within the community, and accountability for spending public dollars in life-enhancing ways.

Self-Determination

Self-Determination is an emerging concept in human services. It builds on the principles of Informed Consent, right to refuse, and consumer empowerment. Self-Determination is really another way of saying individual freedom. In many ways, the concept is a fresh reminder that people with disabilities (whether physical, mental or cognitive) have rights and authority over how, where and with whom they live.

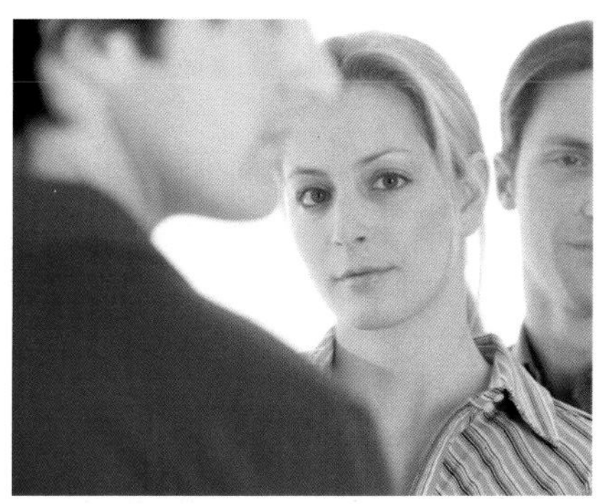

In the recent Olmstead Decision, the Courts have made it clear that people with disabilities have the right to equal, community based options and that States must make these options available. It also means that people have increased control of the resources needed for their support and may participate in advocating more directly for their interests (Bambara, Cole & Koger, 1998).

Recently, a number of states have begun to incorporate the concept of Self-Determination into the public funded human service system. They recommend these key actions to achieve Self-Determination:

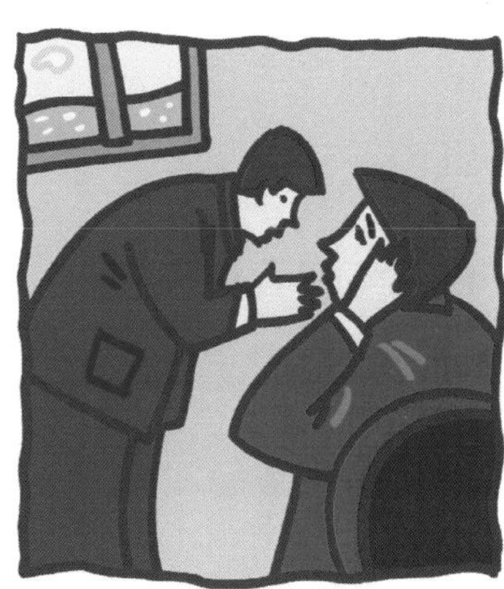

- Transfer financial control to the consumer through individual budgets.
- Use person centered planning to identify, organize, and communicate choices.
- Promote cooperation and collaboration.
- Revise community awareness activities of resources.
- Communicate and share information.
- Change laws, rules, policies and procedures to empower people.
- Train, educate and develop leadership among people with disabilities.
- Gather and analyze data.
- Quality enhancement and evaluation of activities.

Self-Determination is a principle that will continue to factor into rehabilitation and will be sure to influence brain injury rehabilitation. We need to listen to TBI survivors and assure that they are heard.

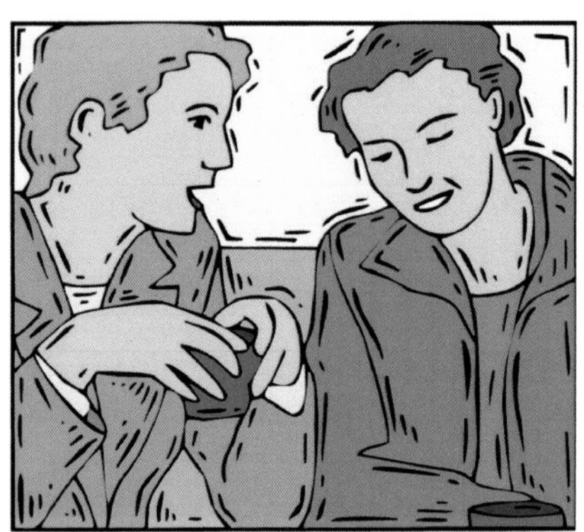

Basis of Interaction within Rehabilitation

The rehabilitation process often involves complex techniques, procedures, or approaches provided by a diverse group of people. They include professionals from various educational disciplines, family members, other concerned citizens and direct care staff. It also involves the creation, adaptation, and use of various community services and supports. The philosophies and principles discussed so far should orient people to the helping role. How can those ideals be realized more consistently? This section highlights particular beliefs and "general interactional styles" that are consistent with the philosophies presented above.

While much of the rehabilitation process can appear quite complicated, it may be important to consider that all rehabilitation is fundamentally based on interactions between two or more people – those providing assistance and those receiving assistance.

There is a very delicate balance between assisting someone by encouraging Inclusion or Self-Determination and interacting in a way that inadvertently contributes to devaluation, social isolation and increased dependency. The best guide to determining what to do in a given situation still may be to consider how you or any individual would prefer to be treated in similar circumstances.

Each person with a brain injury has experienced an unexpected life event that may impact every aspect of their being – living arrangements, family relations, vocation, friendships, sexuality, emotions, ability to benefit from experience, mobility, finances, and sense of self. For virtually all participants, a day in rehabilitation is remarkably different than anything ever experienced before. They are poked and prodded, evaluated and observed. They are often provided with instruction and feedback about how they are doing throughout the day. Rehabilitation can be an extremely invasive and public process.

Empathy is the ability to identify with and understand another person's feelings or difficulties. Having empathy may impact our interactions with those we assist in general ways. However, one probably needs to go beyond having empathy in order to impact interactions in a noticeable, consistent, and effective way. Why be involved in providing assistance? Why stay involved? What gives the greatest sense of satisfaction and joy from the work that is done? How can those things be continued in the midst of the difficult, troubling, and even traumatic circumstances that can occur while providing assistance to others? What is it that those people have, whose interactional style is admired, that allows them to continue acting that way? How can those things be described and learned so that others

Basis of Interaction

While much of the rehabilitation process can appear quite complicated, it may be important to consider that all rehabilitation is fundamentally based on interactions between two or more people – those providing assistance and those receiving assistance.

can interact more successfully in the rehabilitation process?

Mutual Reinforcement and Reciprocity

Behavioral research suggests that:

- Human behaviors often develop and continue because of their "desirable" effects for the individual who performs them.
- People probably have a tendency to treat others as they are treated.
- Self reports of interactional satisfaction (e.g., friendship, love, joy) appear related to the concept of "Mutual Reinforcement."

When there is an ongoing exchange of desired events between people, it can develop into a positive reciprocal relationship.

Mutual Reinforcement is characterized by an exchange of reinforcers or desired events between two or more people (Azrin, Naster & Jones, 1973). It is hypothesized that most continuing relationships involve a regular exchange of reinforcers or desired events between the persons involved. When an exchange of reinforcers develops into a consistent pattern, it can be called a Positive Reciprocal Relationship or positive reciprocity.

Of course, some relationships appear to involve ongoing exchange of unwanted events between people. When this occurs, it can be referred to as a Negative Reciprocal Relationship or negative reciprocity (e.g., as if to "pay back" for each perceived wrongdoing delivered by the other party). Both types of relationships are considered reciprocal (i.e., "you pat my back and I'll pat yours" or "eye for an eye"). We can spot these types of relationships in our lives, as well as in the world around us.

Many conclusions and extrapolations can be made from consideration of these principles. They help explain some of our behavior, as well as the behavior of those around us (e.g., behavior continues for a reason). They may help explain why people sometimes treat each other poorly and continue to do so in spite of the damage done (e.g., negative reciprocity). Striving toward the development of mutually reinforcing relationships or positive reciprocity may help the persons being helped have a greater sense of success in rehabilitation and life. In addition, developing such ongoing relationships may help those giving assistance gain deeper satisfaction and joy from their work. In many ways, these concepts represent the interactional root of the Interdependent Model and the experience of community it proposes.

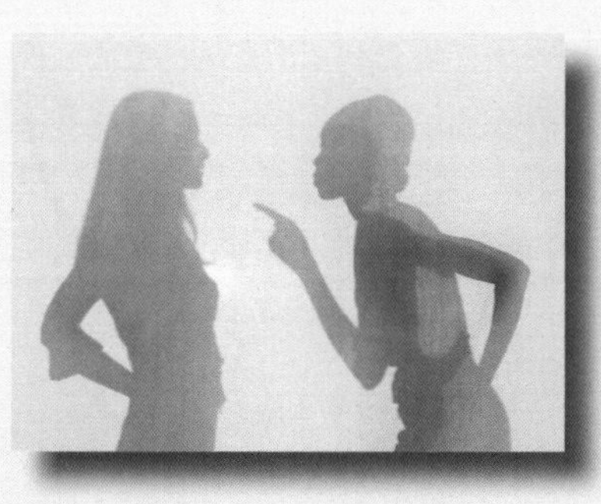

When there is an ongoing exchange of unwanted events between people, a negitive reciprocal relationship can form.

Mutually reinforcing interactions are needed for meaningful rehabilitation outcomes, for satisfaction among those who assist, and for the creation of interdependent communities. The more these types of interactions can be promoted, the greater the likelihood of accomplishing the ultimate goals of rehabilitation.

Promoting Mutually Reinforcing Interactions

What is <u>not</u> wanted in interactions between persons in rehabilitation includes:

- Insensitivity to differences (e.g., particularly those that are unlikely to change)
- The creation or prolonging of negatively reciprocal interactions (e.g., overly corrective, disempowering, or unnecessarily restrictive comments or actions).

So, how can we promote the development of mutually reinforcing interactions in the rehabilitation process?

Active Treatment Interaction

Historically, the term "active treatment" has had many definitions in the human services field.

The preferred definition clarifies that active treatment is an interaction between two people that is intended to result in greater independence, autonomy, empowerment, or Inclusion for one of those people.

For the sake of contrast, Active Treatment Interaction does not promote caring for a person in a custodial sense or behaving in ways that are likely to increase dependency within the relationship. The term is intended to imply directed action, teaching, and a certain degree of risk taking. This very broad concept can be broken down into five desired interactional components, called "PEARL", as defined in the box below.

Responding to opportunities to acknowledge people for "doing things well," rather than waiting for them to fail or correcting their "mistakes," can have a dramatic impact on rehabilitation interactions. It also can affect the participant's self-esteem. Active Treatment Interaction is not a style to use sometimes and not other times. On the contrary, it is recommended that it be the basis of every interaction throughout the rehabilitation process (McMorrow, 1994; Softpath Habilitation, 1994).

P - E - A - R - L

Positive	Is upbeat, enthusiastic, requesting rather than demanding, actively prompting and encouraging participation.
Early	Is proactive when difficult or troubling situations arise, intervening early to facilitate problem solving, and interrupting or redirecting behavioral consequences that could lead to more serious problems.
All	Acts these ways all the time, with all participants, and in all daily situations.
Reinforce	Is consistently recognizing, acknowledging, and socially reinforcing participant accomplishments.
Look	Looks for situations or opportunities to facilitate independence, autonomy, empowerment, or inclusion.

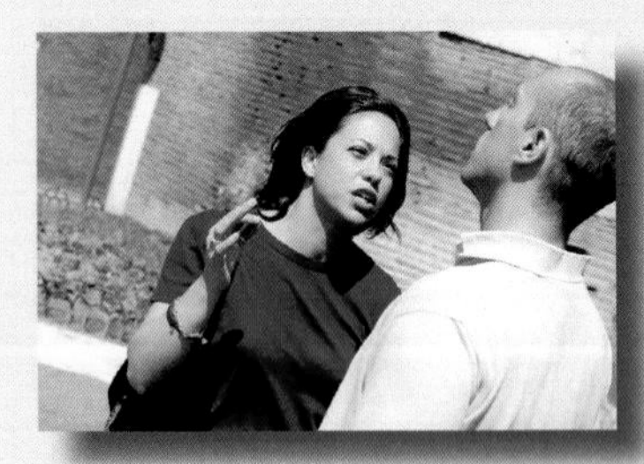

Because we are all predisposed to act in particular ways, blaming people for unwanted actions makes little sense.

No Blame

Each individual is predisposed to act in particular ways in particular situations. This is based on the individual's experience, level of skill, motivation, level of assistance received, and a host of other factors. Predispositions include all the medical, cognitive, physical, biochemical, and environmental factors that influence actions in a given situation. For example, a person in pain may be more likely to be irritable or resistant to touch in a particular area. In the simplest way, predispositions are everything the person brings to the table. Considering various predispositions helps understanding why a person behaves in a particular way. It also helps find better ways to help the person respond differently to the same situation in the future.

It is potentially useful to take the notion of predispositions a step or two further. This may impact how individuals interact during rehabilitation. Put simply, the concept of "No Blame"

Example of *No blame*

Following Bill's third episode of incontinence on her shift, Sharon becomes frustrated and verbally corrects him in a loud voice. She publicly proclaims to her co-workers that "he is doing it on purpose."

proposes that if people are predisposed to behave in certain ways in certain situations, then holding them at fault or blame for unwanted actions does not make good sense. The concept of No Blame is potentially important, because blame often appears to be at the root of some of the most indignant or hurtful things people do to one another. For illustration of this concept see the box above.

Curiously, Sharon's conclusion that Bill is being incontinent on purpose appears to provide her with the reason to treat him in an indignant manner. Sharon would act differently if she considered that Bill is predisposed to incontinence due to his injury, that up until yesterday he wore diapers to address the problem, and he has yet to toilet independently without prompting from others.

If Sharon held the perspective of "No Blame" she would be likely to treat Bill in a way that provides him with the assistance that he needs. More importantly, she might treat him as a dignified adult person, who is also incontinent.

No Blame is probably at the basis of the differences in the way that staff interacted with Lee in the examples at the beginning of this chapter. In the first example, staff viewed Lee as being in control of his behavior. As a result, they labeled certain of his characteristic actions (e.g., he was "psychotic") and interacted with him in a very corrective fashion (e.g., as if all he needed to do was listen to their directions to have his life be different). Once they discovered the extent of his confusion and disorientation (i.e., the predisposing factors for his behavior), they dropped the blame and began to provide assistance that made a difference for everyone.

Can vs. Can't

The concept of "Can vs. Can't" is another important consideration for interactions in rehabilitation. Despite the obligation to protect persons being served from harm, this rationale cannot be used without regard for the person's interest, choice, or preference.

Too often, providers get in the way of assisting increased autonomy by failing to consider the participant's interest in the matter. They fail to consider what is possible (instead of what might possibly happen) and the potential benefit of doing rather than preventing. Instead of focusing on ways to restrict the individual's independent access to the community, how can the focus shift to helping the individual reenter the community safely?

Operating from the stance of "Can vs. Can't" staff are more likely to encourage Inclusion rather than finding themselves in a situation where they must manage exclusion. They can increase mutually desired actions, rather than decrease unwanted behaviors. Staff can also find ways to support a person's interests, rather than constantly refusing requests. When treatment implementation is guided by the "Can vs. Can't" orientation, it offers an individual the dignity of risk that is a vital part of learning, growth, and development for all human beings.

Example of Can vs. Can't

While a participant may not be able to independently arrange getting to and from the shopping mall, purchases at the mall may be able to be made independently with transportation assistance and a reminder note of what to purchase.

Outcome, Partnerships and Agreements

The rehabilitation process calls for the development of partnerships between many different people to accomplish the various goals (e.g., medical stability, increased utilization of support, semi-independent living, etc.). An Outcome Oriented Model is designed to identify areas of agreement between people that are related to the goals of their assistance. This is critical to the development of partnerships. Without clear and meaningful goals, individuals often find themselves "doing what they do" without considering what others are attempting to accomplish and how they are going about it. Partnerships are needed between rehabilitation professionals, between professionals and paraprofessionals, and between professionals and family members.

Most importantly, partnerships are needed with the person who has sustained the injury. These partnerships must be established very rapidly after the injury and must be maintained at every point in the process.

While partnerships may seem less relevant during medical stabilization or post-injury amnesia, it is possible that interactions that occur at these points impact the future likelihood of other constructive partnerships. For example, what really is the long term impact of physically restraining a person who is tremendously confused?

An outcome orientation, combined with a goal of establishing partnerships through agreement may include all the necessary ingredients of a mutually reinforcing rehabilitation relationship. All who are involved need to explore and discover the potential joy that is possible in this work.

Summary

- Avoid promoting a rehabilitation culture that devalues persons who behave differently.
- The Medical Model is particularly useful to address sickness or medical instability.
- The ultimate goal of brain injury rehabilitation is to return people as fully as possible to their communities.
- Establishing a philosophy of rehabilitation that addresses medical instability and returns people to the community needs to go beyond the Medical model.
- The Interdependent paradigm and the principles of Inclusion and Self-Determination represent contemporary rehabilitation philosophies that help persons with brain injuries realize their goals and impact the how persons interact with others who have experienced brain injury.
- The concepts of Mutual Reinforcement and Reciprocity represent ways to organize the interactional basis of rehabilitation relationships.
- Active Treatment Interaction with PEARL (positive, early, all, reinforce and look components). No Blame, and Can vs. Can't are interactional styles that are intended to facilitate the accomplishment of outcome goals, partnerships, and agreement within the rehabilitation process.

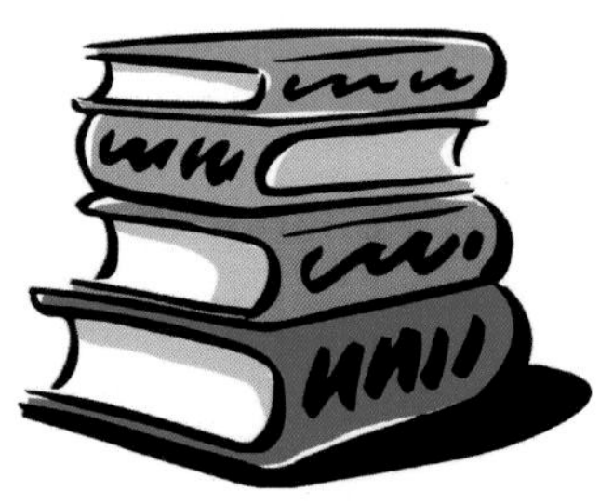

References

Azrin, NH, Naster, BJ, and Jones, R (1973). Reciprocity Counseling: A rapid learning-based procedure for marital counseling. Behaviour Research and Therapy. 11: 365-382.

Bambara, L, Cole, C, and Koger, F (1998). Translating self-determination concepts into support for adults with severe disabilities. The Journal of the Association for Persons with Severe Handicaps. 23 (1), 27-37.

Condeluci, A (1991). Interdependence: The route to community. Boca Raton: St Lucie Press.

McMorrow, MJ (1994). Active Treatment: Putting the concept into practice. Carbondale, IL: Center for Comprehensive Services, Monograph Vol. 1:3.

McMorrow, MJ (2003). Getting ready to help: A Primer on interacting in human service. Baltimore: Paul Brookes Publishing.

Softpath Habilitation. Active Treatment with PEARL. Cobden, IL. Softpath Habilitation, 1994.

Wolfensberger, W. The new genocide of handicapped and affected people. Syracuse, NY.

Training Institute for Human Service Planning, Leadership and Change Agency, 1987.

Zolla, I. The medicalization of aging and disability: Problems and prospects. In C. Mahoney, C. Estes and J. Heumann (Eds.), Toward a Unified Agenda. Berkeley: World Institute on Disability.

Chapter 3

Understanding the Brain and Brain Injury

Learning Objectives

By the end of this chapter, you will be able to:

- Identify basic brain structures and functions.
- Describe brain-behavior relationships
- Describe how an injury to the brain can result in various behaviors and challenges

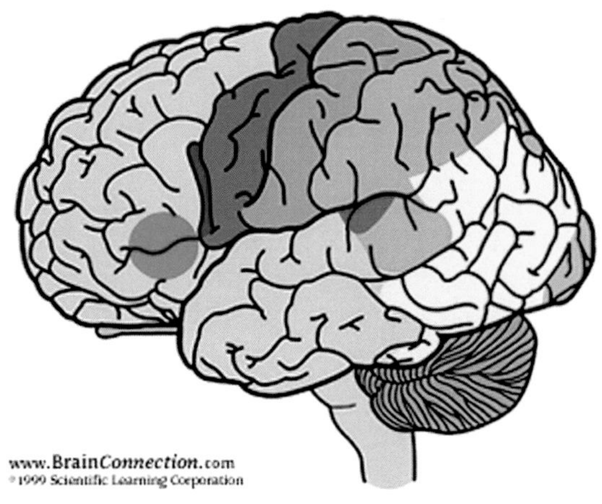
www.BrainConnection.com
©1999 Scientific Learning Corporation

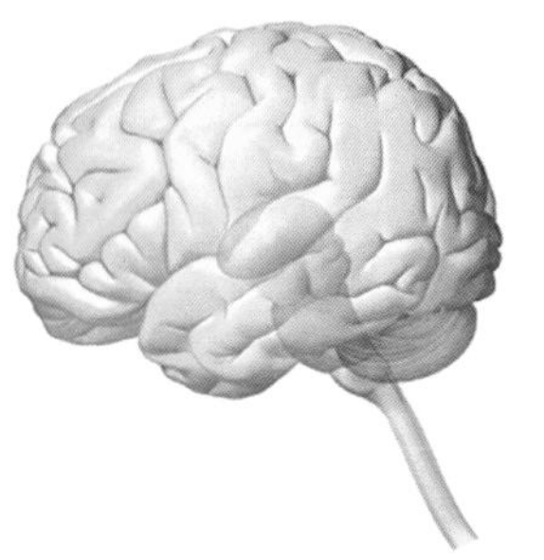

Introduction

The brain is the main organ of learning. It makes it possible for us to think, communicate, act, behave, move about, and create. All that we were, all that we are, and all that we will be – comes from our brain. This chapter describes how the human brain works and what happens when it is injured.

The Brain and Its Parts

The brain is not hard like the muscles in an arm or leg. It is a soft organ, like the consistency of gelatin, that weighs less than one pound at birth and grows to about 3 pounds in an adult. The brain sits inside a rough and bony skull and is bathed in cerebrospinal fluid (CSF). The brain receives oxygen and glucose through a sophisticated system of blood vessels that carry blood to and from the heart.

There are three membranes called meninges that cover the brain. There is the outer dura mater or hard matter, which is like a heavy plastic covering. Then there is the arachnoid which is like a spiderweb that bridges the brain's many wrinkles and folds. Finally there is the pia mater or tender matter which molds around every tiny crook and crevice on the brain's surface.

Between the pia mater and the arachnoid, there is a teacup full (145cc) of cerebrospinal fluid. This fluid flows like millions of little streams and becomes a cushion that protects the nerve tissue.

Inside the brain, there are four different reservoirs or ventricles which make, store, and circulate cerebrospinal fluid. These ventricles are like tiny lakes within the brain that pool the fluid. They help cushion the brain and protect brain tissue when swelling occurs.

When the Brain is Injured

If the brain is injured by a sudden jolt or bang, it reverberates or bounces around like "jello" in a plastic bag. This movement often rips, tears, and stretches the blood vessels and delicate nerve tissues. The inside of the skull is ragged with sharp bony ridges, so major bleeding can occur when the brain rubs against it.

The brain can bleed and/or swell with blood and fluid when it is injured. But unlike other body parts like an arm or leg that swells when twisted or broken, the skull is closed and has no extra room for swelling or fluid. Tremendous pressure can build within the skull after an injury and compress

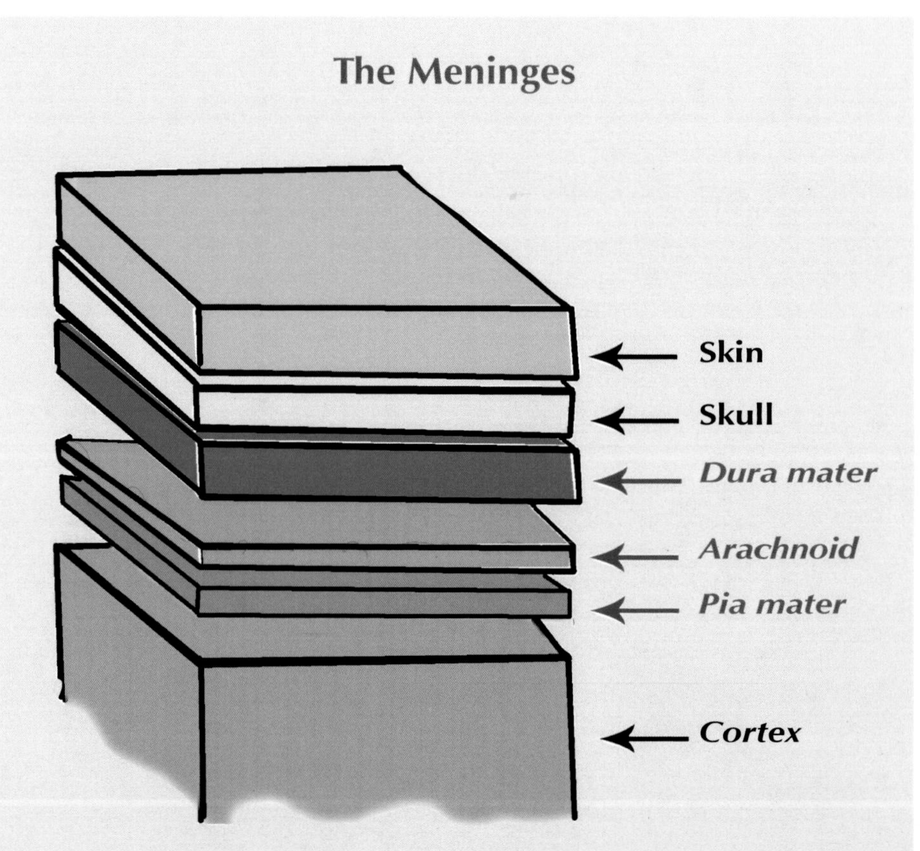

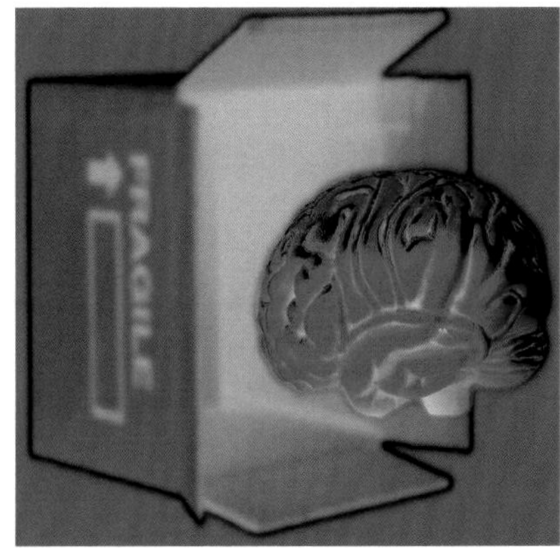

brain tissue and blood vessels. This can deprive the brain of oxygen and create an additional or secondary brain injury.

As the brain swells, pressure builds up inside the skull. Physicians often relieve this pressure (intracranial) by inserting special devices into the skull to monitor it. If the pressure gets too high, surgery may be needed to remove any accumulation of blood (hematomas) or excess cerebrospinal fluid (hydrocephalus).

In some cases, the bleeding may be so slow that the pressure on the brain builds up over time. It may go unrecognized until the person starts to show symptoms (e.g., passes out or has severe headaches). A prominent feature of persons with slow bleeds is disorientation, confusion, forgetfulness and possibly the experience of severe headaches or brief loss of consciousness. This is common with subdural hematomas (bleeding into the space between the dura mater and the arachnoid layers of the meninges).

A brain injury is often the result of two injuries – the "primary injury" caused by the initial blow or insult to the brain, and the "secondary injury" caused by the swelling, bleeding, compression and contusions (bruises) to the brain.

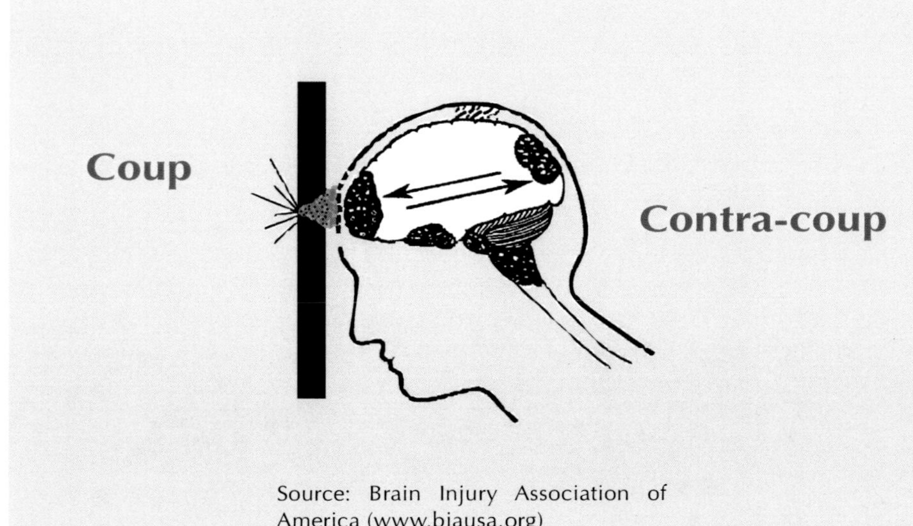

Source: Brain Injury Association of America (www.biausa.org)

A brain injury is often the result of two injuries – the "primary injury" caused by the initial blow or insult to the brain, and the "secondary injury" caused by the swelling, bleeding, compression and contusions (bruises) to the brain.

Other Brain Injuries

An injury to one side of the brain can create a "coup-contra-coup" effect (side-to-side or back-to-back). This means that if the back of the head is struck, the front of the brain can also be injured by this bouncing back and forth or coup-contracoup effect.

Severe brain injuries can happen even without a lot of bleeding into the brain. This can happen when individual nerve cells throughout the brain are stretched and break. These injuries are called diffuse axonal injuries (DAI). They result in extensive injury to the entire brain.

Injuries that cause severe blood loss anywhere in the body can decrease the amount of oxygen getting to the brain (hypoxia) or stop oxygen from getting to the brain (anoxia). This may cause brain cells to die. There are many other causes of anoxia that can result in brain injuries, including near drownings, heart attacks, suffocation, smoke inhalation, asthma attacks, and strangulation.

Severity of Brain Injuries

There are many definitions describing the levels of severity of brain injury. However, they are often classified into three kinds: mild, moderate and severe brain injuries. Listed below are some symptoms of each level.

The Glasgow Coma Scale (GCS) is one measure frequently used. Scores range between 3 and 15. The lower the score, the more severe the brain injury. There are three parameters for eye, verbal and motor responses. The GCS is computed by adding the score from each category:

Eye + Verbal + Motor = GCS.

See below for the definitions of brain injury severity and their corresponding GCS scores.

While these definitions "medically" describe the severity of a brain injury, they may not describe the challenges that the person will experience. For example, a mild brain injury may have a significant impact on a person's life by causing personality changes that in turn cause problems at home, at work, and in the community. If these problems are not addressed through rehabilitation or therapy, they may severely alter a person's abilities to function successfully at work or in social situations.

Many professionals and family members feel that the severity of the actual injury and the severity of the problems or consequences do not necessarily match the strict definitions of mild, moderate and severe.

Post-Concussion Symptoms

- Headache
- Dizziness
- Changes in personality
- Memory problems
- Vomiting
- Depression
- Sleep disturbance
- Difficulty problem solving
- Irritability
- Diminished attention span

Severity Definitions

Mild Brain Injury

- Loss of consciousness for less than 30 minutes (possibly no loss of consciousness).
- Glasgow Coma Scale of 13-15.
- Post-traumatic amnesia less than 24 hours.
- Temporary or permanently altered mental or neurological state.
- Post-concussion symptoms.

Moderate Brain Injury

- Coma more than 20-30 minutes, but less than 24 hours.
- Glasgow Coma Scale of 9-12.
- Possible skull fractures with bruising & bleeding.
- Signs on EEG, CT or MRI scans.
- Some long term problems in one or more areas of life (i.e., home, work, community).

Severe Brain Injury

- Coma longer than 24 hours, often lasting days or weeks.
- Glasgow Coma Scale of 3 to 8.
- Bruising, bleeding in brain.
- Signs on EEG, CT or MRI scans.
- Long term impairments in one or more areas of life (i.e., home, work, community).

Glascow Coma Scale

Eye Opening		Verbal Response		Motor Response	
4	Spontaneous	5	Oriented to person, place, month & year	6	Obeys commands
3	Eye opening to verbal command	4	Confused	5	Localizes pain
2	Eye opening to pain	3	Inappropriate words	4	Withdraws to pain
1	No eye opening	2	Sounds, but words not understandable	3	Abnormal flexion to pain
		1	No verbal response	2	Abnormal extension to pain
				1	No motor response

Neurons

Knowing how the brain communicates with itself helps a person understand how an injury affects it. There are billions and billions of tiny brain cells making up the nervous system. Neurons are the cells which "communicate." Glial cells are non-communicating cells that support and nourish the neurons. There are about 100 billion neurons in the brain, with about 10 to 50 times that many glial cells.

Each neuron has three main parts: cell body, axon (a long, slim "wire" that transmits signals from one cell body to another via junctions known as synapses), and dendrites (networks of short "wires" that take in information at the synapse from other neurons).

The neurons communicate with each other via a unique "electro-chemical" process. The neurons receive and transmit information in a relay where electrical impulses alternate with chemical messengers (neurotransmitters). When these electrical impulses reach a junction between the axon of one neuron and the dendrite of another neuron called a synapse, it triggers a neurochemical response. The electrical impulses flow through the axons and dendrites. Neurochemical transmitters leap the synaptic gaps between each neuron's axon and the other neurons with which an axon makes contact.

Each neuron is its own miniature information center that decides to fire or not fire off an electrical impulse. This decision depends on the numerous signals it receives every moment. After a person sustains a brain injury, many of these pathways may be torn apart or stretched so that information transmission is no longer possible between affected neurons.

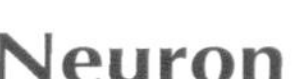

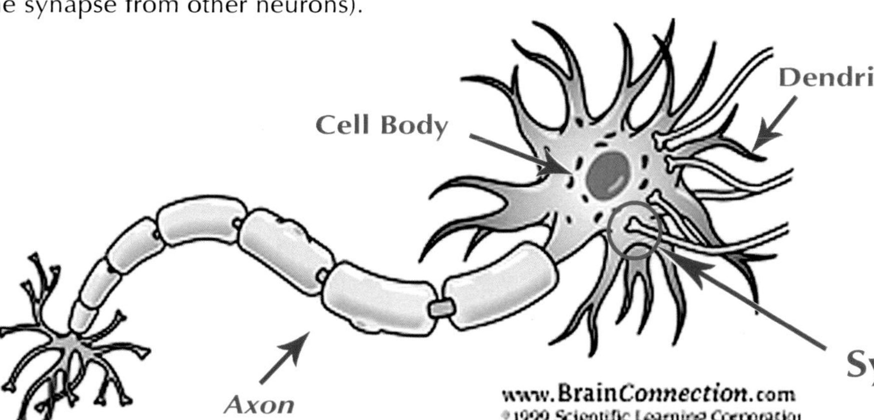

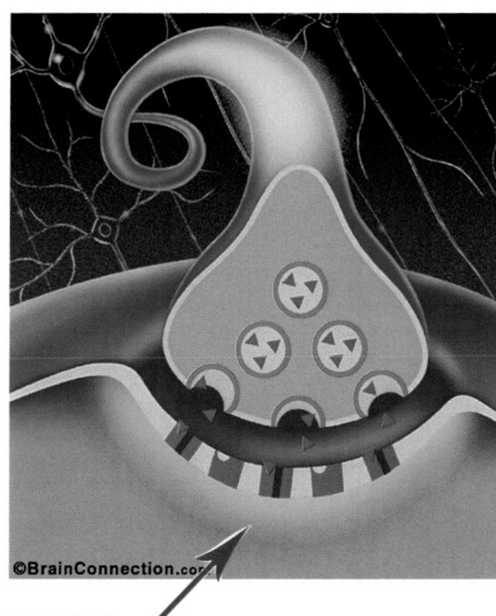

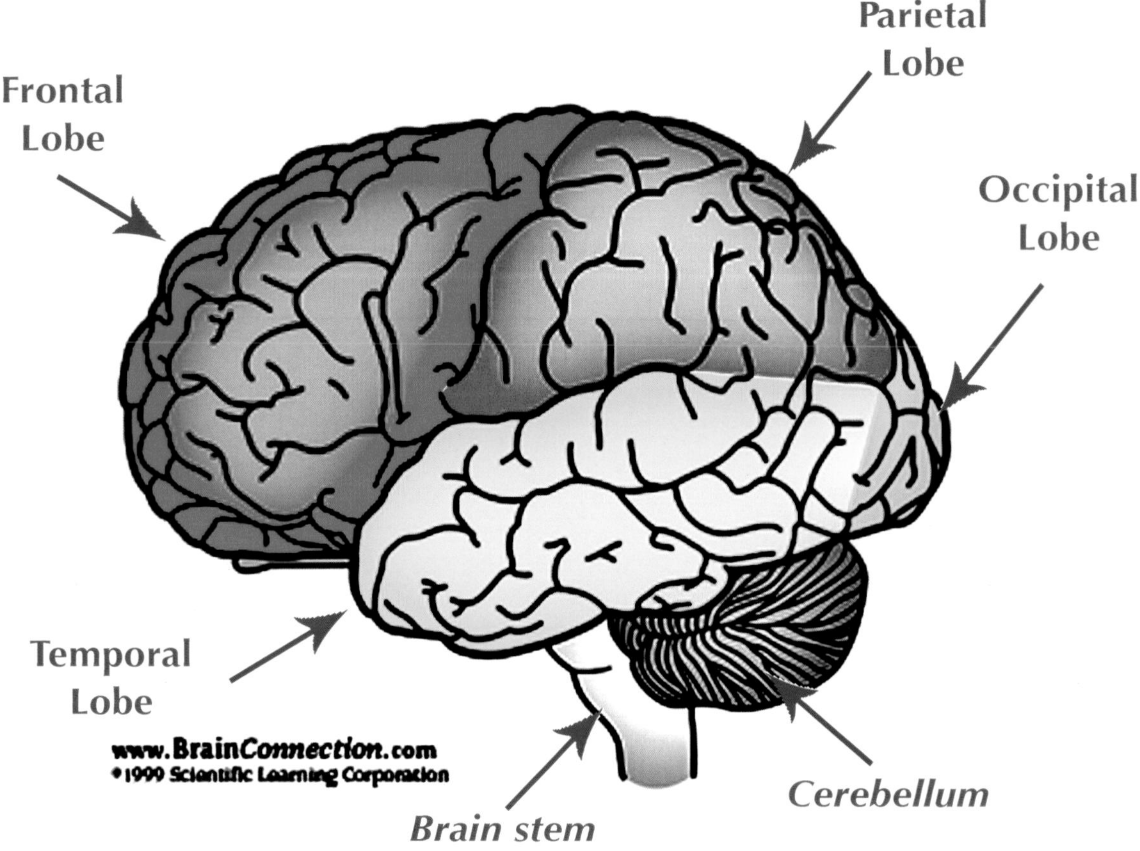

Brain Geography

Some basic neuro-anatomy provides a geography lesson on the brain. It is helpful to understand how the brain helps a person to think, move, and act.

To visualize the brain's geography, take a "road trip" of the human brain from the bottom to top. The major parts include the:

Brain stem

Located at the top of the spinal column, the brain stem relays information in and out of the brain. The brainstem is like the "point person" for all incoming and outgoing information and basic life functions.

Diencephalon

The diencephalon is made up of the thalamus, hypothalamus and other structures (see page 44). Located centimeters above the midbrain, the diencephalon is a master relay center for forwarding information, sensations, and movement.

Limbic System

The limbic system is in the middle section of the brain. It sits on top of the brain stem. The limbic system is involved in emotions and basic feelings (see illustration on page 45).

Cerebellum

Located in the lower back section of the brain, the cerebellum coordinates, modulates, and stores all body movement.

Cerebral Cortex

The cerebral cortex is divided into two hemispheres dedicated to the highest levels of thinking, moving, and acting. The right and left hemispheres are further divided into four lobes – frontal, parietal, temporal and occipital.

The Brain Stem

A more detailed look at the central nervous system reveals a major trunk at the top. This is the brainstem which evolves from the spinal cord. The brainstem is made up of three integral areas called the medulla, the pons, and the midbrain. The brainstem also contains many of the centers for the senses of hearing, touch, taste, and balance, though it does not affect sight and smell.

Within the brainstem, there is a collection of nerve fibers and nuclei called the reticular activating system (RAS). This system modulates or changes arousal, alertness, concentration, and basic biological rhythms. If a person is getting sleepy or having trouble attending to information in this chapter, the reader needs to "turn up" the RAS. It is much like the dimmer switch on a light that can be turned up to make the light brighter, or turned down to make it darker.

After a brain injury, many individuals lose consciousness, which can result in coma. Because of the severity of the injury or the brain swelling, their "dimmer switch" may be turned down. This leaves them unaware of their surroundings and unable to respond to even simple commands. Unfortunately, the RAS can be depressed to a point where a person even dies because all main body functions are shut down permanently.

Medulla

The first area in the lower part of the brain stem is the medulla. This is involved in many basic living functions. The medulla is about one inch of brain tissue that is vital to life and death. It contains reflex centers which control many involuntary functions such as breathing, heart rate, blood pressure, swallowing, vomiting, and sneezing. The medulla is where the polio virus struck, resulting in many children being placed in the "iron lung" machines of the 1950s. When the medulla is injured, as with any area of the brainstem, life is immediately threatened.

Pons

Just above the medulla is the pons. This important part of the brainstem is essential for facial movements, facial sensation, hearing, and coordinating eye movements. Like the other parts of the brainstem, it transmits all the sensations from the body up to the brain, and all of the movement signals down from the brain to the body. It also serves as a bridge of nerve fibers that connect the cerebral cortex and the cerebellum. This bridge enables the "thinking" part of the brain (cortex) to work with the "movement" (cerebellum) part of the brain. Disruption to the pons can cause a complete loss of ability to coordinate and control body movements. As a result, a person may be partially or totally paralyzed.

Midbrain

The smallest part of the brainstem is the midbrain. Yet as small as the midbrain is, elementary forms of seeing and hearing are possible. More

The Reticular Activating System

The RAS modulates or changes arousal, alertness, concentration, and basic biological rhythms. It is much like the dimmer switch on a light that can be turned up to make the light brighter, or turned down to make it darker.

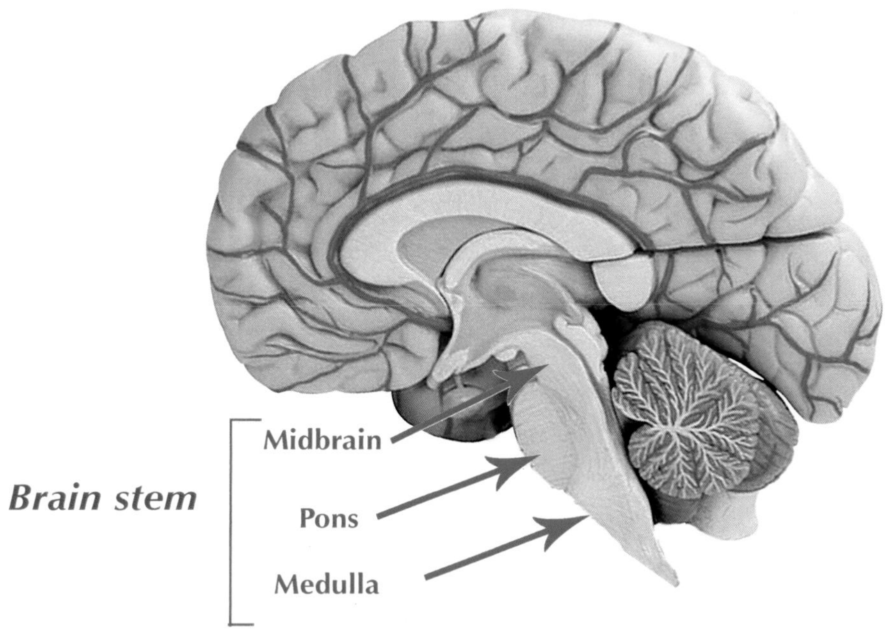

importantly, it is responsible for alertness and arousal.

Sometimes the cerebral cortex (hemispheres and lobes) of the brain can sustain catastrophic injury that renders this "thinking" part of the brain unresponsive; however, the person continues to live. Because of the functioning of the brain stem, "vegetative body functions"(e.g., breathing, heart rate, blood pressure and even sleep-wake cycles) may return since they are controlled by the brain stem.

These individuals still can breathe and their hearts still beat, even without life supporting equipment. In this situation, the person is in a prolonged coma or minimally conscious and this condition often is called a vegetative state. This condition is better referred to as coma and/or low level of consciousness.

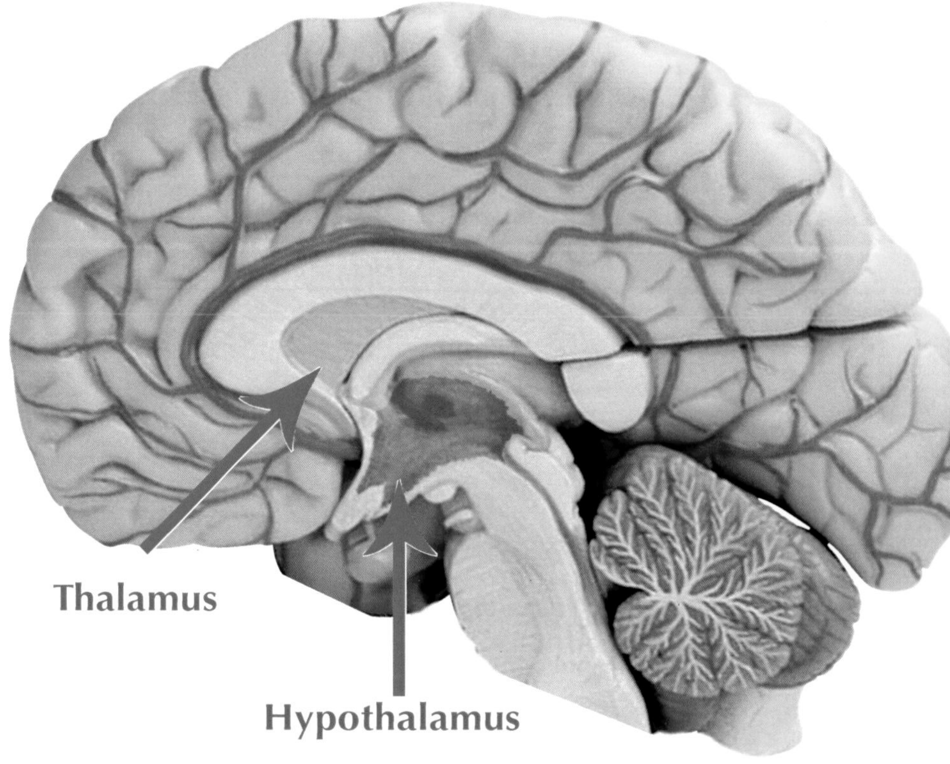

Diencephalon

The diencephalon is made up of the thalamus, hypothalamus and other structures.

The thalamus sits on the very top of the brain stem just beneath the cortex. It acts as a major relay station for incoming and outgoing sensory information. Each sense (except smell) relays its impulses through the thalamus.

Individuals who have an injury to their thalamus can have severe attention and concentration problems, difficulty with memory storage and retrieval, weakened mental stamina, decreased sensory information, difficulty in reacting to stress, difficulty with excessive or not enough emotional responses, and disorders in eating/drinking, sleeping, and sexual functioning.

The hypothalamus, in particular, is the control center for hunger, thirst, sexual response, endocrine levels, and temperature regulation. It is also involved in many complex responses like anger, fatigue, memory, and calmness. It serves as the "conductor" of a person's emotional orchestra.

Since the hypothalamus is the major brain region that manages the release of body hormones, individuals who have this part of their brain injured may have many complex problems. The brain is also the largest "chemical" factory in the body. Disruption to the hormonal, endocrine, and/or neurochemical systems can be just as devastating as an injury to the neural network. Physicians may prescribe medications to enhance the effectiveness of certain neurotransmittors and/or hormones.

The Limbic System

Situated above, around, and interconnected with the diencephalon is the limbic system. Many neurosurgeons, neurologists, and neuro-psychologists argue about which particular areas of the brain best fit into certain systems. Is the diencephalon with its thalamus and hypothalamus part of the limbic system or the upper brain stem? It is easier to understand if the brain is viewed as a highly interconnected organ with complex systems that control all internal and external responses and actions.

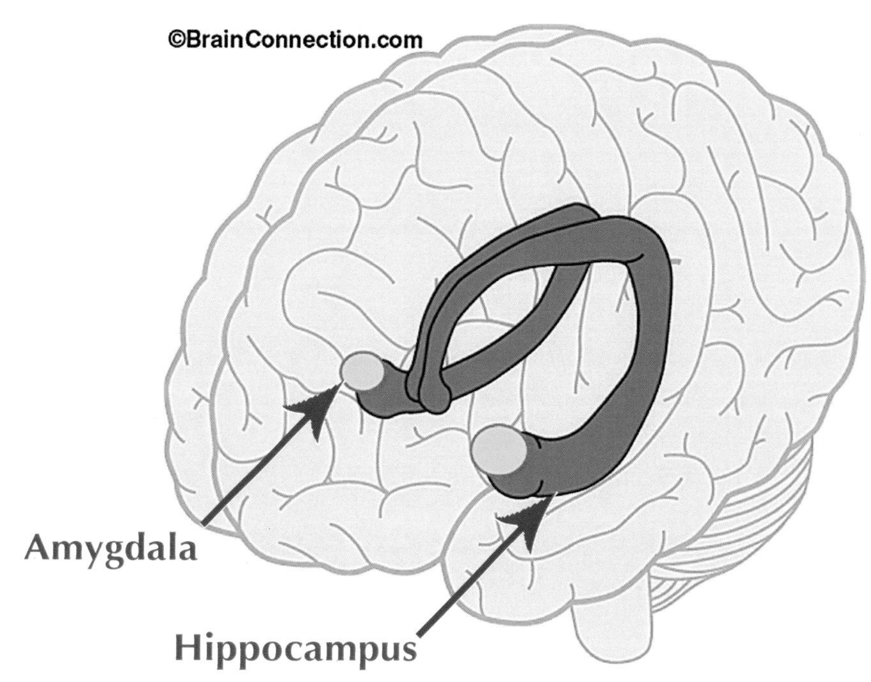

Taking a more detailed look at the limbic system, there is increasing complexity and connectiveness with other parts of the brain, especially the cerebral cortex. Some brain researchers have referred to the "middle" (limbic) part of the brain as the "mammalian brain", the evolutionary, animal like part of the brain that houses basic elemental drives, emotions, and survival instincts.

Injury or disruption to the limbic system can produce serious problems involving basic emotional perceptions, feelings and responses to the world and oneself. One's actions, so often guided by emotions, can become uncontrollable. A person can become locked into over or under reacting to the simplest situation. One minute everything is all right, the next the world seems to be crashing down. Individuals may feel that they no longer have any control over their actions. They become impulsive, haphazard, disconnected from their family and friends.

When the cerebral cortex is injured, the limbic system seems to run wild. An individual, who is usually able to balance emotions and control as well as the expression of emotions, now loses that ability. As thinking, feeling, and social beings, if an individual is not in "balance", these actions may bring only further complications.

The two major structures usually associated with the limbic system include the hippocampus and the amygdala. Injury or damage to any of these structures can leave long–term and devastating problems for individuals.

Hippocampus

The hippocampus is a paired–organ, one on each side of the brain. It sits within the temporal lobes, "between your ears" so to speak. The hippocampus is most commonly associated with memory functioning. It is particularly susceptible to loss of oxygen. Injury to the hippocampus causes individuals to have a great deal of difficulty with short term memory, turning short term memories into long term memories, and organizing and retrieving stored memories.

The hippocampus is like the pole in the closet where clothes are hung. If the pole is pulled out, the clothes fall into a heap on the floor. The entire system of hanging similar clothes in particular places (structure and organization) is completely disrupted. As a person tries to store new clothes, there is no pole (organizational structure) to help. So clothes end up in a mess on the floor, which makes it difficult to find anything. Even when a piece of clothing is found, like a shirt, it has taken longer to find and it is wrinkled. Memories, like clothes, may be poorly stored, hard to retrieve, and not accurate (messy) when produced.

Amygdala

Close to the hippocampus is the amygdala. This is a "fight or flight" structure that seems to be more closely tied with emotional memories and reactions. It is like the "front door" to a person's emotions.

Neuroscientists speculate that when a perception reaches the cerebral cortex, it is transmitted to the amygdala where the stimulus is evaluated for emotional content. For example, hidden fears of snakes, spiders, and creatures of the night may cause a person to "flee" or "fight" depending on the emotional response from the amygdala.

Interestingly, both the hippocampus and amygdala are directly tied with the olfactory fibers (smell). While all sensations — sight, sound, taste, touch — evoke memories, both smell and taste seem to be the most powerful stimulants for recollection.

Basal Ganglia

Another group of brain structures that works together as an integrated system is called the basal ganglia. The four nerve cell clusters of the basal ganglia or "nerve knots" help handle physical movements by relaying information from the cerebral cortex to the brainstem and cerebellum.

The most important function of the basal ganglia centers is to act as a "checking" system that comes to attention when something is not working the way it should be. An injured or diseased (Parkinson's disease) basal ganglia affects voluntary motor nerves. This results in slowness and loss of movement (akinesia), muscular rigidity, tremor, and can be focal or diffuse. The neurons in the basal ganglia respond when someone loses balance and sends a signal to the muscles to restore lost equilibrium.

The Cerebellum

The interconnectedness of the brain makes it difficult to separate it into distinct working units, since the brain is a complicated organization of multiple systems. The cerebellum is wedged between the brainstem and the cerebral cortex and "hitched" to the back of the head. It is about 1/8 of the brain's mass and has its own distinctive arrangement of brain cells.

The cerebellum has been referred to as the tree of life, because the layers of cells fan out in a striking pattern like the leaves of a tree. The cerebellum governs a person's every movement. It monitors impulses from the motor and sensory centers (brainstem, basal ganglia, motor/sensory cortex) to help control direction, rate, force and steadiness of a person's movements. It enables us to develop and store the motor skills to play sports, ride a bike, do aerobic exercises, perform martial arts routines, drive a car, and to train the "mind and body" to accomplish amazing athletic feats.

Injury or disease to the cerebellum can produce problems with coordination, fine motor movements, equilibrium (balance) and one's sense of where the body is in space. A person with a damaged cerebellum may look "drunk" when they walk. The person may not even be able to walk a marked straight line or sit without support. The eye and hand coordination so necessary in life may be disabled to the point that the person cannot even reach out and pick up a glass of water. Likewise, the person's movement may become so awkward that trying to brush one's teeth results in a blow to the face.

Since the cerebellum is responsible for coordinating muscle tone, posture, and eye/hand movements, damage can seriously inhibit a person's movement within their community. Once common routines such as getting dressed, writing one's name, and getting from class to class in a school become frustrating and impossible to control.

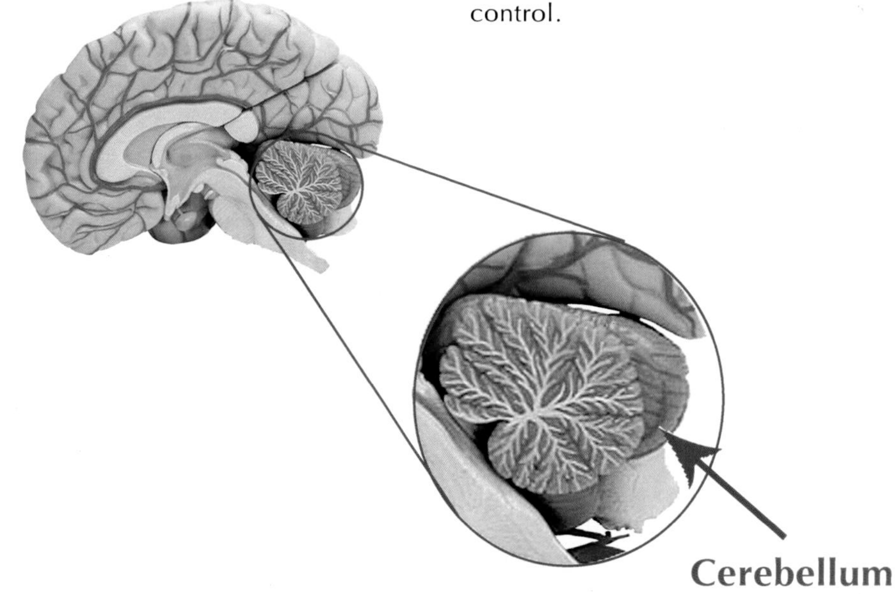

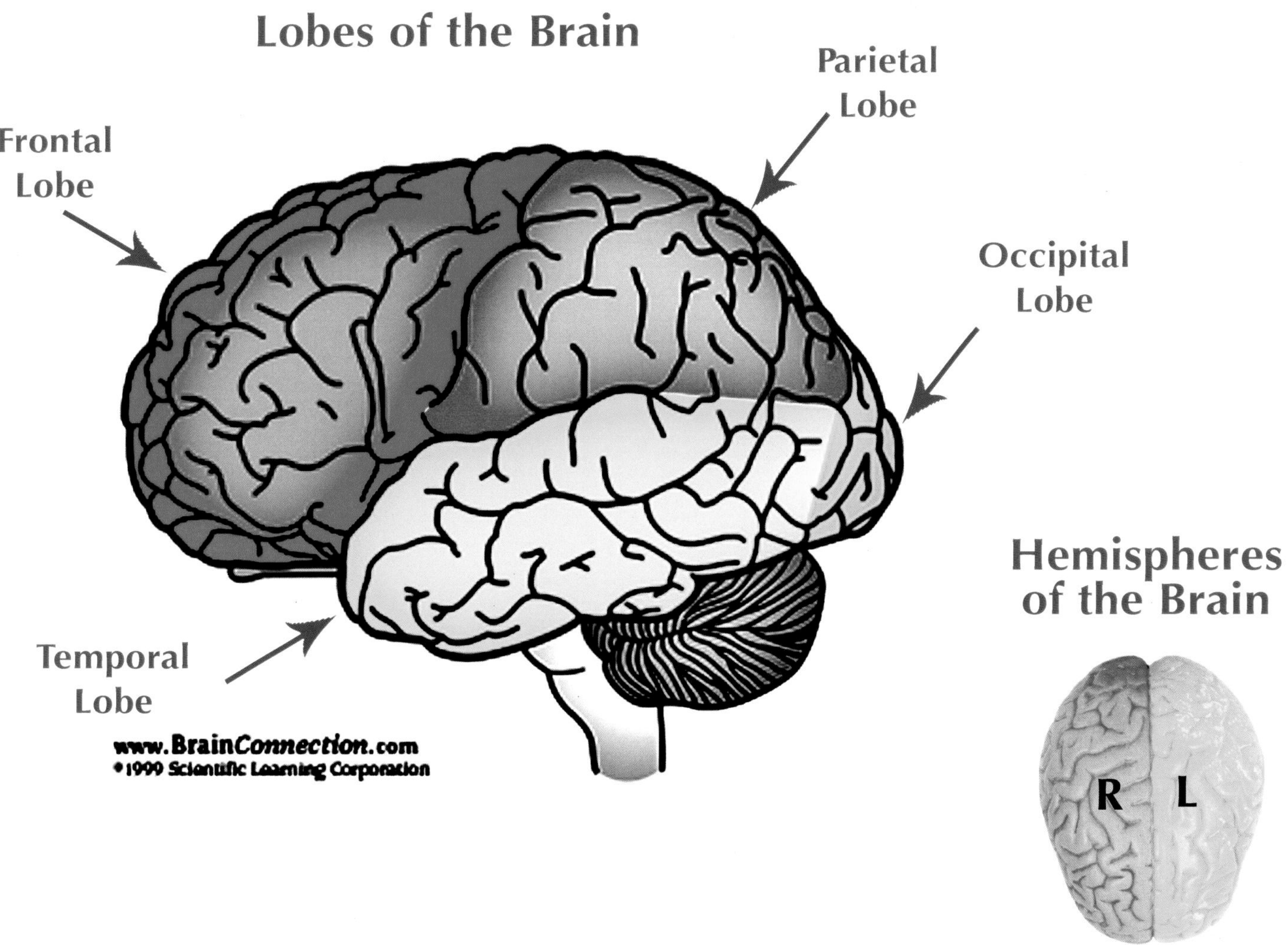

The Cerebral Cortex

By far the most complicated structural component of the brain is the cerebral cortex made up of the right hemisphere and the left hemisphere. Each hemisphere has four lobes including the frontal, parietal, temporal and occipital lobes.

The cortex is full of wrinkles and folds. If you took out and flattened the cortex, it would be the size of a pillowcase. The wrinkling and folding helps pack much more brain mass into the skull. It is the fact that we have "two brains", or rather two hemispheres, that leads neuroscientists to marvel at information processing abilities and differences of the cortex.

History abounds with references to the "duality of the mind", but it wasn't until the 1960s when Dr. Roger Sperry and Dr. Joseph Bogen gave detailed reports of their patients who had undergone surgery to alleviate their seizures by cutting the corpus callosum. The corpus callosum is a complex band of nerve fibers that exchange information between the two hemispheres. This groundbreaking surgery began the "right brain — left brain" differences and stimulated topics for common discussion.

The Bogen/Sperry studies showed that the two hemispheres of the brain, while seeming alike, had unique ways of processing information. The right hemisphere is more holistic, visual–spatial, and intuitive. The left hemisphere is more linear, verbal–analytic, and logical.

From a geographical perspective, comparing the two hemispheres is like comparing the two halves of the United States. They have a major river, the Mississippi, running between them (like the corpus callosum) that serves as a major divider and connector at the same time. While they have similar "rules and regulations", they also have their own distinct styles (East Coast versus West Coast). The similarities and differences between Californians and New Yorkers exemplify this.

Interestingly, the cerebral hemispheres control opposites sides of the body. Thus, if a person receives an injury to the right hemisphere, there will be difficulty controlling the left arm or leg.

The left hemisphere processes information in a logical and linear manner which helps a person better understand and use language (speaking, reading, writing, calculations).

The right hemisphere responds to information in a more holistic and spatial sense (shapes, faces, music, art).

The left and right hemispheres have processing differences as well as similarities. This is evidenced by modern brain scanning, electroencephalograph (EEG) research, and studies of people who have had their hemispheres separated by surgically sectioning the corpus callosum.

While the left hemisphere is responsible for most language functions, the right hemisphere recognizes simple words like "book" and "dog." Words of higher conceptual demand like "honesty" or "perseverance" are recognized by the left hemisphere.

The uniqueness of the cerebral hemispheres is that they do communicate with each other a thousand times a second through the corpus callosum. This 4 inch long, pencil thick band of complex nerve fibers allows the two hemispheres to work in tandem. When an individual sustains a brain injury, the impact or swelling may seriously damage this precious relay system and result in impaired processing of information. Individuals can have major damage to one hemisphere, plus have damage to the corpus callosum pathway. Such injuries create very complex cognitive difficulties for people and many compensatory strategies are needed to help them live effectively.

In order to fully understand the impact of an injury to the brain, it is important to remember that when one part of the brain is impacted or struck, it reverberates throughout the brain like shock waves through a "jello" mold.

Each brain injury is very different, depending on the type and severity of the injury and the age of the person when injured.

Hemispheres of the Brain

Back

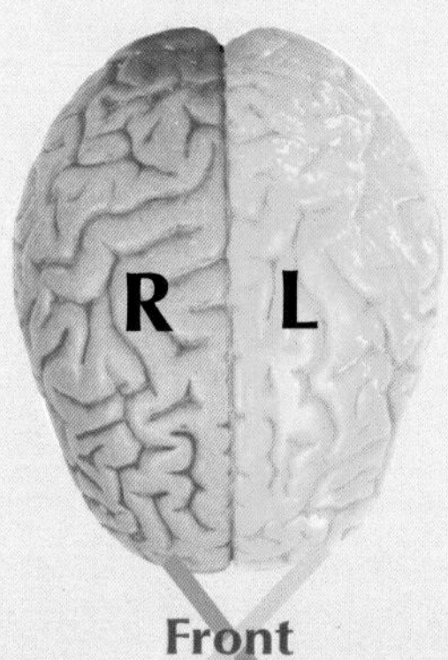

The right side of the brain (right hemisphere) controls the left side of the body.

The left side of the brain (left hemisphere) controls the right side of the body.

Front

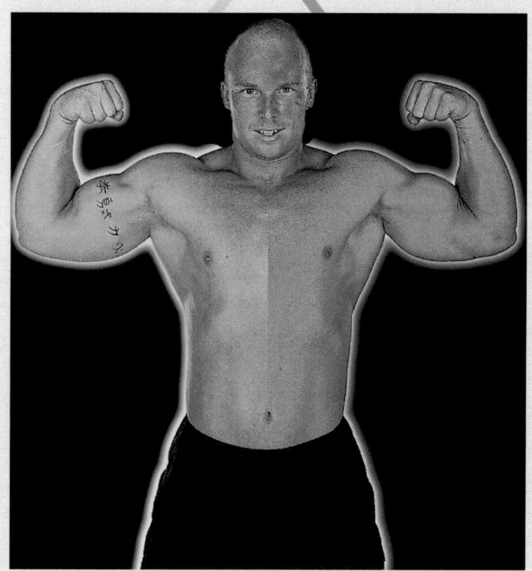

Lobes of the Brain

The functions of the four lobes of the cerebrum — frontal, parietal, temporal, and occipital — must be understood to appreciate the effects of an injury. Because there are two hemispheres, the lobes comprise both a left–side and a right–side involvement. Thus, there is a left frontal lobe and a right frontal lobe, each working together, yet displaying many processing differences just like the left and right hemispheres.

These four lobes or areas of brain anatomy are named after the main skull bone that covers them. These landmarks help map the surface of the brain, but the lobes do not necessarily match brain areas designated for different tasks. Like the hemispheres with its corpus callosum, the lobes are interconnected by complex neural fibers. The projection fibers fan out from the brainstem and relay impulses and information to and from the cortex. The association fibers loop and link together different sections of the same hemisphere and modulates the cerebral cortex. These two neural fiber systems help the four lobes of the cortex work together and keep it intricately connected with both the limbic system and the brainstem.

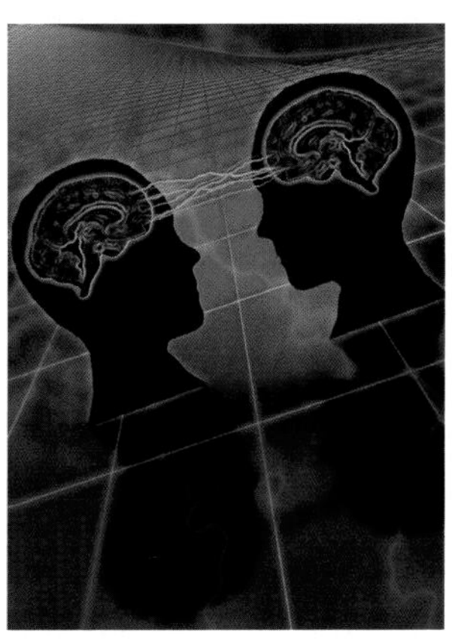

Brain & Behavior Relationships

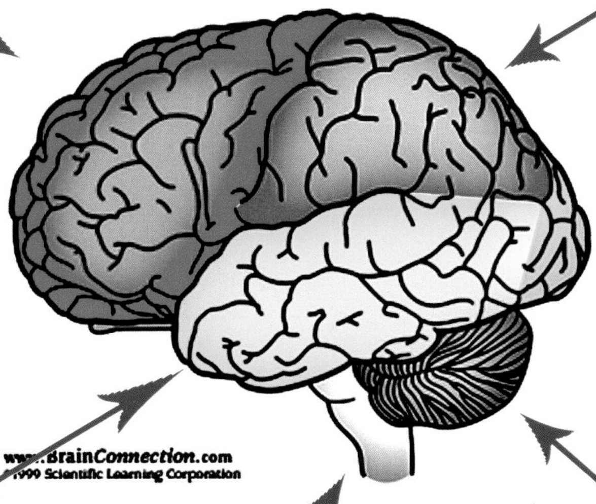

Frontal Lobe

Initiation
Problem-solving
Judgment
Inhibition of behavior
Planning/Anticipation
Self-monitoring
Motor planning
Personality/Emotions
Awareness of abilities/Limits
Organization
Attention/Concentration
Mental flexibility
Speaking

Parietal Lobe

Sense of touch
Differentiation of size, color, shape
Spatial perception
Visual perception

Occipital Lobe

Vision

Temporal Lobe

Memory
Hearing
Understanding language
Organization & sequencing

Brain stem

Breathing
Heart rate
Arousal/Consciousness
Sleep/Wake functions
Attention/Concentration

Cerebellum

Balance
Coordination
Skilled motor activity

www.BrainConnection.com
©1999 Scientific Learning Corporation

Frontal Lobes

The frontal lobes of the brain can be divided into a narrow motor "strip" which curves over the top of the head like a hairband, and the prefrontal cortex, which are the much larger parts of the frontal lobes, anterior to the motor strip. At the very front of the lobes sit the frontal poles— regions that are particularly vulnerable to injury since they sit just inside the front of the skull near a rough bony area. The frontal lobes have extensive connections with many brain regions, especially with the parietal lobe and the limbic system (emotions).

The motor strip sends signals down to the muscles of the body, telling them what to do. For the most part, the right frontal lobe controls the muscles on the left side of the body and the left frontal lobe controls the muscles on the right. For this reason, injury to one side of the frontal lobe often causes weakness or even paralysis on the opposite side of the body. Yet there is much more to the human frontal lobes, since the prefrontal cortex contains many of the neurons we associate with the broad spectrum of human behavior.

Before a final "decision" is made about a motor action, the prefrontal cortex judges options, predicts likely outcomes, and decides the best course of action for the body to take. When the prefrontal cortex is injured or damaged, an individual's ability to synthesize signals from the environment, assign priorities, make decisions, initiate actions, control emotions, behave and interact socially, make plans, and utilize other executive functions is severely compromised.

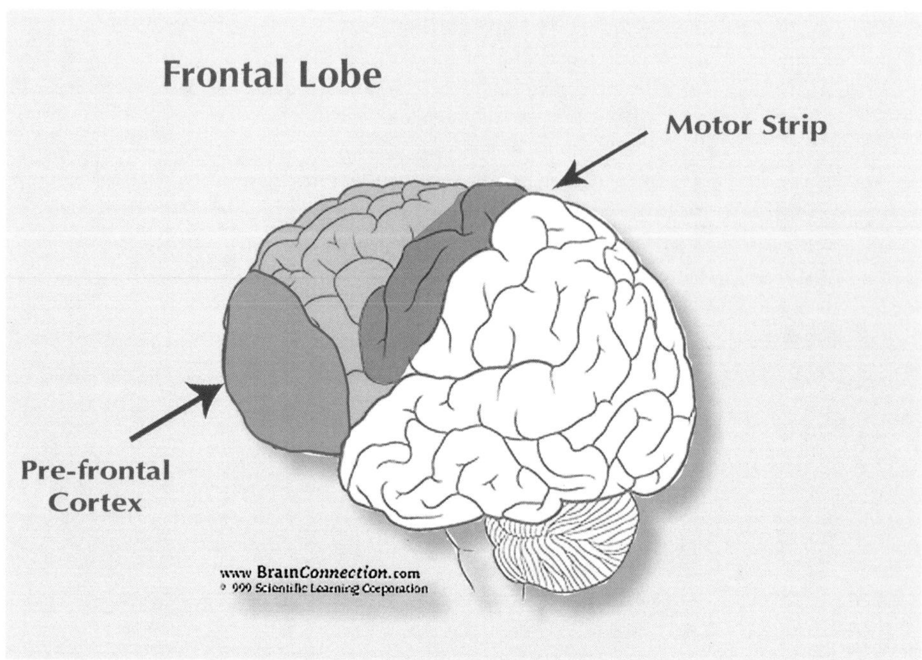

While injury to any specific area of the brain creates problems, injury to the prefrontal lobes is especially debilitating since the frontal cortex is responsible for so many of our executive functions and many aspects of our personality. When damage occurs, it may seem as if the entire personality changes; a person does not seem to be the person they once were. The prefrontal lobes are also responsible for motivation. Since so much of everyday life involves movement and motivational states, individuals with injured prefrontal lobes may exhibit a host of complex problems in their activities of daily living.

The prefrontal cortex also helps hold information in memory for several minutes—so-called "working memory." Damage to this region makes it more difficult for a person to keep their mind focused on a task, or pay attention to more than one task.

For example, staff may sometimes find that warning a person with prefrontal lobe damage about the consequences of a behavior works less well than helping them see the circumstances that usually come before that behavior – that is, using an "antecedent" based behavior model (i.e., what is happening before the water goes over the dam). Once the antecedents are known, the events that can lead up to an unwanted behavior can sometimes be eliminated or modified, thus, preventing the unwanted behavior from occurring in the first place. Trying to manage behaviors consequentially after the "water is over the dam" or "the horse is out of the barn" may be less effective for some individuals with prefrontal lobe injuries.

Prefrontal lobe injuries in young children sometimes go unnoticed, since they are at an age when parents and teachers function as their frontal lobes in a sense. Teachers and parents organize, plan, and direct children's lives. As children get older and enter early ado-

lescence, they are expected to be more independent and learn to manage themselves over time. For the child with a brain injury, the capability for more independent frontal lobe functioning has been diminished by the earlier injury.

Located at the anterior part of the frontal lobes (right over one's eyebrows) is the prefrontal cortex. The prefrontal cortex, in particular, is responsible for various emotional responses to circumstances. Rather than just responding to situations intellectually, individuals respond with delight, anxiety, hope, pessimism or a range of other higher level emotions. Neuroscientists are telling us that the prefrontal cortex is responsible for the ability to learn from consequences. If the frontal lobes are injured, the person may not be able to "learn from mistakes" and repeat unwanted behaviors over and over again.

Children may begin to experience a lack of control over a wide range of behaviors not because they are misbehaving, but because their frontal lobes are not responding at a level that is developmentally appropriate. Attempts to merely discipline or punish children with frontal lobe injuries do not help them understand or compensate for their loss. Ways to deal with complex behaviors using antecedent management strategies need to be taught to children just like new learning or memory strategies would be introduced and taught.

Parietal Lobes

The parietal lobes sit behind the frontal lobes where we find the primary sensory cortex poised like another hair band, posterior to the motor strip. The primary sensory cortex is the first part of the brain to consciously register physical sensations, but, there's much more to the parietal lobes. They respond to sensory information such as touch, heat, cold, pain, and are responsible for one's sense of body awareness. Injury to the parietal lobes can cause a loss of these sensing abilities.

A person with damage to the right parietal lobe may not even recognize that anything is wrong with movement of the body's left side. This is not because of "psychological denial" but rather because of neurological damage. More complex functions like attention and awareness can also be affected by damage to the parietal lobes.

Occipital Lobes

The occipital lobes are a person's primary visual center. Yet, they are located far away from the eyes, in the posterier section of the skull. This is why when a person falls and hits the back of the head, the person often sees "stars" — in effect, the occipital lobes have been stimulated.

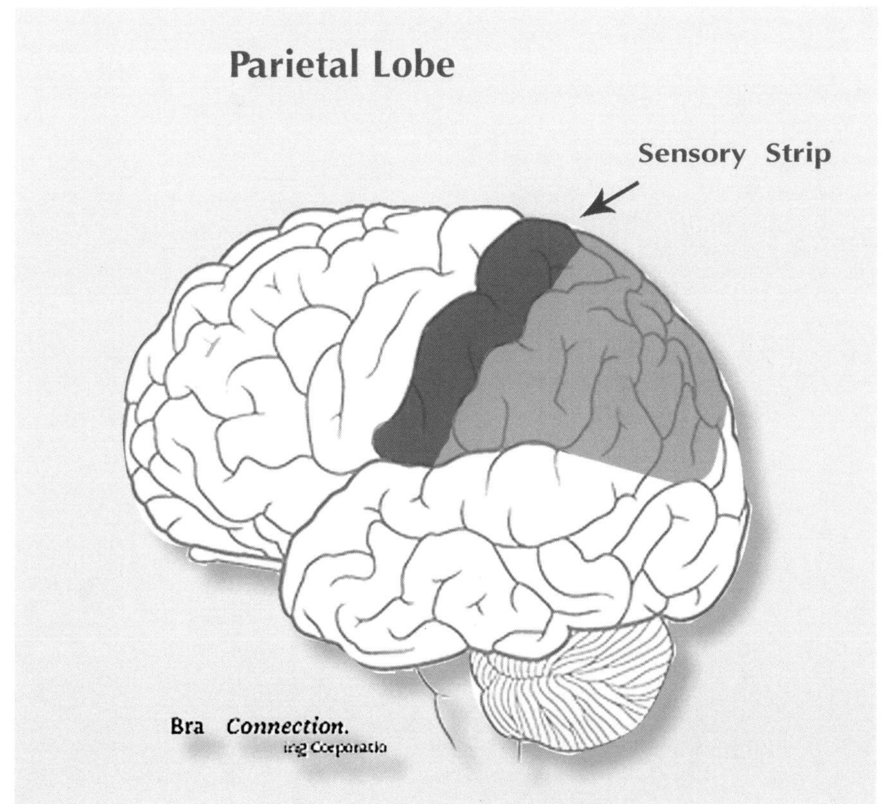

The visual cortex is connected to the eyes by optic nerves. No other sense involves so many nerve cells. Vision, neurologically speaking, is a complex process. As incoming light rays pass through the eyes and are changed into electrochemical impulses, nerve fibers arrange and code these impulses. Near the back of the eyes, the optic nerves carrying these signals meet at a "crossing" called the optic chiasm. At this cross–point, optic fibers from the inner half of each retina cross to the opposite hemisphere of the brain. The left optic track carries signals from the right–side field of vision, and the right optic track takes signals from the left. This results in the both sides of the brain "seeing" or perceiving the same stimuli.

After these signals pass through a relay station in the thalamus and reach the left and right occipital cortex, the whole image is reassembled and processed by different visual areas for size, shape, position, recognition, color, etc. Most of what a person "sees" derives its meaning from prior learning and symbolic representations. To separate vision from movement, or sound, does not really describe vision in its broadest sense. Unfortunately, injury to the brain often disrupts "what we see" because of the complexity of this sense. Thus, visual–perceptual–motoric damage can create many problems for individuals.

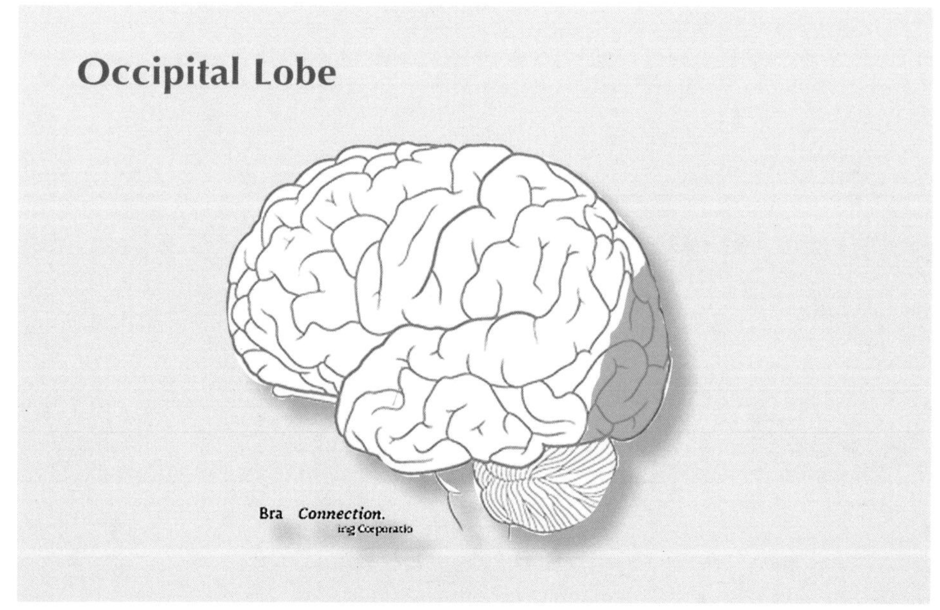

Temporal Lobes

The temporal lobes rest on both sides of the brain and are the centers for language, hearing, and may be where memories are permanently stored. More than a century ago a French surgeon, Paul Brocca, and a German neurologist, Karl Wernicke, discovered that damage to particular areas of the left temporal and parietal lobes left people unable to speak or understand language.

The Brocca's area of the brain is located in the lower portion of the motor cortex in the left frontal–temporal lobe. This area controls the muscles of the face and mouth and enables the production of speech. Individuals with damage to Brocca's area speak with a halting, labored, dysarthric spech largely comprised of action words. An example might be "I . . . w e n t . . . home."

Wernicke's area, located in the left temporal–parietal lobe area, governs a person's understanding of speech and the ability to make sense of the thoughts that are spoken. Together these two areas direct the smooth transfer of thought and expression into speech. Individuals with damage to Wernicke's area speak fluently but do not make sense. An example might be "I bent the pool but the car is not."

The process of hearing, like vision, is also very complicated. As sound waves are picked up and passed through the outer and middle ear to the inner ear, a series of events take place. The transmitted sound waves vibrate thousands of tiny sensitive hairs in the organ of Corti. Each hair is connected to thousands of nerve fibers which send signals through the eighth cranial (acoustic) nerve to the brainstem. There, many of the nerve fibers cross over before taking signals up to the tops of the temporal lobes for analysis.

A brain injury can produce a breakdown of this process, either neurologically or mechanically. While many "mechanical" disruptions to the outer and middle ear can be restructured, damage to the inner ear and temporal lobes can produce more serious consequences.

The memory processing and storage capacities of the temporal lobes are not entirely understood. While the brain can store short–term memories in the hippocampus, long–term memories seemed to be holistically stored throughout the brain. The temporal lobes, with their connections to the hippocampus, help in the long–term storage of permanent memories (where someone went to school; names of friends and families; knowing how to play a game). Memories having to do with meaningful content are more likely stored as long term in the temporal lobes as well as throughout the brain.

Individuals with brain injuries often have difficulty with new learning while exhibiting good memory for information learned previous to the injury.

The memory system for understanding, storing, and/or retrieving new information in individuals with temporal lobe injuries has been disrupted by the injury to their brains. When attention, concentration, and memory problems go hand–in–hand, individuals have difficulty connecting new information with prior knowledge and their everyday life functioning may be affected.

Although we've discussed the lobes of the human brain individually, virtually every behavior depends on the interconnectedness of the brain. For example, when a person smells food, it triggers a response in the temporal lobe. Visual attention may be drawn towards the source of the smell by the parietal lobe, and the food will be seen with the occipital lobe. The sights and smells of the food may trigger memories stored in multiple cortical regions, may provoke anticipatory pleasure in the limbic system, and may lead to increased arousal in the brain stem. This complex array of responses is sent to the frontal lobes for consideration, and a motor plan may be generated making the person more likely to move toward the food. Because of the interconnectedness of brain and behavior functions, even an injury that is relatively mild in severity or small in size may lead to many distressing symptoms.

Summary

In this chapter, you have learned about various brain-behavior relationships and how an injury to the brain can affect overall functioning. By knowing how the brain works and the neurological changes that can occur to individuals with brain injury, you will be better able to understand their challenges. Other chapters in this manual will help you use cognitive and behavioral strategies to help people function better in life.

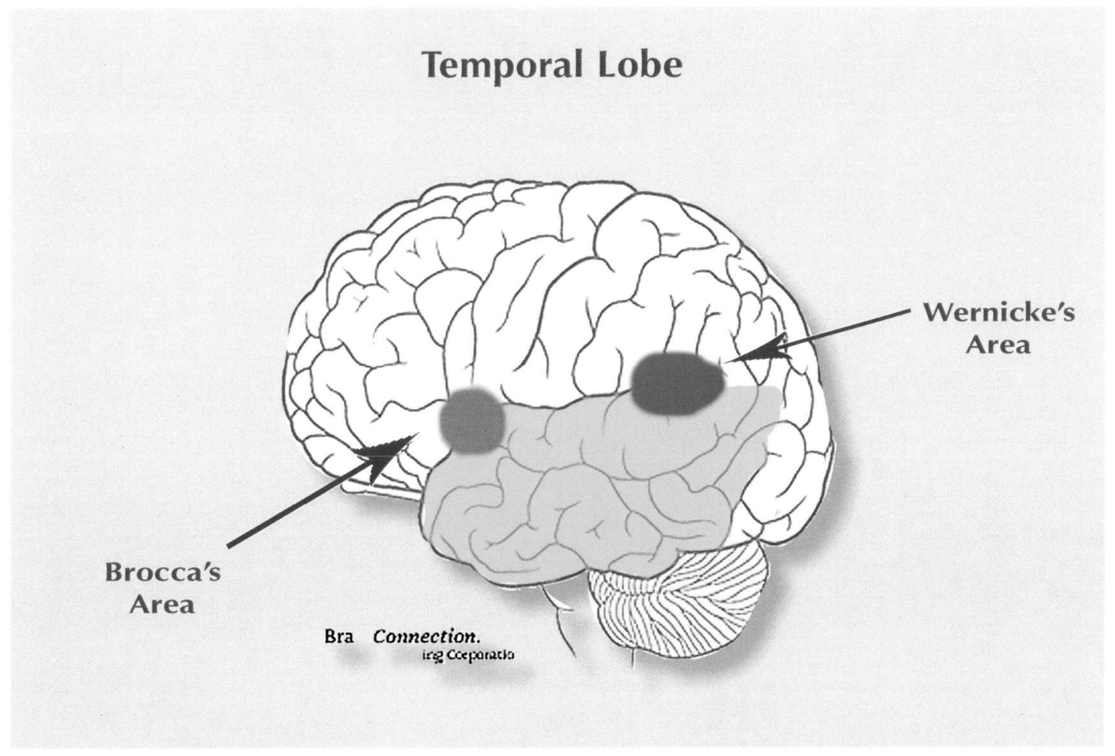

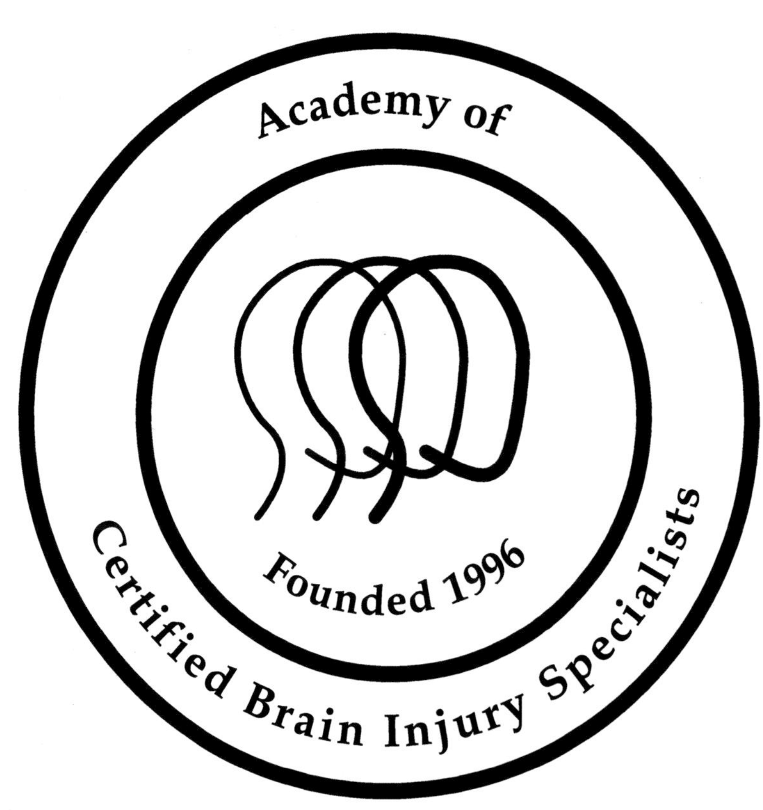
Academy of
Founded 1996
Certified Brain Injury Specialists

Chapter 4

Health, Medication and Medical Management

Learning Objectives

By the end of this chapter, you will be able to:

- Understand the uniqueness of an individual with a brain injury by gathering information about the person's background, injury, treatment and current factors that impact their potential for optimum recovery.
- Understand, identify and report signs and symptoms of potential medical complications that are commonly encountered in persons after a brain injury.
- Demonstrate knowledge of the most commonly prescribed medications used after brain injury.
- Understand the effects of alcohol and substance abuse in brain injury.
- Identify aspects of aging with brain injury.

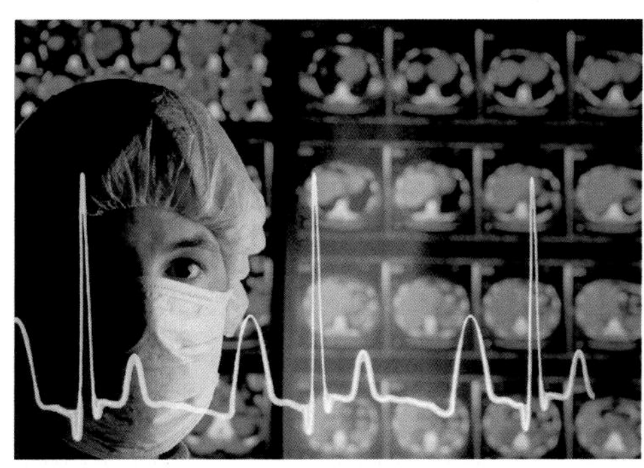

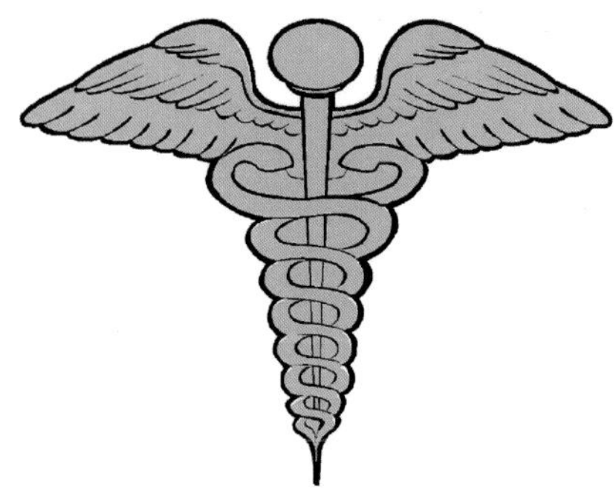

Introduction

The brain is a complex and vulnerable organ. Injury can result in a multitude of physical and psychological impairments as well as medical complications. The need for rehabilitation should be assessed, and if clinically appropriate, begun in the intensive care unit (ICU). Once a person has been deemed "medically stable" by the acute care hospital staff, transfer to either medically-based or community-based rehabilitation programs, or even to home, may occur. The current trend in healthcare involves transferring patients sooner than ever before. Post-acute programs may be admitting patients with medical complications, thus requiring more staff training to safely treat these persons.

Just as each person's injury is unique, each person's recovery is also unique. Treatment interventions must be highly individualized to best meet the needs of the person with the brain injury and the family.

It is important that all staff members understand the medical factors which affect a person's health and ability to achieve individualized goals. In particular, it is the direct care staff, who provide direct care and spend the majority of time with the person, who often first identify possible conditions and complications that affect a person's medical stability.

Health and freedom from medical problems were the most important issues related to satisfaction with quality of life cited in a 1998 community integration outcome study of persons with brain injuries (cited in Bogner, 1995).

The goal of rehabilitation is to help an individual regain the most independent level of functioning possible. The rehabilitation process is different for every person who has sustained a brain injury.

Treatment must be individualized in accordance with each person's unique needs.

The first step in assisting the person on the road to recovery is a thorough review and assessment of factors which have impacted the whole person. In addition, well documented information on the health status of the individual when admitted is important. It is a baseline for comparison with later changes in health status.

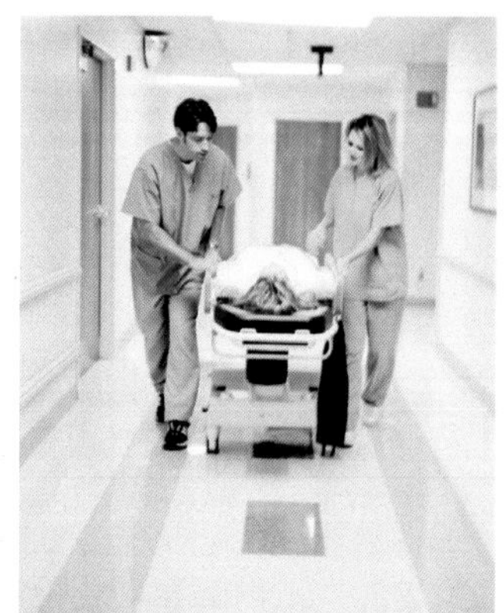

The goal of rehabilitation is to help an individual regain the most independent level of functioning possible.

Initial Assessment

Participate in the pre-admission process and review past medical history, including:

- How the injury happened.
- Time elapsed since injury.
- Age at onset of injury.
- Physical or mental health problems prior to the injury.
- History of loss of consciousness or brain injury prior to this injury.
- Major hospitalizations and surgery.
- Determine right or left handedness.
- Sleep habits.

Review historical information including:

- Developmental / psychosocial / behavioral history.
- Educational history including evidence of learning disability, Attention Deficit Disorder or Attention Deficit Hyperactivity Disorder.

- Work history/socioeconomic status.
- Military service.
- Marital history.
- Legal record.
- Substance abuse.
- Cultural, religious, and language background.
- Sexual orientation.
- Recent life stressors (i.e. deaths, family, marital, financial, academic, vocational).
- Nature and extent of financial resources.
- Family support systems.

Review information about the accident/injury and subsequent treatment including:

- Area of the brain injured.
- Etiology of the injury (e.g., traumatic, anoxic).
- Severity of the injury (Glasgow Coma Scale scores, length of coma, duration of post traumatic amnesia).

- Presence of multiple injuries.
- Acute medical/rehabilitative course of treatment including complications and coexisting medical conditions.
- All current assessments including medical, physiatric, nursing, neuropsychological, neuropsychiatric, physical therapy, occupational therapy, speech language therapy, social and vocational history.
- Interviewing available family members not only about the injury, but especially about who the person was before the injury .
- The need for assistive devices and durable medical equipment.
- Medical, psychological, behavioral and neurocognitive health issues.
- Current functional status.

Review current medications, dosages and side effects.

- It is important that information about medications be available to direct care staff since they may be responsible for monitoring, and sometimes helping people take medication if the patient is unable or unwilling.
- It is important to stress the five R's- right med, right person, right dosage, right route of administration and right time.
- It is essential to talk to the person about medications and be aware of any allergies, possible drug reactions, and potential interactions with food and other medications. Pharmacy instructions regarding crushing medications and emptying capsules must be followed. Crushing may cause drug interactions, stomach upset and a premature increased effect of drug therapy. If a medication error is made, it should be immediately reported to a physician/nurse.

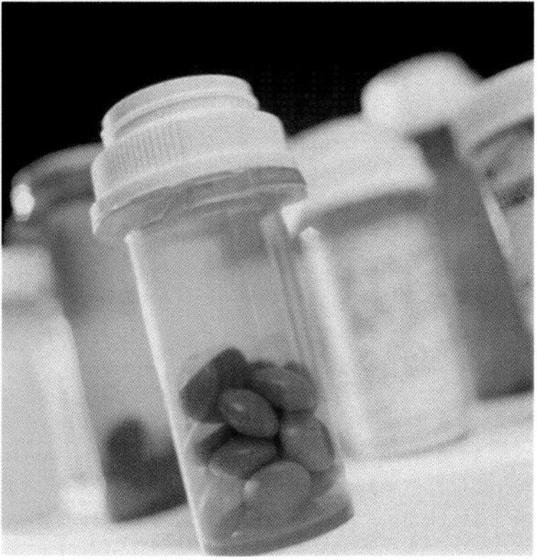

Throughout this chapter, medications are listed with the generic name first followed by the brand name. The information on medications is meant to be a general overview and is not all inclusive. This information is not

The 5 "R's" of medication passing

- **Right Med**
- **Right Person**
- **Right Dosage**
- **Right Route**
- **Right Time**

intended to review every use, direction, precaution, adverse effect or interaction that can occur and information on medications is constantly changing. Any questions should be addressed to the physician in charge of the person's treatment.

In addition to information provided by the physician, pharmacies provide educational handouts with information which may include indications, precautions, contraindications, proper use, possible adverse reactions and drug interactions. Staff should also have access to reference information sources such as the U.S. Pharmacopeia DI (USP DI), the Physician's Desk Reference (PDR), Mosby's Nursing Drug Reference, or other comparable references.

If in doubt, ask! Careful observation of the patient and immediate reporting of adverse medication effects to the physician is imperative.

It is clearly well beyond the scope of this manual to extensively discuss predictive factors of recovery. However, it is important that the reader be aware that examples of factors influencing the long-term outcome from brain injury may include age, socioeconomic status, education, financial resources, family and vocational support systems, motivation and coping skills, work history, spiritual beliefs, history of substance abuse, psychosocial issues, and medical factors (e.g., injury severity, hypotensive and hypoxic episodes, increased intracranial pressure, anoxic injury, medical complications, seizures, multisystem trauma, etc.).

Medical Conditions and Complications

The medical management of brain injury is complex. It often presents a continuing challenge throughout the person's life. Space does not permit an inclusive list of all possible conditions nor highly technical, specific and detailed discussion. Rather, an organ systems approach is provided to help all levels of staff identify complications promptly and initiate early treatment.

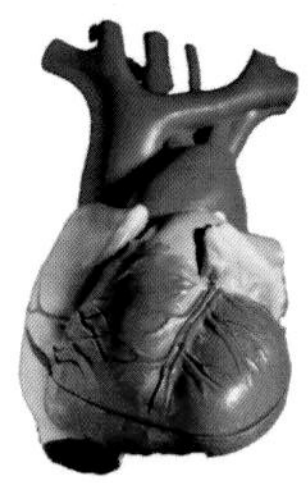

Cardiopulmonary

Heart (cardiac) or respiratory (breathing) abnormalities have been reported in up to one third of persons with brain injuries (Kalisky et al, 1985). Individuals who sustain damage to the respiratory center in the brain stem require immediate life support. They may remain dependent on a ventilator indefinitely. Even if brain stem injury has not occurred, other complications such as spinal cord injury, infection, airway obstruction, and trauma to the larynx (voice box), trachea (wind pipe), chest, and lungs can further affect the respiratory system.

In the acute care setting, persons with severe injuries often need to have a tracheostomy (surgical opening made through the neck with a tube inserted into the trachea to help with breathing). Closure of the tracheostomy is a goal as soon as medically feasible; however, it is increasingly more common for patients to go to a rehabilitation setting with a tracheostomy in place, due to earlier discharges from more acute settings.

Other related problems may include weakened cough and gag reflex, difficulty swallowing, narrowing of the trachea, and recurrent regurgitation (the return of swallowed food into the mouth). These problems can be very serious because of the increased risk of aspiration (inhaling foods, liquids or vomitus into the lungs) and subsequent pneumonia or other respiratory infections. It is important that these individuals be monitored for abnormalities in respiration rate (normal adult rate 12- 20 breaths per minute), depth and pattern of respirations and for signs of respiratory distress.

Cardiac abnormalities may be caused by direct trauma to the heart, complications from trauma, and damage to parts of the brain that control the functioning of the heart. The person should be routinely monitored and abnormal heart rates (normal rate 60-90) beats per minute), rhythm, and complaints of chest pain immediately reported.

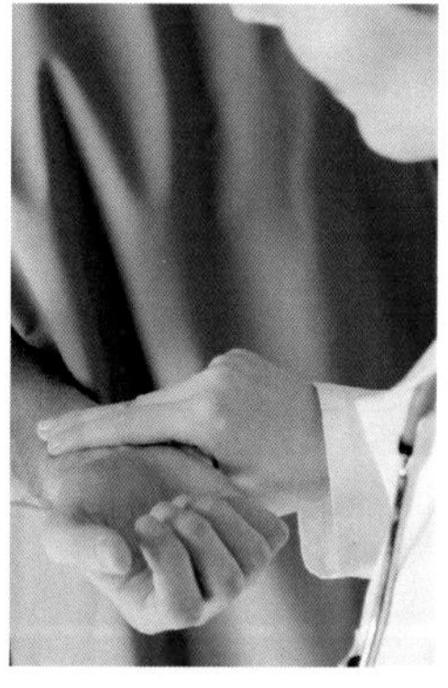

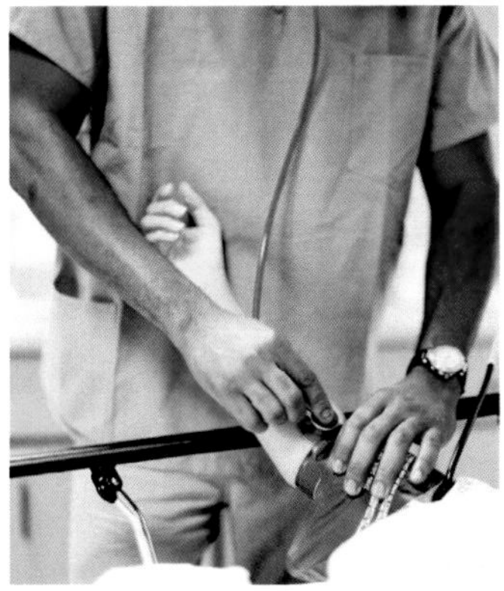

Hypertension (elevated blood pressure exceeding 140/90 mm Hg.) has been reported in an estimated 11 to 25% of individuals in the acute and subacute period following TBI (Kalisky et al,1985; Jennett & Teasdale, 1981). These patients are often started on medications which lower blood pressure; however, only 45% require these medications when discharged from rehabilitation (Labi& Horn,1990). If an individual becomes dizzy or lightheaded, especially just after standing, blood pressure medications may need to be adjusted. Routine monitoring of blood pressure (optimal 120/80 mm Hg) should occur along with follow up with the physician regarding the need for these medications.

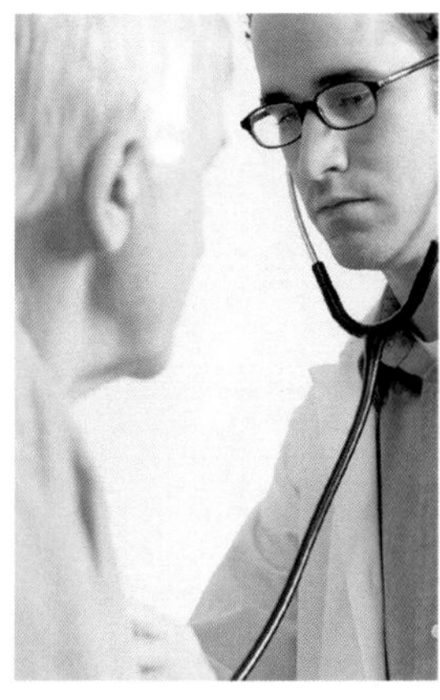

Musculoskeletal

Muscle and skeletal complications are commonly seen after brain injury. The actual diagnosis, however, may be delayed. Whenever a person sustains a brain injury, achieving medical stability becomes the first priority in the acute care setting. Studies have reported that 11% of people later admitted to rehabilitation programs had fractures and/or dislocations that were previously undiagnosed (Garland&Bailey,1981). Accurate diagnosis of spinal injuries is particularly critical and fracture stabilizations should occur as soon as clinically appropriate.

Like fractures, peripheral nerve injuries are commonly seen after brain injury with an estimated 34% incidence in persons with severe brain injuries. Causes include trauma, improper positioning, heterotopic ossification (see page 60), and postoperative complications. Unfortunately, 11% (Garland & Bailey, 1981) of these persons also present to a rehabilitation program undiagnosed. It is important for staff to pay particular attention to the signs of peripheral nerve injuries which include weakness, numbness, muscle wasting, and uncoordinated, uncontrollable twitching of a single muscle group.

Spasticity is an involuntary increase in muscle tone (tension) that causes the muscle to resist being stretched. Flexor and extensor muscles of the arms, wrists and fingers and extensor muscles of the legs are most commonly affected. Movement may be painful and require great effort.

Early detection of spasticity enhances the person's chance for successful treatment. If spasticity goes undetected, the person is at increased risk for skin breakdown, bone fractures and progressive deformities. Problems with the use of upper extremities, walking and running may also occur.

Contractures (abnormal, usually permanent condition of a joint characterized by flexion and fixation due to wasting away and abnormal shortening of muscle fibers and loss of skin elasticity) are particularly problematic. Whenever a person has a severe contracture, the hands, wrists, knees, ankles, lower and upper extremities can appear to be frozen into a nonfunctional position.

Treatment options include splinting devices, casting, and positioning exercises to normalize tone and improve flexibility and mobility. Oral anti-spasticity medications such as baclofen (Lioresal®), diazepam (Valium®) and dantrolene sodium (Dantrium®) are sometimes prescribed. However, their effectiveness in reducing spasticity in persons with brain injuries is questionable. In addition, these medications may produce serious adverse effects such as confusion, memory impairment and sedation. Some positive results have been reported with the use of tizanidine (Zanaflex®). Other treatment alternatives include phenol

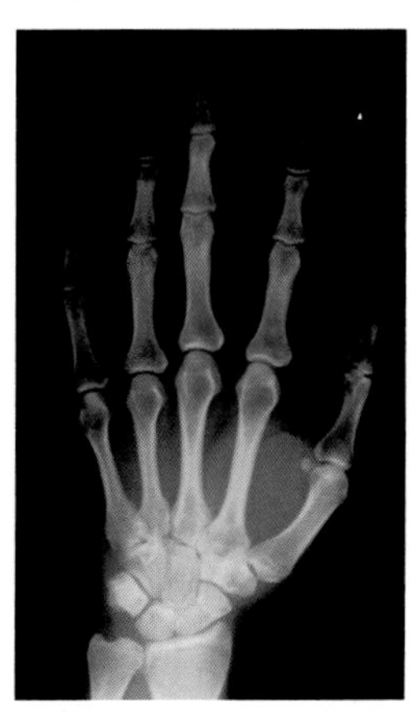

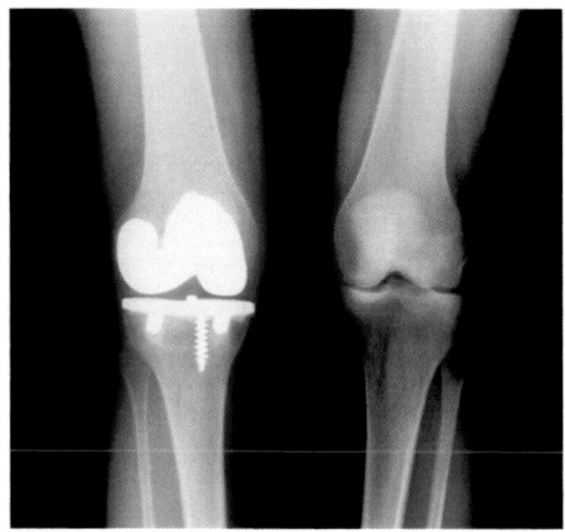

and/or botulinum toxin (Botox,) nerve blocks, orthopedic management and surgically implanted baclofen pumps. If a baclofen pump has been implanted, it is important to know that periodic refills are needed.

Heterotopic ossification (HO) is the creation of abnormal growth of bone in soft tissues or around joints. Symptoms may not appear immediately. However, as calcification of the bone continues, pain, inflammation, swelling and decreased range of movement occurs. This is followed by loss of functional mobility, nerve compression and pain. In persons who sustain brain injury, HO is most commonly seen in the hip, followed by the elbows, shoulders, and knees.

Persons with a history of prolonged coma, immobility and spasticity of the limbs are most at risk, particularly during the first 3 to 4 months post injury. HO can significantly limit a person's functional abilities, particularly in activities of daily living, hygiene, sitting, positioning, and ambulating. Persons who present in the rehabilitation setting with HO may be taking anti-inflammatory medications and require specific range of motion exercises and possible surgery.

Staff members need to notify medical personnel if they observe, or if the individual complains of limb pain accompanied by swelling, redness, warmness and sensitivity to touch. Clinical assessment and diagnosis can be challenging in persons with altered consciousness or impaired communication. These signs and symptoms can signal several serious and possibly life threatening conditions such as deep venous thrombosis (DVT), (a blood clot in one of the deep veins of the body), reflex sympathetic dystrophy (RSD - a painful and debilitating condition which can result in damage to tissue, muscle and bone), phlebitis (inflammation of a vein) or cellulitis (inflammation of the skin). Early detection is critical to successful treatment outcome.

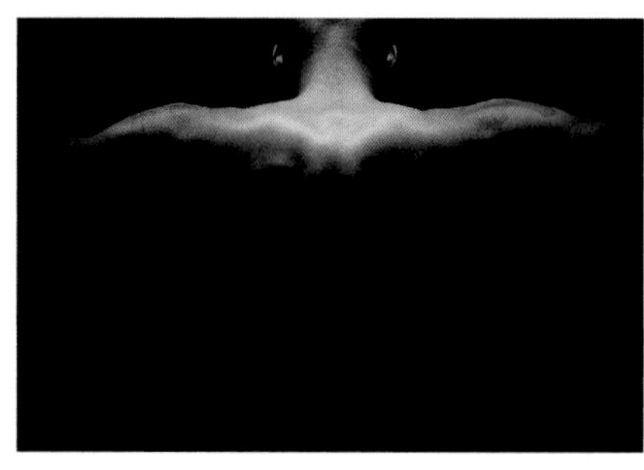

Skin

The most frequently seen skin complications after brain injury are lacerations and abrasions. Acne and profuse sweating may appear or be worsened by a brain injury. In addition, medication reactions may produce rashes or worsen skin conditions.

Unfortunately, people may also acquire pressure ulcers. Pressure ulcers are the most frequent complication of chronic illness and physical disability. If a person lays in bed or sits in a wheelchair and does not reposition or receive assistance from staff to reposition, soft tissue is compressed between the bony prominences of the body and external surface of the wheel chair or bed. The blood supply to the area is compromised and the tissue reddens. If the pressure is not relieved, skin-break down occurs and can progressively deteriorate to become deep, crater like ulcers that extend through the skin and muscle tissue, right down to the bone (Antoinette, 1996).

Bony prominences such as hips, coccyx, heels, elbows, shoulder blades and the back of the head are the most common areas for pressure ulcers to develop. Persons using wheelchairs must be closely observed for pressure ulcers of the ischium (the back lower portions of the hip bones). These pressure ulcers may be caused by seating issues, lack of pressure relief cushions and/or lack of mobility. It is important to assure that the person is provided with a pressure reduction or pressure relief mattress/bed as deemed clinically appropriate.

Casts and splints can also be a source of pressure against the skin and lead to the development of pressure ulcers. Proper application of casts and splints is crucial. Schedules for splint removal must be adhered to and frequent skin checks performed (Antoinette, 1996).

The American Health Care Policy and Research (AHCPR) Guidelines on Pressure Ulcers is an excellent resource on prevention and appropriate treatment. Antiseptic agents such as peroxide, betadine, iodine, and Dakin's, which were historically used, are no longer recommended. These products can cause further skin damage (Agency for Health Care Policy and Research, 1994).

Prevention of further skin breakdown is imperative. Even in the post-acute setting, factors which place persons at high risk for skin breakdown include sensory impairment, immobility, contractures, and spasticity. Incontinence and poor nutritional status are also considered high risk factors. Staff must frequently examine skin, promptly report any skin abnormalities, use proper transfer techniques, frequently reposition, and provide adequate nutrition and hydration. All are instrumental in preventing this debilitating complication.

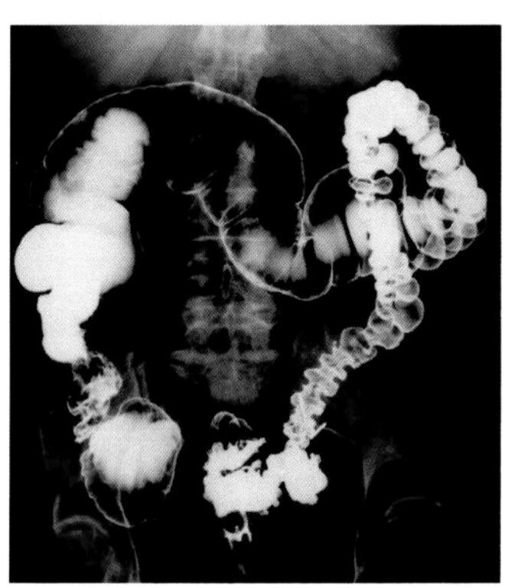

Gastrointestinal

Injury to the brain directly affects a person's nutritional needs. A person's metabolism may increase after brain injury, which in turn causes the body to need increased energy and increased caloric needs (Pepe and Barba (1999). A study by Brooke and Barber reported an average weight loss of 29 pounds prior to admission to a rehabilitation hospital (Brooke, Barbour & Cording, 1989). The requirement for increased calories can persist indefinitely.

Problems such as poor hand to eye coordination, difficulty swallowing, diminished attention and impaired cognition can further compromise a person's nutritional intake. An

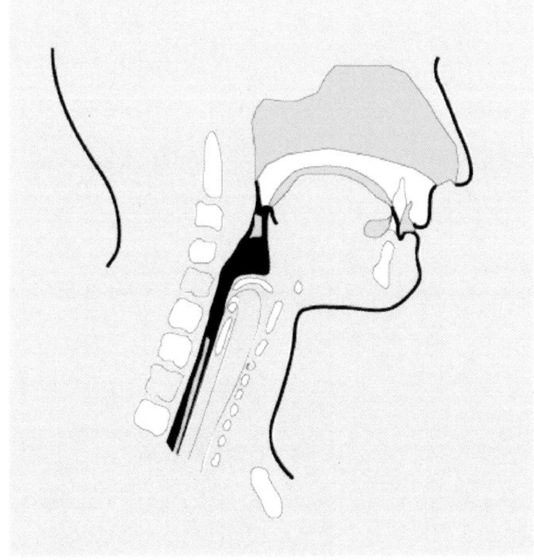

individual's weight must be accurately taken and nutritional intake closely monitored.

Swallowing disorders after brain injury are common. Swallowing disorders after brain injury are common. Incidences range from 25-42% in inpatient rehabilitation (Field and Weiss, 1989, Weinstein, 1983) up to 61 % in acute care (Mackay, Morgan, Bernstein, 1999). The most common abnormal swallowing characteristics include: loss of bolus control, reduced lingual control, and decreased tongue base retraction (Logeman, Pepe and Mackay, 1994: Mackay, Morgan and Bernstein, 1999; Lazarus and Logeman, 1987). In a 1999 study, utilizing multivariate models, admitting Ranchos Los Amigos levels, CT scan results, ventilation time and aspiration emerged as a significant independent predictors of impaired oral intake (Mackay, Morgan and Bernstein, 1999).

Persons with brain injuries may have had modified barium swallows while in the acute care hospital. This specialized x-ray study provides serial images of barium mixed with food of different consistencies. This helps the speech therapist determine the specific nature of the swallowing problem. It is especially important that swallowing ability be carefully monitored to assure that food does not enter the trachea and travel to the lungs.

Persons sometimes present in the rehabilitation setting with a gastrostomy tube (g-tube; a tube placed through a surgical opening into the stomach to administer liquid feedings). They need to be closely observed for nausea, vomiting, swollen stomach, constipation, fecal impaction and diarrhea. The skin at the site where the tube enters the body must be kept clean and dry. The site must be monitored for redness, heat, swelling, crusting or oozing fluid. Specific instructions for checking tube placement should be followed and the person's head elevated 30-45 degrees or more as tolerated to prevent aspiration pneumonia.

Medications used to treat gastrointestinal problems may include metoclopramide (Reglan®), cimetidine (Tagamet®), famotidine (Pepcid®), and ranitidine (Zantac®). These agents can also impair cognition (the conscious process of knowing or being aware of thoughts or perceptions, including understanding and reasoning). More recently, omeprazole (Prilosec®) and rabeprazole (Aciphex®,) have been prescribed in some settings with limited cognitive impairments anecdotally reported.

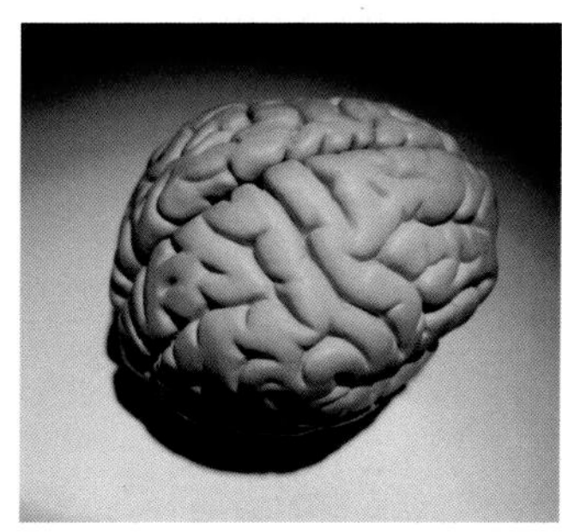

Elimination

The brain is the control center for bowel and bladder function. When the brain has been injured, these regulatory systems may be disturbed. An individual may be unaware of the need to have a bowel movement in an appropriate and timely fashion.

Regardless of the person's cognitive status, a daily bowel training program should be developed. The program is based on information obtained from present elimination patterns, physical assessment, bowel habits prior to injury, amount of assistance needed, activity level, life style, preferences and the individual's level of abilities. Inactivity, diet and medication side effects may cause problems with constipation or diarrhea.

Dietary and fluid intake should be monitored to assure adequate intake of bulk, roughage and fluid. A regular schedule of toileting should be established, ideally 15 to 30 minutes after a meal. Medications such as stool softeners and bulk laxatives, combined with a regularly scheduled suppository, usually produce adequate emptying of the bowel without accidents. Harsh laxatives and enemas should not be used on a regular basis and can actually worsen the problem.

Urinary incontinence can be an embarrassing and disruptive problem. An injury may affect areas of the brain involved in urination, which may affect the person's ability to control when to empty the bladder. Normally, stretch receptors in the bladder carry information to the brain that alerts the person to the need to empty. The external sphincter, under voluntary control, allows the person to remain continent. If it were not for this voluntary control, the bladder would empty when the stretch signals cause the involuntary response of bladder contraction and bladder sphincter relaxation.

The most common type of bladder incontinence after brain injury is a disinhibited type of neurogenic bladder. This refers to a neurological impairment (central or peripheral nervous system) that affects bladder function. The person may have normal bladder sensation, but decreased bladder capacity, urgency (sudden urge to urinate), frequency and incontinence. The person is not able to inhibit, or stop, the urge to void (urinate). That is why this condition is referred to as a disinhibited neurogenic bladder. In addition, a bladder may be hyperreflexive, which means that the need to empty is triggered easily.

Other types of injuries, such as spinal cord injury or direct trauma to the bladder and medical conditions, such as an enlarged prostate in the older adult male, may cause additional problems with urination.

The person may enter a rehabilitation setting with a Foley catheter. This catheter is an indwelling catheter, which means that it remains in the bladder and drains urine continuously. The catheter should be removed as soon as possible because it increases the possibility of urinary tract infections. Bladder training should begin as soon as the person is oriented and has sufficient short term memory to participate in a timed voiding schedule or specific program based on the person's type of incontinence.

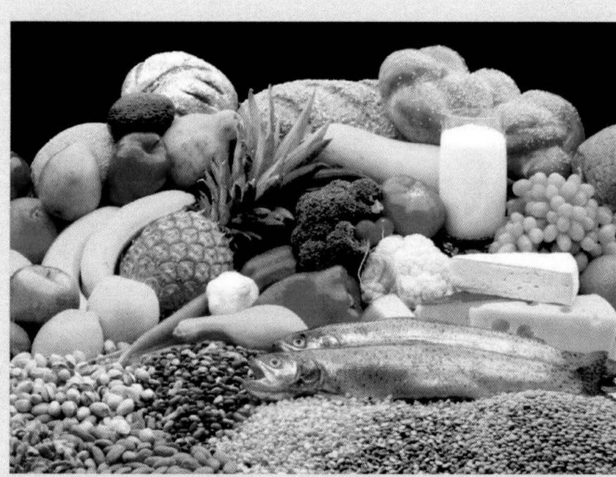

Dietary and fluid intake should be monitored after brain injury to ensure adequate intake of bulk, roughage and fluid.

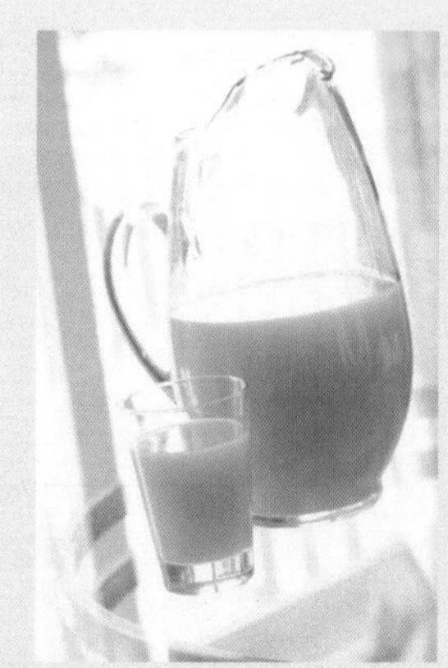

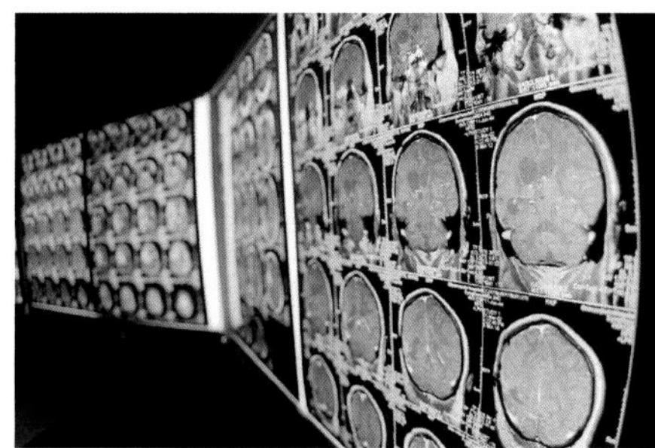

Neurological System

After brain injury occurs, there are a variety of physical effects that can occur as a result of neurological damage to the brain. The changes are the focus of this section of chapter four.

Effects Within the Brain

Headache is the most common neurological condition reported after brain injury. Post-traumatic headaches may be accompanied by memory impairment, dizziness, fatigue, difficulty concentrating and cognitive impairment (difficulty with perception, memory, attention and reasoning skills). Although most persons improve in 6 to 12 months (Packard & Ham, 1994), persistent headaches may continue in 15-20% of persons with brain injuries (Speed, 1991).

Hydrocephalus, the enlargement of fluid-filled cavities (ventricles) in the brain, caused by excess CSF, can present either acutely after injury or as a chronic complication. Symptoms of post-traumatic hydrocephalus usually occur within one year post injury, and include impaired consciousness, ataxia, behavioral changes, and incontinence. Early diagnosis and placement of a shunt (a tube that moves excess spinal fluid out of the skull) may be required to improve outcome and to slow further deterioration.

Motor and sensory impairments can have a profound effect on rehabilitation outcomes. An individual may present with weakness, paralysis, ataxia, spasticity or movement disorders, as well as vision and hearing deficits.

Seizures

Seizures are caused by an abnormal, disorderly discharge of electrical activity in the nerve cells of the brain. The probability of a person having a late seizure (those which occur after the first week post injury) is variable, depending on the nature of the person's injury. A study by Yablon reported the overall incidence of late seizures in persons with traumatic brain injuries to be approximately 5%. However, this rate may increase depending on the cause, such as gunshot wounds (33% to 50%), intracranial hematoma (25-30%), prolonged coma and post-traumatic amnesia (35%) and other variables. Of those persons who develop post traumatic seizures from brain injury, the seizures occur within one year after injury in 50-66% of the persons and by two years after injury in 75-80% of cases (Yablon, 1993). Seizures are categorized as either partial or generalized.

Partial Seizures

Partial seizures arise from disturbances in specific, localized areas of one hemisphere of the brain. Symptoms are linked to the area of the brain that is affected. Partial seizures are further sub-classified as follows:

Seizures

Seizures are caused by abnormal disorderly discharge of electrical activity in the nerve cells of the brain.

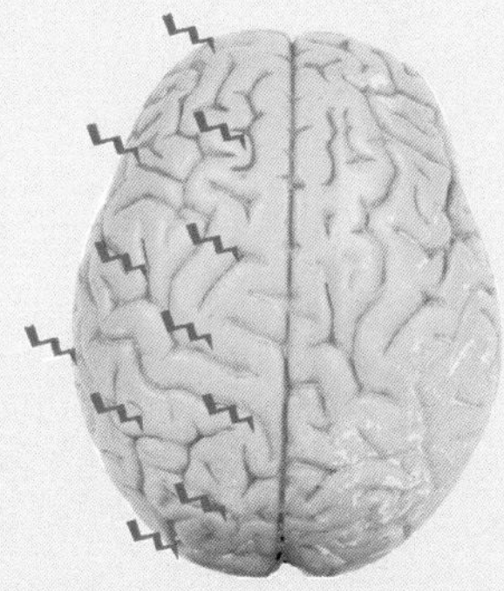

Partial seizures arise from disturbances in specific, localized areas of one hemisphere of the brain.

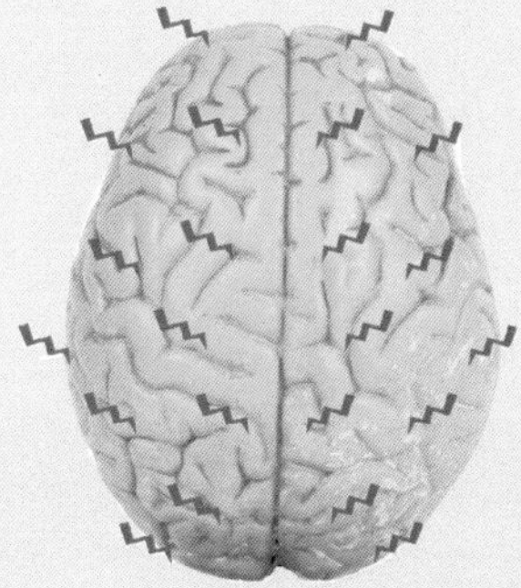

Generalized seizures are a sudden burst of abnormal discharges that usually affect both hemispheres of the brain.

Simple partial seizures (focal seizures) have no alteration or loss of consciousness. Abnormal, localized electrical activity in the motor area of the brain may result in motor symptoms such as stiffening or jerking of muscles (e.g., face, hand, side of mouth, finger, foot). The person may move the eyes from side to side, and have unusual movement of the tongue, blinking and facial twitching. Abnormal movements of one part of the body sometimes spread or "march" to arms, legs or other muscles on the same side of the body (Chipps, Clanin & Campbell, 1992).

Abnormal electrical activity in a localized area of the sensory strip of the cortex may produce sensory symptoms such as numbness, tingling, abnormal sensations, buzzing, ringing sounds, and unpleasant tastes. Psychic symptoms may include hallucinations, sudden feelings of fear or anger, and sensations of déjà vu. Most simple partial seizures last 30 seconds or less with no post-seizure confusion (Chipps, Clanin & Campbell, 1992).

Complex partial seizures (formerly known as psycho-motor or temporal lobe seizures) impair consciousness. At the onset, the person may experience a warning sign or aura (e.g., headache, ringing sound, dreamy sensation, nausea, numbness, unpleasant taste, irritability, "strange" feeling all over). This alerts the person that a seizure is about to occur. They may engage in semi-purposeful and inappropriate actions, such as compulsive patting or rubbing body parts, lip smacking, walking aimlessly, or picking at clothing. The person may seem to be dreaming with open eyes and a vacant stare. The person may even speak, but the words may not make sense. The person may appear to be conscious, but is only partially aware of surroundings and will not remember details of the incident. These seizures usually last one to three minutes and may be followed by some confusion (Chipps, Clanin & Campbell,1992).

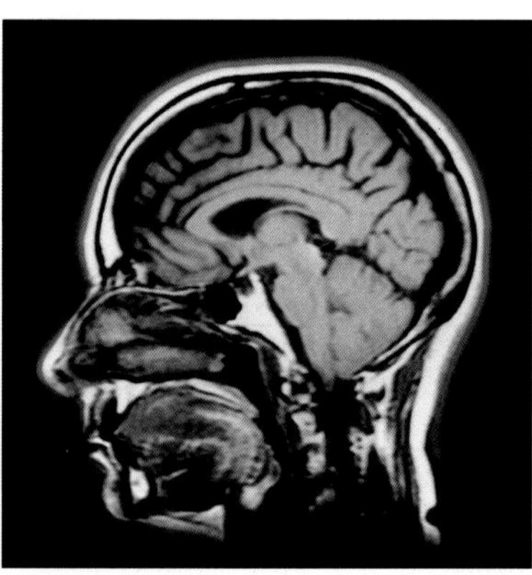

Generalized Seizures

Generalized seizures are a sudden burst of abnormal, generalized discharges that usually affect both hemispheres of the brain. Many adult seizures begin as focal seizures, then spread through the brain to become generalized. Generalized seizures are further sub-classified as follows:

Tonic-clonic seizures, formerly known as grand mal, have abrupt loss of consciousness. At the onset, the body stiffens in tonic (excessive muscle tone) contraction (5-30 seconds). The person may cry out as a result of air forced through the vocal cords. The person drops unconscious to the ground, eyes may roll up or turn to the side and the tongue may be bitten (Chipps, Clanin & Campbell, 1992).

The clonic (alternating contraction and relaxation of muscles) phase consists of violent jerking of the head, face and extremities with gradual slowing in frequency and intensity. Incontinence, noisy respirations, and confusion may follow. The person may fall into a deep sleep. Seizures typically last a total of two to three minutes with consciousness slowly returning over a 10-30 minute period. The person typically awakens to a state

Precipitants that may increase the potential for a seizure include:

- Fatigue and illness.
- Consumption of drugs or alcohol.
- Elevated body temperature.
- Flashing lights (e.g., strobe, television, computer terminals).
- Agitation or emotional distress including hyperventilation.
- Decreased oxygen/hypoxia (e.g., lack of adequate amount of oxygen).
- Dehydration due to sweating (e.g., chemical/electrolyte imbalance).
- Alcohol or drug withdrawal.
- Hypoglycemia (low blood sugar).
- Medications (e.g., antidepressants, anti-psychotics and others that lower the seizure threshold).

of confusion, extreme fatigue and no memory of the seizure (postictal state; Chipps, Clanin & Campbell, 1992).

Absence seizures (formerly known as petit mal) have transient loss of consciousness for several seconds. The person may cease physical movement, have a loss of attention or stare vacantly, neither speaking nor appearing to hear what is said. There may be excessive eye blinking, staring or chewing movements. The seizures may be of such short duration that they are not recognized by observers or even the individual experiencing the seizure. The impairment then quickly "lifts" and the person continues the activity. The individual is unaware of what happens during the seizure, but quickly returns to full awareness once the seizure stops. As many as 50 to 100 absence seizures can occur a day (Chipps, Clanin & Campbell, 1992).

Myoclonic seizures are sudden, brief contractions of muscle groups which produce rapid, jerky movements in one or more extremities. Persons may report spilling beverages held in their hands or violent falls.

Status epilepticus has varying definitions. For the purposes of this chapter, it is most practically defined as a

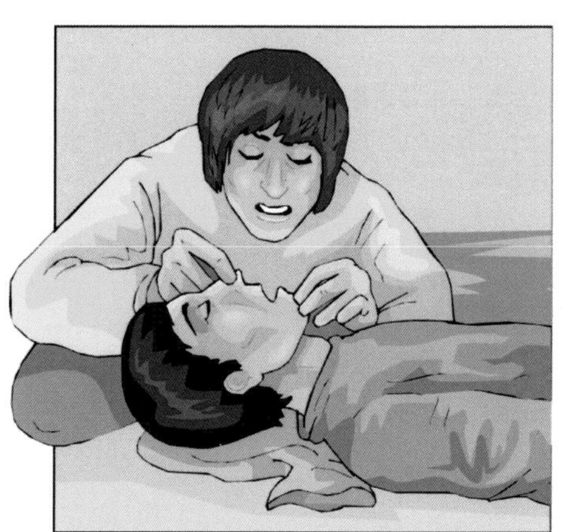

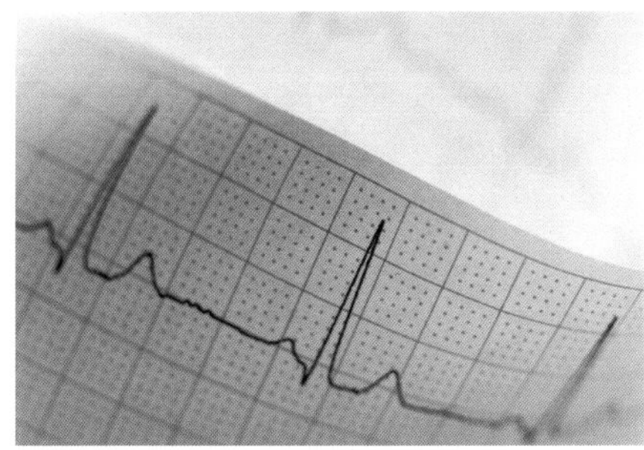

continuous type of seizure that lasts 5 minutes or longer, or two or more seizures without time between for the person to recover consciousness. Status epilepticus is a medical emergency! If the seizure is not treated effectively, brain damage or death can result. The longer the seizure lasts, the greater the danger.

First Aid Procedures for Seizures:

- Do not force any object into the person's mouth!
- Clear the environment of harmful objects.
- If possible, ease the individual to the floor to prevent injury from falling.
- Turn the person to the side to keep the airway clear.
- Remove eyeglasses or hearing aids while turning the head to one side to allow saliva to drain from the mouth.
- Do not try to hold the tongue.
- Put something soft under the head if possible.
- Place pillows or padded side rails along bedrails, if in bed.
- Loosen tight clothing around the neck.
- Do not attempt to restrain the person.
- Do not give liquids during or just after the seizure.
- Continue to observe the person until fully alert and check vital signs such as pulse and respirations periodically.
- Give artificial respiration if the person does not resume breathing after the seizure.

If a generalized tonic-clonic seizure lasts longer than five minutes, or two or more seizures occur without time between for the person to recover consciousness, seek medical help immediately. Be prepared to describe the seizure activity in detail (see section below on documentation of the seizure). Medical personnel may

Documentation of the seizure

Any time seizure activity occurs it is important to record information about:

- Time the seizure begins and ends.
- Level of consciousness.
- Parts of the body involved.
- Type of movements or other symptoms
- If bowel and bladder incontinence occurred.
- Possible causes.

ask questions regarding the person's past medical history, possible drug withdrawal, low blood sugar, infection, substance abuse (particularly cocaine) or eclampsia if the person is pregnant. It is also important to report the medications the person is receiving and when they were last taken.

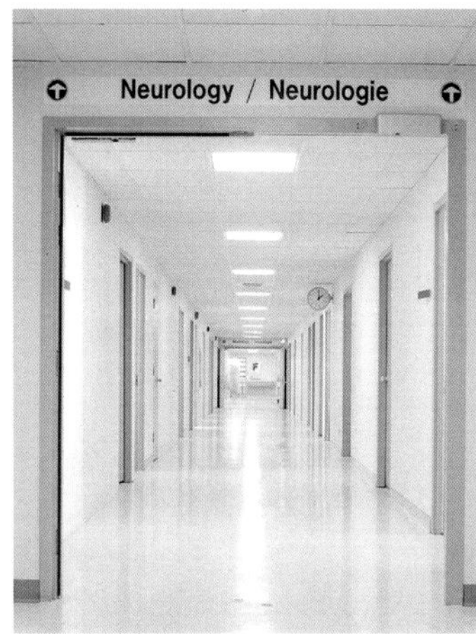

Drug Treatment of Seizures

After an initial seizure occurs, the physician typically performs a detailed neurological examination and orders blood studies, an EEG or other brain imaging study such as a CT or MRI scan. The individuals's current medications are reviewed, since some medications may increase the likelihood of a seizure. The physician may reduce or discontinue some medications.

The decision as to whether or not to start a person on anticonvulsant medication and the period of time the medication is to be maintained for seizure prophylaxis (prevention) is one that the physician makes based on a multitude of clinical variables. Practice management guidelines have been promulgated by the Brain Injury Special Interest Group of the American Academy of Physical Medicine and Rehabilitation and by the Brain Trauma Foundation in conjunction with the American Association of Neurological Surgeons and the Joint Section on Neurotrauma and Critical Care. (Brain Injury Special Interest Group of the American Academy of Physical Medicine and Rehabilitation, 1998, Bullock, Chestnut and Clifton, 2000).

Once the decision is made to start an anticonvulsant medication, the physician must weigh its potential risks (e.g., blood, liver, endocrine and skin disorders, cognitive impairment) versus its potential benefits. If the person has experienced a seizure it is important that an accurate description of the seizure be relayed to the physician since this information may influence the decision regarding the choice of which anticonvulsant medication may be prescribed.

Once an anticonvulsant medication is prescribed, the patient , their family and any caregivers must be educated to observe for potential complications and adverse reactions that may require physician notification.

It is important for staff to closely observe the person for signs and symptoms of additional seizures, as well as potential medication side effects and signs of toxicity.

It is beyond the scope of this text to discuss the uses, side effects/ adverse reactions, contraindications and dosages of the medications used for seizures and specific conditions. It is essential that prior to administering any medication that staff members have a thorough understanding of the medications their patients are receiving. Any questions should be addressed to the physician in charge of the person's treatment.

Anticonvulsant medications most commonly prescribed for *seizures* include:

- Carbamazepine, (Tegretol®).
- Valproic Acid (Depakote®).
- Phenytoin (Dilantin®).
- Phenobarbital.
- Clonanzepam (Klonopin®).
- Gabapentin (Neurontin®).
- Topiramate (Topamax)
- Lamotrigine (Lamictal®).

Summary of Signs and Symptoms Requiring Attention of a Physician or Nurse

Since medical personnel are often not present 24 hours a day in the post-acute setting, it is imperative that direct care staff identify and report symptoms that require medical attention. Astute observation and reporting can mean the difference between life and death.

Listed to the right is a summary of signs and symptoms for each bodily system which must be monitored, identified and reported to medical personnel:

Respiratory System

- Difficulty breathing, painful, noisy respirations.
- Shortness of breath.
- Cough.
- Increased production of sputum.
- Cyanosis (bluish discoloration of the skin and mucous membranes).
- Abnormal respiratory rate (normal 12-20 breaths/minute).

Musculoskeletal System

- Swelling, discoloration, limited range of motion.
- Stiff, tender or painful joints.
- Pain and/or altered sensation.
- Inability to bear weight.
- Abnormal shape of arm or leg.
- Falls.
- Increased muscle tone.
- Severe pain upon forcible movement of joints.

Urinary System

- Pain or burning upon urination.
- Foul smelling urine.
- Urinary frequency.
- Urinary retention.
- Blood in the urine.
- Lower abdominal pain/ discomfort.
- Incontinence.
- Fever, chills.
- Flank, back or abdominal pain.
- Nausea/vomiting .

Integumentary (Skin) System

- Increased sensitivity or pain.
- Any reddened area of the body that does not return to original color after repositioning.
- Severe skin tears.
- Rash, raised and reddened bumps.
- Severe itchiness.
- Pressure ulcers

Cardiovascular System

- Chest pain/palpitations.
- Abnormal pulse rate or rhythm (normal 60-90/minute).
- Abnormal blood pressure (optimal 120/80).
- Edema (swelling) of leg and ankles.
- Cyanosis and painful noisy respirations.
- Painful, swollen, red and warm to touch extremity.
- Profuse sweating, clammy skin, pallor.
- Extreme fatigue, dizziness.
- Nausea/vomiting.

Gastrointestinal System

- Severe constipation.
- Abdominal pain/tenderness.
- Abdominal distension, gas, complaints of feeling bloated.
- Severe loss of appetite.
- Cramping.
- Frequent watery stool.
- Nausea/vomiting.
- Fecal impaction.
- Pain when attempting bowel movement.
- Rectal bleeding/ tar-like stools.
- Fever.

Neurological System

- Vision impairments/neglect of visual space, blurred or double vision.
- Hemiparesis (weakness of one side of body).
- Hemiplegia (paralysis of one side of body).

- Aphasia (difficulty underst-anding speech and/ or difficulty expressing thoughts).
- Dysphagia (difficulty swallowing).
- Vertigo/dizziness.
- Sensory impairment, numbness, tingling.
- Loss of perception of body and environment.
- Ataxia (muscular incoordination when voluntary movements are attempted).
- Memory deficits.
- Apraxia (inability to conduct purposeful movement).
- Change in mental status.
- Decreased level/loss of consciousness.
- Motor weakness.
- Headache.
- Seizure.
- Tremors.

Infection

- Redness.
- Drainage.
- Warm to touch.
- Fever.

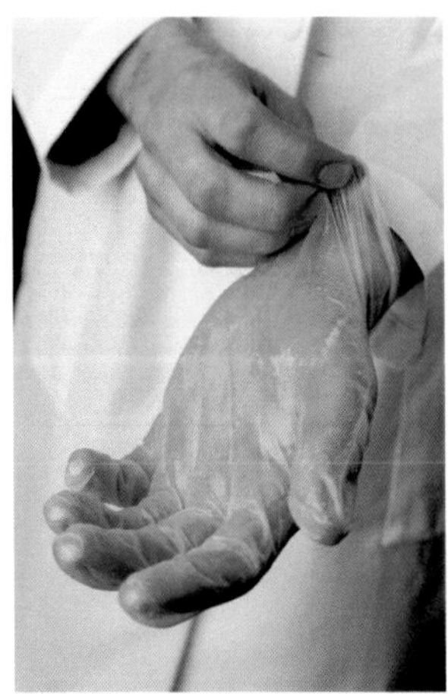

Use of Standard Precautions

Infections are easily spread in an environment where multiple people are in daily contact. Hand-washing and follow up monitoring for compliance is critically important for staff and for the persons receiving care.

Standard precautions is an approach to infection control that helps prevent transmission of blood-borne pathogens. Blood and certain body fluids and tissues have the possibility of being contaminated with Human Immunodeficiency Virus (HIV), Hepatitis-B, Hepatitis-C and other blood-borne pathogens.

There is a risk of exposure to blood-borne pathogens when contact occurs with another person's blood or body fluids through touching, splashing, splattering or spraying. Exposure can occur, for example, when changing bed linen contaminated with bloody stool, suctioning, flossing teeth or changing dressings.

Staff members are required to wear personal protective equipment whenever a person's skin or mucus membranes can come into contact with blood and body fluids. The personal protective equipment puts a barrier between the staff person and potentially infected fluids. This protection blocks dangerous contact and transmission of blood-borne pathogens. Personal protective equipment includes gloves, masks, gowns, aprons, goggles and shoe covers. In addition, all staff who work closely with patients should receive the hepatitis vaccine.

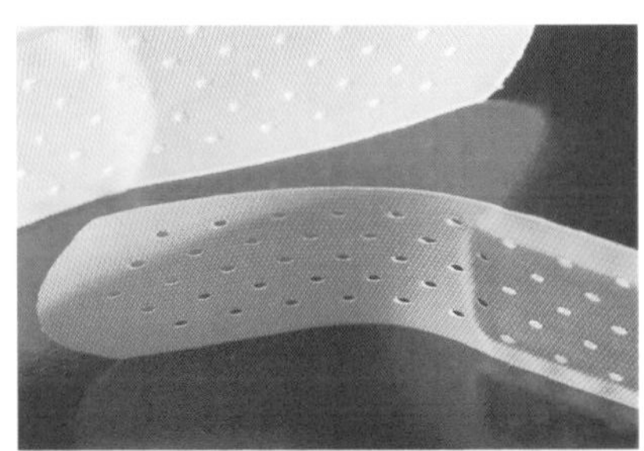

General First Aid

All staff in a facility should be trained to administer first aid (e.g. minor cuts, burns, insect bites, bleeding, etc.), and know how to contact medical personnel, poison control centers, and the closest emergency room immediately. In addition, certification to perform the Heimlich maneuver and cardiopulmonary resuscitation (CPR) should be mandatory for all direct care staff.

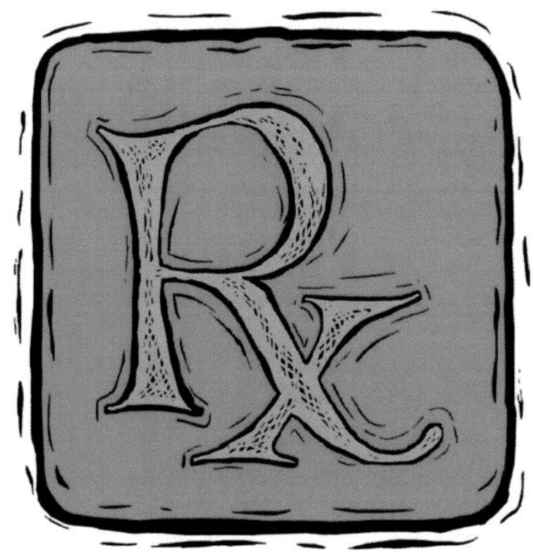

Pharmacology and the Treatment of Brain Injury

The effect of a brain injury on a person's cognition and behavior is variable, complex, and often enduring. Not only is the individual with the brain injury affected, but so are family, friends, community and society in general. Persons with brain injuries report that their cognitive and behavioral problems profoundly impact their quality of life and are more disabling than the residual physical deficits (Jennett, Snoek & Bond, 1981).

Whenever a person sustains a brain injury, many damaging changes occur. These changes can affect axons, neurons and the production, release, or absorption of neurochemical transmitters. Because these changes alter the brain's ability to process information, many bodily functions are subsequently affected. Medications work by either facilitating or inhibiting neurochemical transmitter activity. The use of medications, for enhanced arousal, behavioral control and/or mood regulation after brain injury can have both positive and negative effects on recovery.

Medications should never be used as a substitute for appropriate treatment planning and levels of staffing.

It is also important to consider the impact of the environment on behavior. If there is not enough environmental stimulation a person with hypo-arousal may not recover to maximum capacity. On the other hand, persons demonstrating irritability, agitation, impulsivity and anxiety may require a more structured and less stimulating environment.

Scientific literature, that is based on well controlled, methodologically sound, prospective studies, specific to pharmacological intervention after brain injury is sparse. The decision to use a particular medication is often based on theoretical rationale, animal models, studies conducted with persons with similar clinical symptoms, case studies and clinical experience.

Before any medication is begun, it is important to assure that the person is as medically stable as possible. Many of the medical problems previously discussed can contribute to changes in cognition. Discontinuation of medications is often the first step in effective pharmacological management of brain injury. If treatment for a particular medical problem is required, it may be possible to substitute equally effective drugs that have fewer or no cognitive side effects.

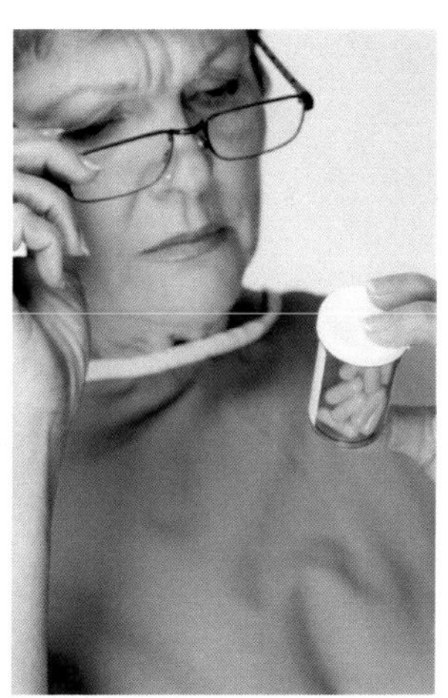

If the decision is made to start medication, continuous monitoring must occur to see if the drug is:

- Producing the intended effect.
- Still needed.
- Causing adverse effects (e.g., sedation, memory dysfunction, decreased arousal) that may impede recovery.

It is also important to provide feedback to the physician. This valuable information can assist the physician to determine whether or not to start, increase, decrease or discontinue medications.

Consideration should also be given to the use of behavioral and social interventions. Neuro-psychologists, neuropsychiatrists, physiatrists (physical medicine and rehabiliation physicians) and neurologists can help staff identify specific cognitive deficits and psychiatric symptoms (e.g., mood swings, depression, anxiety, paranoia, psychosis). They can implement neuropsychological/neuropharmacological interventions so that the person with a brain injury can obtain optimum therapeutic gains.

Medications Used to Potentially Facilitate Cognitive Recovery

The most common cognitive consequences of brain injury include impairments in memory, attention, concentration, problem solving, abstract reasoning, information processing, organization, insight and judgement. Scientific studies of the effects of medications to treat cognitive deficits after brain injury are in their infancy.

Every brain injury is different and every person's response to injury and to medication is unique. It is important to remember that the person may have had pre-existing conditions such as a learning disability, attention deficit disorder, dementia, psychiatric history, substance abuse or previous injuries. It is also important to understand that brain injury can sometimes magnify these conditions. These issues can impact how medications are utilized by the body.

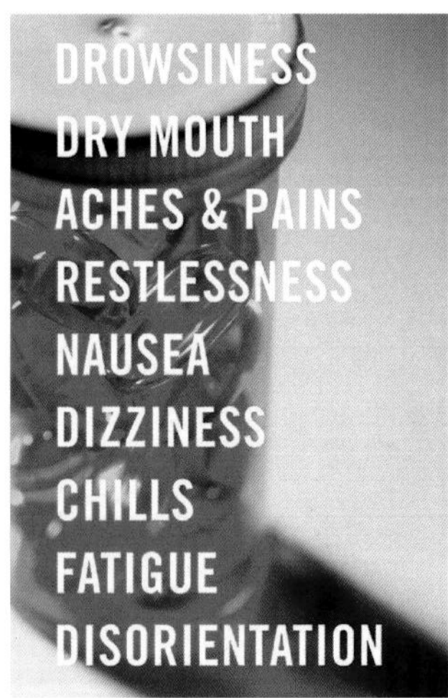

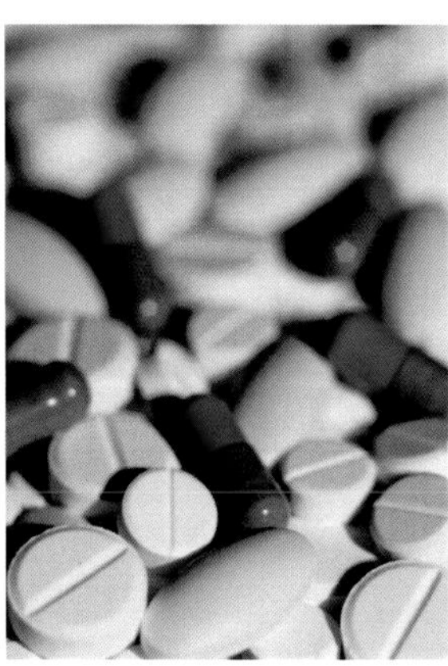

It is certainly beyond the scope of this manual to have an exhaustive discussion of the pharmacological management of brain injury. The reader is referred to the references at the end of this chapter particularly Zafont, Elovic and Mysiw et.al. and Wiercisiewski. This section is a general overview on the most commonly used medications and is certainly not all-inclusive. Candidates for the basic ACBIS certification are not expected to be experts, but familiarity with specific information regarding indications, efficacy, dosage, precautions, contraindications, adverse reactions, safety and drug interactions specific to each medication can be life-saving knowledge. Please discuss any questions or concerns with the patient's physician.

Arousal, as defined, by John Whyte M.D., (Whyte, 1992) is the "general state of readiness of an individual to process sensory information and/or organize a response."

Medications that are sometimes used for deficits in arousal that are being studied for possible benefit after TBI include the following anti-parkinsonian and stimulant medications (Zafonte, Elovic & Mysiw, 1999):

Antiparkinsonian Medications

- Carbidopa-levodopa (Sinemet®).
- Bromocryptine (Parlodel®).
- Pergolide (Permax®).
- Amantadine (Symmetrel®).
- Selegiline (Eldepryl®).

Stimulants

- Methylphenidate (Ritalin®).
- Dextroamphetamine (Dexedrine®).
- Adderall.
- Modafinil (Provigil®).

Alzheimer's Medications for use in TBI

Medications used to treat Alzheimer's disease that are being studied for possible benefit after TBI include:

- *Donepezil (Aricept®).*
- *Rivastigmine (Exelon®).*

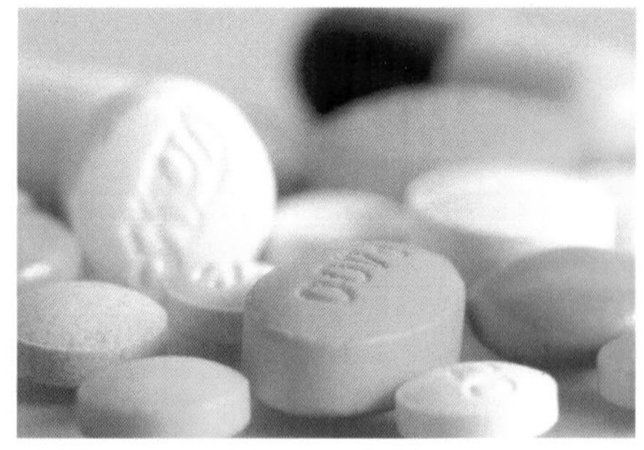

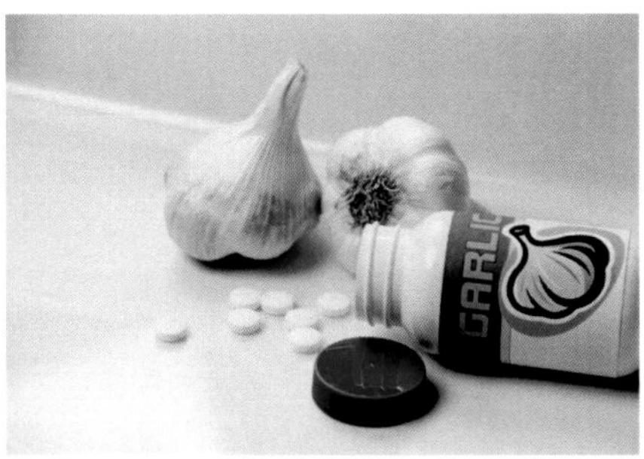

Alternative Medications/ Vitamins

Although there is reason to hope that herbs, natural supplements or vitamins (e. g., ginko, ginseng, melatonin, thiamine, zinc, or B12) will eventually be shown to be safe and effective, there is still a lack of controlled, high-standard clinical trials which show a benefit for persons who have sustained a TBI. In addition, the quality of preparations of the substances is highly variable and serious side effects and medication interactions can occur.

The use of alternative medications, vitamins and over-the-counter medications should be avoided unless specifically recommended by a physician. Even common cold and cough medications contain ingredients that may not be well tolerated by persons with a brain injury. Caution must also be exercised due to possible drug interactions with other medications the person is receiving.

Medications to Treat Neuro-behavioral Symptoms

Injury to the frontal lobes, temporal lobes and limbic system can result in undesirable behavior. Behaviors may include:

- Anxiety.
- Emotional outbursts.
- Poor impulse control, hostility.
- Verbal and physical aggression.
- Akathisia (motor restlessness).
- Disinhibition.
- Emotional lability.
- Personality changes.
- Apathy.
- Withdrawal.
- Sexual dysfunction.

Psychiatric manifestations including major depression, bipolar disorder, psychoses and anxiety disorders (panic attacks, phobias, obsessive compulsive disorder) may also occur after a person has a brain injury. Individuals with severe brain injuries are most at risk for developing and sustaining these symptoms.

It is important that the interdisciplinary team identify specific behavioral symptoms to target for treatment. Rating scales, such as the Agitated Behavior Scale (Corrigan 1989) and Overt Aggression Scales (Yudovsky, 1986) are instruments that help team members objectively define behavioral symptoms and reach consensus about behaviors to target.

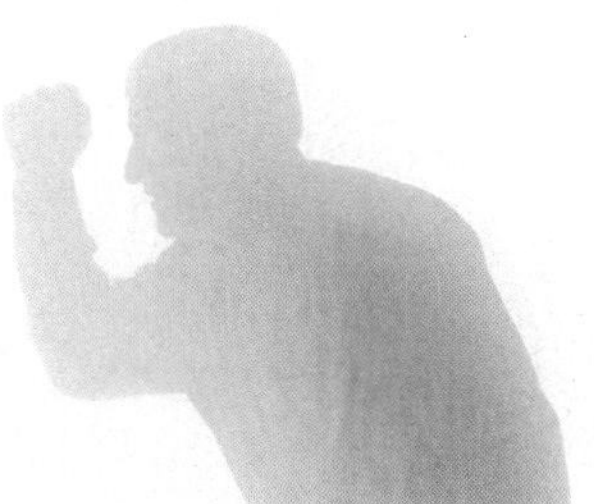

Medication use factors for treatment of neuro-behavioral symptoms

The person's current medications should be reviewed and unnecessary medications discontinued or substituted before considering medication to treat neuro-behavioral symptons.

Factors requiring consideration in medication use include:

- Age.
- Type and location of the injury.
- History of previous brain injury.
- Injury severity.
- Medical complications.
- Nutritional deficiencies.
- History of substance abuse.
- Pre-injury coping strategies.
- Psychosocial and cognitive development.
- History of psychiatric illness.

Aggravating factors in the environment, such as noise levels and distractions, should be assessed and

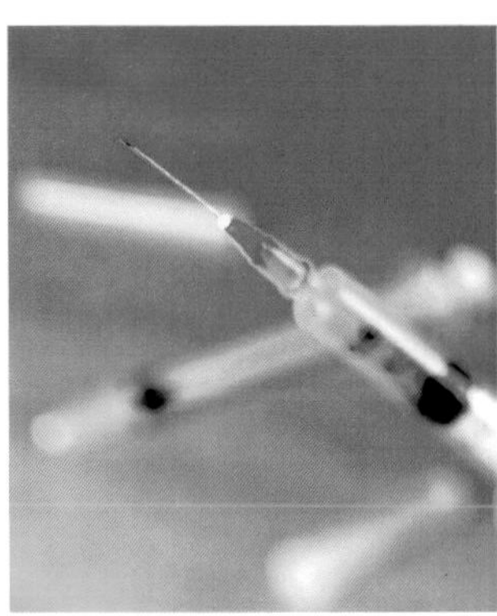

eliminated if possible. De-escalation techniques, relaxation training, and behavior therapy should also be implemented as deemed clinically appropriate.

Once specific target symptoms are objectively identified and it is determined that medication is the most appropriate intervention, decisions must be made about medication choice, dosing, drug interactions and potential side effects. Medication is typically started at a low dosage and increases are dependent upon improvement, tolerability, or deterioration. If the medication is effective, the necessity for the medication is continually assessed and reassessed. When appropriate, it is tapered and discontinued. If one medication is ineffective, another may be appropriate for trial. It is best to make only one medication change at a time, so that behavioral changes can be more closely correlated with the use of that particular medication.

There are few prospective studies and only a few case reports and retrospective studies of medication interventions for neurobehavioral sequelae in persons with brain injuries. However, medical practitioners have described the successful use of some of the following medications to treat post-traumatic agitation.

The anticonvulsant, carbamazepine, (Tegretol®) is the most commonly used medication to treat post-traumatic agitation, aggression and bipolar illness precipitated by brain injury. The anticonvulsant, valproic acid, (Depakote®) is also being assessed in this population for post-traumatic agitation particularly with psychotic features.

Relatively little research has been done to determine whether antidepressants are helpful for treating behavioral dyscontrol after brain injury. Anecdotal experience suggests that trazodone (Desyrel®), because of its sedating properties, may be beneficial. The class of antidepressants known as selective serotonin reuptake inhibitors (SSRIs) are more commonly used to treat behavioral dyscontrol rather than tricyclic antidepressants or MAO inhibitors. Tricyclic antidepressant use may be associated with side effects such as sedation, lowered seizure threshold and cardiac effects. An overdose can be particularly lethal.

The oldest class of antidepressants used to treat post-traumatic agitation were the monamine oxidase inhibitors (MAOIs). Use of these agents is now discouraged due to the need

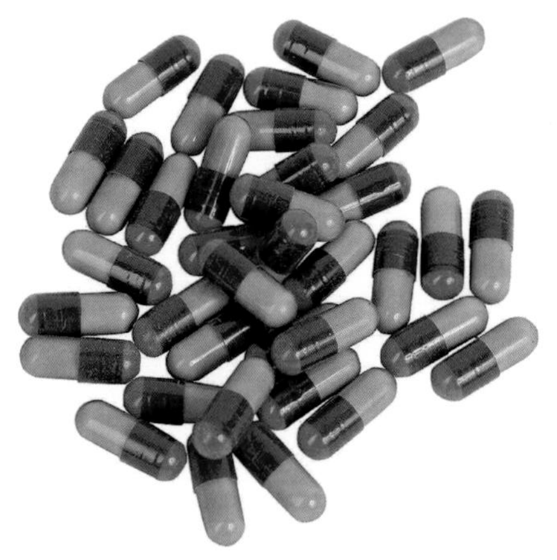

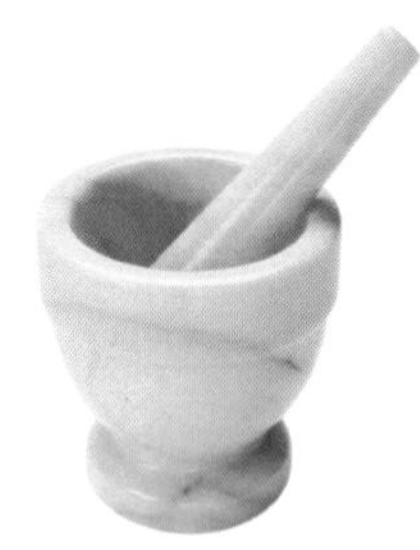

for dietary restrictions of foods that contain high levels of tyramine (e.g. cheese, red wine, beer, sardines, sauerkraut, liver, aged meats) as well as problems with interactions with cold medications, antiparkinsonian drugs and meperidine (Demerol®). If these foods or medications are taken, a hypertensive crisis characterized by increased blood pressure, severe headache, heart palpitations, cardiac effects and stroke can occur.

Some miscellaneous medications, which may be considered, include antihypertensive (blood pressure) medications such as propranolol (Inderal®), which is sometimes effective in reducing restlessness and irritability, aggression and explosive disorders. Clonidine (Catapress®), also an antihypertensive medication, has been used to treat motor restlessness, hypervigilance and hyperactivity seen with severe orbitofrontal lesions.

Lithium, which has been traditionally used to treat bipolar disorder, may sometimes be utilized for post-traumatic agitation, however, its use is rare due to serious central nervous system side effects. In addition, blood levels must be closely monitored because there is only a small difference between doses that are therapeutic and those that are toxic.

Anti-anxiety medications, (also known as Anxiolytics), have been historically used to treat agitation, although they now have a limited role in the treatment of post-traumatic agitation. Side effects including cognitive and memory impairment, confusion, respiratory depression, sedation, increased potential for addiction and an increased propensity toward falls, are particular concerns for persons with brain injury.

Administration of these anti-anxiety drugs in some individuals can even precipitate worsening agitation and belligerence due to their effect of increasing disinhibition. One relatively recent exception has been the use of buspirone (Buspar®), for the treatment of chronic anxiety. This medication differs from the more traditional anti-anxiety medications, in that the side effect profile is far more favorable. It may take several weeks, however, for the anti-anxiety effect to stabilize.

The traditional use of antipsychotic medications, although once the primary drugs of choice for treating agitated and aggressive behaviors, is controversial and these medications are not considered to be agents of first choice. Antipsychotic medications have been reported to delay recovery, impair learning and memory, and lower seizure threshold. Anticholinergic side effects (e.g., drowsiness, agitation, urinary retention, tachycardia, confusion, dizziness dry mouth, constipation, delirium, insomnia, confusion, palpitations, blurred vision, GI upset) are more common with phenothiazines.

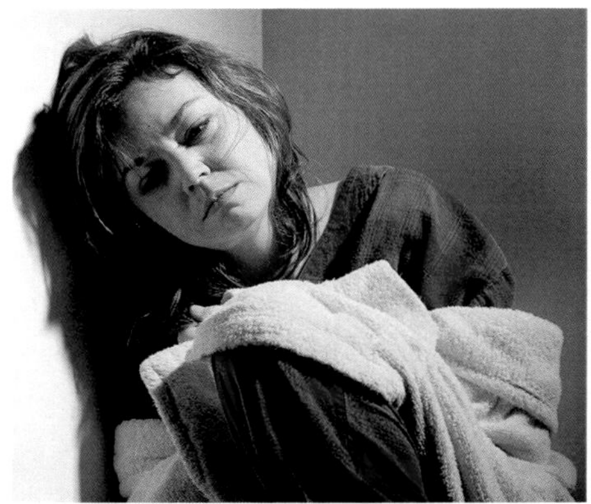

Extrapyramidal effects such as muscle tremors, masked facial appearance, cogwheel rigidity (rigidity with little jerks when the muscle in the arms and legs are stretched by the examiner), shuffling gait, drooling, akathisia (inability to sit or stand still), dystonic reaction (spasms of neck, tongue, or facial muscles), grimacing, abnormal eye movement, torticollis (twisted position of the neck) are more common with the older conventional agents (especially haloperidol and thiothixene) and less common with the new atypical agents. Tardive dyskinesia, (which may be irreversible) is a very serious side effect. This involuntary movement disorder is characterized by lip smacking, rhythmic darting of the tongue, chewing movements, aimless movements of the arms and legs and in severe cases, difficulty breathing and swallowing.

There may be times, however, when antipsychotics are clinically indicated and a risk versus benefit decision must be made. For example, antipsychotic medications may be prescribed for persons with a pre-injury diagnosis of schizophrenia or who present with hallucinations, delusions, paranoia, physical aggression, and danger to themselves or others. If it is deemed necessary to use antipsychotics, "atypical antipsychotic" agents such as risperidone (Risperdal®), olanzapine (Zyprexa®), and quetiapine (Seroquel®) may have more favorable side effect profiles than conventional typical antipsychotics.

It is certainly beyond the scope of this manual to have an exhaustive discussion of medications used to treat neurobehavioral sequelae which arise after brain injury. The medications listed are examples of medications previously described and are certainly not all-inclusive. It is essential that specific information regarding dosage, precautions, contraindications, adverse reactions and drug interactions specific to each medication be reviewed by all staff members responsible for the person's care. Please discuss any questions or concerns with the physician.

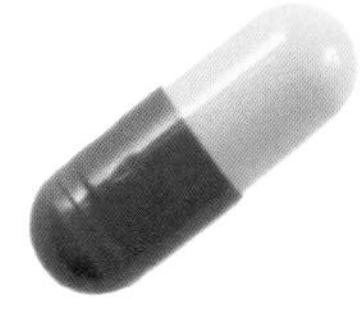

Anti-Depressants: Selective Serotonin Reuptake Inhibitors (SSRIs)

- Paroxetine (Paxil®).
- Sertraline (Zolof®).
- Fluoxetine (Prozac®).
- Citalopram (Celexa®).
- Escitalopram (Lexapro®)

Anti-Depressants: Serotonin Norepinephrine Reuptake Inhibitors (SNRIs)

- Duloxetine (Cymbaltal®).
- Venlafaxine (Effexor®).

Other Antidepressants

- Trazodone (Desyrel®).
- Bupropion (Wellbutrin®).

Tricyclic Antidepressants

- Nortriptyline (Pamelor®).
- Imipramine, (Tofranil®).
- Amitryptyline,(Elavil®).
- Desipramine (Norpramin®)
- Clomipramine, (Anafranil®).
- Doxepin(Sinequan®).
- Protyptoline (Vivactil®).

Monamine Oxidase Inhibitors (MAOIs)

- Tranylcypromine (Parnate®).
- Phenelzine (Nardil®).

Anti-anxiety Medications

- Lorazepam (Ativan®).
- Alprazolam (Xanax®).
- Oxazepam (Serax®).
- Clonazepam (Klonopin®).

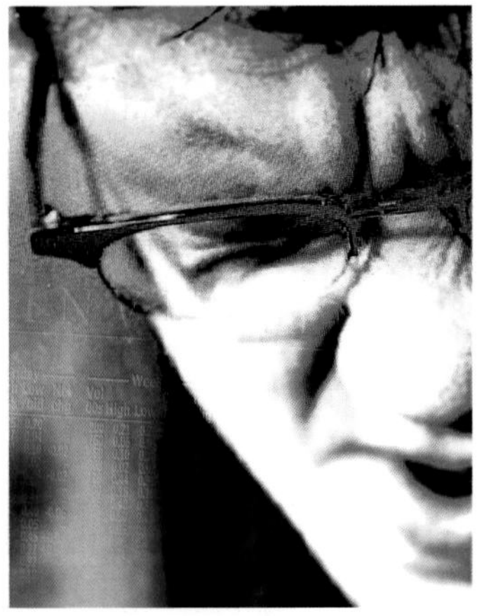

Atypical Antipsychotics

- Risperidone (Risperdal®).
- Olanzapine (Zyprexa®).
- Quetiapine (Seroquel®).
- Clozapine (Clozaril®).
- Ariprazole (Abilify®).

Conventional Antipsychotics

- Chlorpromazine (Thorazine®).
- Thioridazine (Mellaril®).
- Mesoridazine (Serentil®).
- Fluphenazine (Prolixin®).
- Perphenazine (Trilafon®).
- Trifluoperazine (Stelazine®).
- Clopromazine (Compazine®).
- Nonphenothiazines.
- Haloperidal (Haldol®).
- Loxapine (Loxitane®).
- Molindone (Moban®).
- [illegible]

Medications to Treat Sleep Problems

Problems falling asleep and/or staying asleep are common complaints after a person has sustained a brain injury. Prior to starting any medication, it is important to complete a medical and clinical evaluation. The person's self-report and observation by direct care staff are crucial. In addition, it may be helpful to use an assessment scale, such as the Pittsburgh Sleep Quality Index Questionnaire (Busseye D, 1989) to better provide objective and measurable information.

Trazadone (Desyrel®) and zolpidem (Ambien®) have been anecdotally reported to produce favorable outcomes in treating sleep disturbances and have low side effect profiles. As previously discussed, anti-anxiety drugs should usually be avoided in this population due to previously mentioned concerns of sedation and cognitive and motor impairment.

Medications to Treat Depression

The most common mood disorder following TBI is depression (Varney, Martzke & Roberts, 1987; O'Donnell, ML. Creamer, M, Pattison, P, Atkin, C, 2004). Estimates of post-traumatic depression range from 10 to 77%. A thorough medical and clinical exam should be followed by behavioral, psychological, and, when necessary, medication interventions. The SSRIs are typically the first medications considered due to their low side effect profile, efficacy, ease of dosing, and low risk of life threatening overdose (Turner-Stokes, Hassan, Pierce & Clegg, 2002; Fann, Uomoto & Kato, 2001; Schmitt, Kruizinga & Reidel, 2001; Lee, Kim, Kim, Shin, & Yang, 2005; Alderfer, Arciniegas, & Silver, 2005). It is important for both the patient and the staff to realize that the antidepressant effect can take 3-8 weeks before a noticeable change occurs.

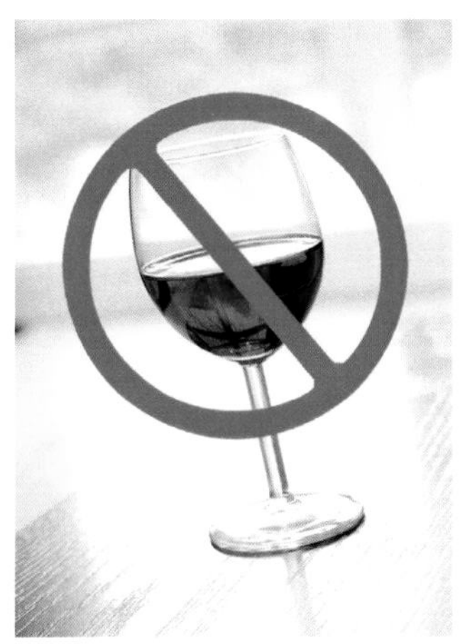

Substance Abuse

There is little debate that acquired brain injury and substance abuse are linked. Several studies suggest that:

- Acquired brain injury and spinal cord injury are the leading cause of death and disability for people under 50. Alcohol is the predominant risk factor for injury and an obstacle to rehabilitation for both brain and spinal cord injury (Marion,1998).
- Nearly 58% percent of individuals with acquired brain injury had a history of alcohol abuse or dependence prior to injury (Kreutzer, Dougherty,& Harris, et al.,1990).
- One-third of ABI outpatients had used illicit drugs prior to their brain injury. Marijuana was used most commonly followed by cocaine. (Kreutzer, Wehman & Harris, et al., 1991).
- As many as 50 percent of individuals with an acquired brain injury will return to using drugs and alcohol post-injury (Sparadeo, Strauss & Barth, 1990).
- The 1988 National Head Injury Task Force on Substance Abuse reported that approximately 40 percent of persons in post-acute rehabilitation facilities have moderate to severe problems with substance abuse, and alcohol is the substance most abused in over 90 percent of the cases.

Pathological changes, some of which are irreversible, have been demonstrated within the brain and the central nervous system of some substance abusers. The absolute amount of brain damage sustained by the chemical abuser depends to a large degree upon the drug(s) utilized, their purity and the frequency and duration of abuse.

Whenever a person sustains a brain injury and is taken to the emergency room of an acute care hospital, it may be difficult to make an accurate diagnosis when the brain injury is accompanied by moderate to high levels of blood alcohol or drugs. When a brain injury occurs in the setting of substance abuse, it is possible that pre-existing biochemical and structural damage to the brain might be added to that caused by the brain injury itself. Further complicating the clinical picture, is the fact that behaviors noted following acute intoxication and overdose are very similar to those following brain injury (lethargy, or agitation, confusion, disorientation, respiratory depression, etc.). It appears that in some emergency rooms, patients may be discharged with a diagnosis of intoxication when they have also sustained an undiagnosed brain injury.

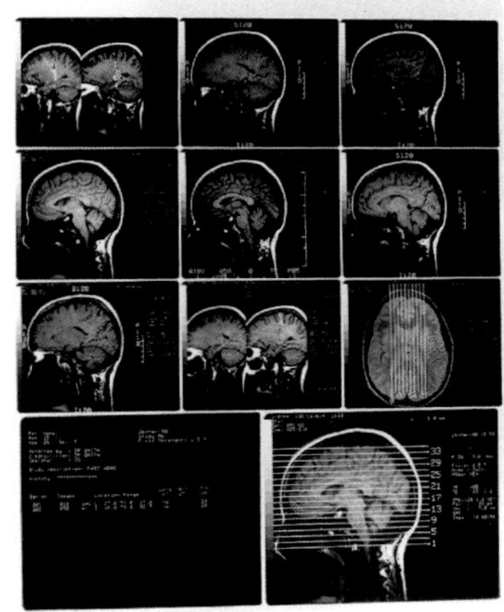

Post Injury Alcohol Use

As many as 50 percent of individuals with an acquired brain injury will return to using drugs and alcohol post-injury (Sparadeo, Strauss & Barth, 1990)

Substance abuse also causes metabolic changes in the body. At the time of hospital admission, alcohol consumption can lead to fluid and electrolyte abnormalities. These can worsen cerebral edema from trauma. Second, the likelihood of developing hematomas (collection of blood trapped in the tissues of the skin or in an organ) is increased in persons with cerebral Atrophy (wasting of size or functional activity) associated with alcohol abuse. This is due to increased fragility of the capillaries, decreased brain counter-pressure to deal with low pressure leaks (Markwalder,1981) and possible alterations in blood clotting mechanisms (Elmer, Goransson & Xoucas, 1984).

In addition, tolerance of blood loss is decreased and blood pressure on admission is decreased (Elmer & Lim, 1985) This is due to dilatation (widening) of peripheral blood vessels. This in turn increases the risk of hypoxia (lack of oxygen) to the brain. It has been suggested that alcohol can cause respiratory depression, which also increases the risk of hypoxia.

By the time the individual with a brain injury enters the rehabilitation setting, physical withdrawal from recreational drugs or alcohol, if present at the time of the injury, has been completed. Unfortunately, psychological dependency has not been addressed so the problem continues to pose a threat. Additionally, within the acute care setting, the stage may have been inadvertently set for later problems with chemical abuse. As previously discussed, individuals may have been prescribed a variety of medications for seizure control, behavioral control, pain management or sleep induction.

The rehabilitation facility may be unaware of pre-existing problems in this area, since neither the person nor family members are likely to voluntarily admit problems for fear of making the person appear a poor candidate for rehabilitation. Accompanying medical records may not include this information.

The physical and medical deficits following brain injury are frequently so wide-ranging that multiple physicians may be involved in diagnosis and management. Significant changes in prescribed medications may occur as health care professionals begin to address long-term issues such as seizure control, incontinence, spasticity and behavioral dyscontrol. Even the individual who has no history of drug use may experiment with alternative medications, nonprescription drugs, and illegal substances (i.e. marijuana) in an attempt to relieve troublesome symptoms.

To forestall the misuse or abuse of both prescription and nonprescription drugs, it is critical that a single physician assume responsibility for the coordination of medication management. This helps minimize undesirable drug interactions and ensures continuity of care.

Aging with Brain Injury

The graying baby boomer generation has placed a national spotlight on issues of aging that bears relevance in the field of brain injury. Since the Vietnam War era, enhancements of the medical emergency response system and advances in trauma care have contributed to a growing population of individuals surviving moderate and severe brain injuries. Many of these individuals experience significant residual disabilities, which persist throughout the aging process.

Studies have reported that during the "normal" aging process, individuals may experience memory impairment, slower learning of new material, gait and balance problems, decreased sensory acuity, diminished executive functions and reductions in appetite and libido (Goldstein and Shelly,

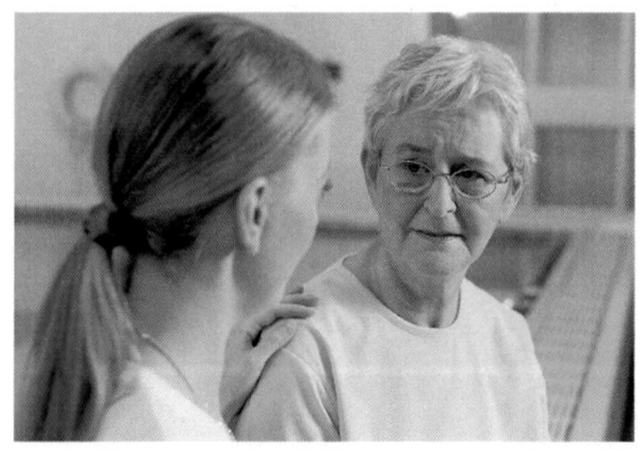

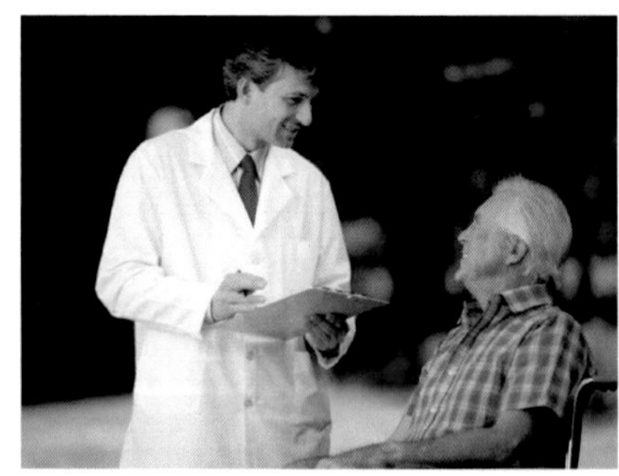

1975). The concept was considered that the relative cognitive impairment of individuals with brain injury would appear less significant with age due to the cognitive decline of their age peers. Goldstein and Shelly (1975) concluded, however, that the differences between individuals with brain injury and their age peers did not decrease with age. Both study groups (those with and without brain injury) demonstrated cognitive decline. More recent studies also strongly suggest that TBI can provoke some of the changes seen in the brain of persons suffering from Alzheimer's disease and can accelerate brain aging (Goldstein et.al., 1996; Klein, Houx & Jolles, 1996; Nemetz et.al., 1999).

Several long-term studies have also reported that after brain injury, persons reported persistent problems with behavior disorders, personality changes, learning and memory deficits, psychosocial readjustment issues, social isolation, chronic unemployment, health, self-awareness, and major psychiatric disorders (especially depression) (Brooks et al, 1987; Burleigh, Farber & Gillard, 1997; Dawson & Chipman, 1995; Hibbard et. al., 1998; O'Neill et. al., 1998; Rothweiler, Tekmen & Dikmen, 1998; Tennant, McDermott & Neary, 1995; Trudel & Purdum, 1998; Trudel, Tryon & Purdum, 1998).

One study reported that eight of the

top ten problems most frequently reported by relatives at five years post-injury were psychological in nature. The most commonly reported symptom, personality change, increased from 60% to 74% at year five. Family subjective burden also increased over time, with researchers noting that the scenario at year five was similar to or worse than that at year one (Brooks, et al,1986).

Psychiatric diagnoses may include major depression, anxiety disorders (Hibbard et al 1998, Rosenthal, Christensen & Ross, 1998; Van Reekum et al., 1996), psychosis (Thomsen, 1984) and other conditions that negatively influence outcome and recovery, presumably on a long-term basis. Interpreting psychiatric data in relation to brain injury is complicated by both pre-existing conditions (particularly substance abuse related) and by disorders that may arise from or be maintained by a combination of neuroanatomic, neurochemical and psychosocial factors.

Post-traumatic epilepsy is associated with many unfavorable long-term consequences (Hernandez,& Naritoku, 1997) including shortened life span, neurotoxic effects of long term anticonvulsant use, increased

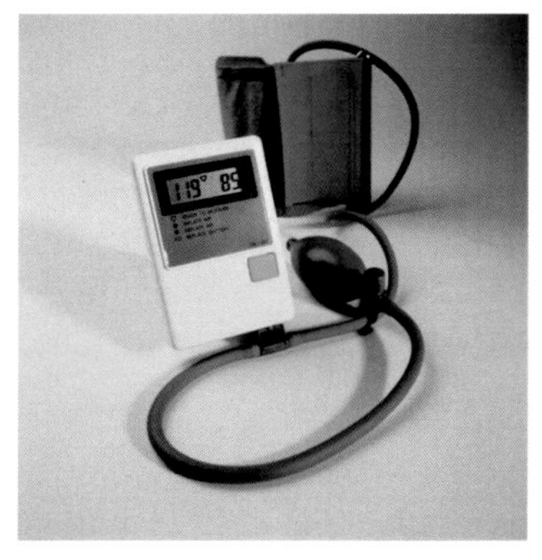

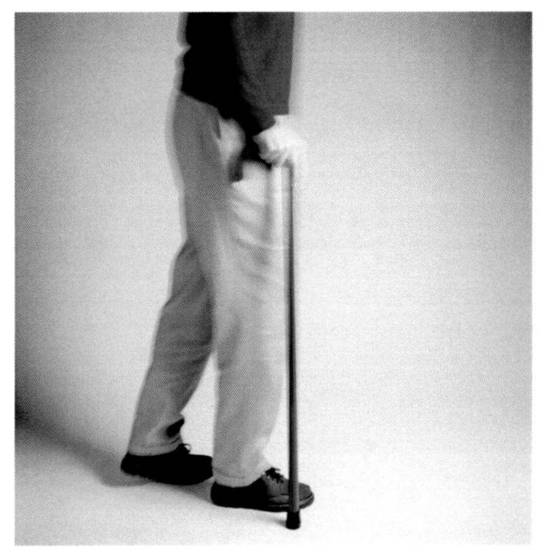

probability of psychiatric complications and in some studies, a reduced overall functional outcome (Gualtieiri & Cox, 1991).

In studying Alzheimer's disease, three risk factors have become evident: age (diagnosis is in part age determined), family history of Alzheimer's disease or Down's syndrome (present in first degree relative and therefore increasing genetic probability) and history of TBI (Gaultieri & Cox, 1991, Sullivan, Pettiti & Barbaccia, 1987). Regarding the theoretical basis for the development of Alzheimer's disease (or Alzheimer's type neurodegeneration) following TBI, Ramusson et al. (1995) discussed the possibilities that brain injury contributes to the death of neurons by axonal shearing, or by weakening the blood-brain barrier thereby exposing the brain to potential neurotoxins.

Other researchers report the significance of finding deposits of beta-amyloid (B-A4 proteins) in the cortex of the brains of both young and old victims of brain injury upon autopsy. Amyloid proteins have been implicated in the formation of the plaques found in the brains of persons diagnosed with Alzheimer's disease.

Other problems which must be considered when examining the problems specific to aging with brain injury include musculoskeletal complications (e.g., arthritis, bursitis, tendonitis) which can result from previous traumatic injuries as well as the stress, wear and tear on joints involved in supporting altered mobility patterns. Many persons also report a general loss of energy after years of living with a disability. Alterations in endocrine and immune systems may affect the person's susceptibility to infection. (Hibbard et al., 1998)

The aging process is inevitable for everyone, but for persons who have sustained brain injuries, this process may occur at earlier ages and be more dramatic. As mobility, energy and physical function decline, activities of daily living may further decline as pleasurable activities are replaced with those that focus on survival.

Currently, the American Congress of Rehabilitation Medicine (ACRM) Brain Injury Interdisciplinary Special Interest Group has undertaken a large scale study examining aspects of aging with brain injury (special focus on health and prevention). It is through research efforts such as this that systems and structures for service provision have and will continue to evolve to meet the needs of persons with brain injuries and their families (ACRM, 2001).

Summary

All staff members need working knowledge of the effects of brain injury on each organ system and the subsequent medical complications that arise as part of the body's response to injury. Astute observation and subsequent reporting of symptoms that require the attention of medically trained personnel can mean the difference between life and death.

Knowledge of medications and subsequent monitoring for effectiveness or adverse effects is critically important for helping the person attain optimum recovery. Substance abuse and the effects of aging further complicate the person's overall health and recovery. The goal of this chapter was to inform direct care providers of the health and medical issues that persons who have sustained a brain injury must face on a daily basis.

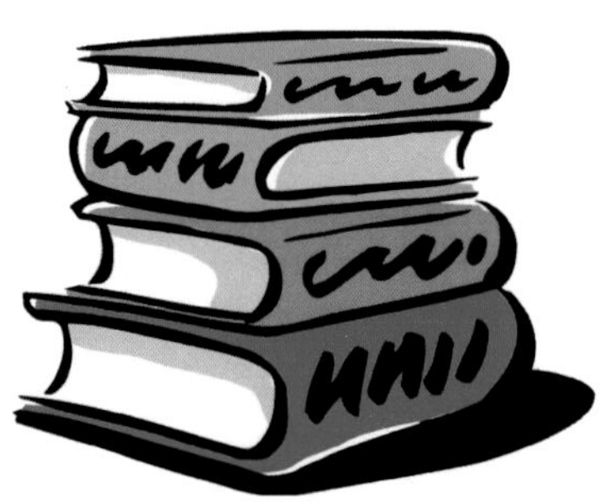

References

Agency for Health Care Policy and Research (1994). Treatment of pressure ulcers. Rockville, MD, U.S. Department of Health and Human Services.

Alderfer, BS, Arciniegas, DB & Silver, JM (2005). Treatment of Depression Following Traumatic Brain Injury. Journal of Head Trauma Rehabilitation, 20:544-562.

American Congress of Rehabilitation Medicine-Brain Injury Long Term Issues Task Force (2001). Brain injury, aging and health: conducting large scale survey research. Rehabilitation Outlook, Summer: 8-9.

Antoinette, T (1996). Rehabilitation nursing management for persons in low level neurologic states. Neurorehabilitation, 6(1),33-44.

Brain Injury Special Interest Group of the American Academy of Physical Medicine and Rehabilitation: Practice parameter: Antiepileptic drug treatment of post-traumatic seizures (1998). Arch Phys Med Rehabil 79: 594-597.

Bogner J (1995). Improving Outcomes Following Brain Injury. A Longitudinal Study at the Ohio Valley Center on TBI Prevention and Rehabilitation. Ohio State University.

Brooke, MM, Barbour PG & Cording LG (1989). Nutritional status during rehabilitation after head injury. Neurorehabilitation, 3: 27-33.

Brooks, N, Campsie, L, Symington, C, Beattie & McKinlay, W (1986). The five year outcome of severe blunt head injury: A relative's view. Journal of Neurology, Neurosurgery and Psychiatry, 49:764-770.

Brooks, N, Campsie, L, Symington, C, Beattie, A, & McKinlay, W (1987). The effects of severe head injury on patient and relative within seven years of injury. Journal of Head Trauma Rehabilitation, 2(3):1-13.

Bullock R, Chestnut RM, Clifton GL, et al (2000). Role of antiseizure prophylaxis following head injury. Journal of Neurotrauma 17:549-553.

Burleigh, S., Farber, RS, & Gillard, M (1997). Community integration and life satisfaction after traumatic brain injury: Long term findings. American Journal of Occupational Therapy, 52(1):45-51.

Busseye D et al (1989). The Pittsburgh Sleep Quality Index: A new instrument of psychiatric practice and research. Psychiatry Res 28; 193-213.

Chipps, EM, Clanin NJ, and Campbell,VG (1992). Neurologic Disorders. St Louis, Missouri: Mosby-Year Book Inc.

Corrigan JD (1989). Development of a scale for assessment of agitation following traumatic brain injury. J Clin Exp Neuropsychol 11:261-277.

Dawson, DR & Chipman, M (1995). The disablement experienced by traumatically brain-injured adults living in the Community. Brain Injury, 9(4):339-353.

Elmer, O, Goransson, G, & Xoucas, E (1984). Impairment of primary homeostasis and platelet function after alcohol ingestion in man. Homeostasis 14:223-228.

Elmer, O & Lim R (1985). Influence of acute alcohol intoxication on the outcome of severe nonneurologic trauma. Acta Chirurgica 151:305-308.

Fann, JR, Uomoto, JM & Katon, WJ (2001). Cognitive Improvement with Treatment of Depression Following

Mild Traumatic Brain Injury. Psychosomatics, 42: 48-54.

Field, LH & Weiss, CJ (1989). Dysphagia with Head Injury. Brain Injury, 3:19-26.

Garland D, & Bailey, S (1981). Undetected injuries in head injured adults. Clinical Orthopedics 155-162.
Gaultieri, T & Cox, DR (1991). The delayed neurobehavioral sequelae of traumatic brain injury. Brain Injury, 5(32):219-232.

Goldstein, FC, Levin, HS, Roberts, VJ, Goldman, WP, Kalechstein, AS, Winslow, M & Goldstein, SJ (1996). Neuropsychological effects of closed head injury in older adults: A comparison with Alzheimer's Disease. Neuropsychology, 10(2):147-154.

Goldstein, G & Shelly, CH (1975). Similarities and differences between psychological deficit in aging and brain damage. Journal of Gerontology, 30(4):438-455.

Hernandez TD & Naritoku, DK (1997). Seizures, epilepsy, and functional recovery after traumatic brain injury: A reappraisal. Neurology, 48:803-806.

Hibbard, MR, Uysal, S, Kepler, K, Bogdany, J, & Silver, J (1998). Axis I psychopathology in individuals with traumatic brain injury. The Journal of Head Trauma Rehabilitation, 13(4):24-39.

Hibbard, JR, Uysal, S, Sliwinski, M. & Gordon, WA (1998). Undiagnosed health issues in individuals with traumatic brain injury living in the community. The Journal of Head Trauma Rehabilitation, 13(4):47-57.

Jennett B, Snoek J, and Bond MR, et al (1981). Disability after severe head injury: Observations on the use of the Glascow Outcome Scale. Journal of Neurology, Neurosurgery, Psychiatry 44:285-293.

Jennett, B, and Teasdale, G (1981). Management of Head Injuries. Contemporary Neurology Series, (20). FA Davis, Philadelphia.

Kalisky, A et al (1985). Medical problems encountered during rehabilitation of patients with head injury. Archives of Physical Medicine and Rehabilitation 66:25.

Klein, J, Houx, PJ & Jolles, J (1996). Long term persisting cognitive sequelae of traumatic brain injury and the effects of age. Journal of Nervous and Mental Disease, 184(8):459-467.

Kreutzer, JS, Dougherty DR, and Harris AZ. et al (1990). Alcohol use among persons with traumatic brain injury. Journal of Head Trauma Rehabilitation 5:9-20.

Kreutzer, JS, Wehman PH & Harris JA et al (1991). Substance abuse and crime patterns among persons with traumatic brain injury referred for supported employment. Brain Injury 5:177-187.

Labi, MC & Horn, LJ (1990). Hypertension in traumatic brain injury. Brain Injury 4:365.

Lee, H, Kim, SW, Kim, JM, Shin, IS & Yang, JM (2005). Comparing Effects of Methylphenidate, Sertraline, and Placebo on Neuropsychiatriic Sequelae in Patients with Traumatic Brain Injury. Human Psychopharmocology, 20: 97-104.

Logeman, JA, Pepe, J, Mackay, LE. (1994). Disorders of Nutrition and Swallowing: Interaction Strategies in the Trauma Center. Journal of Head Trauma Rehabilitation, 9:43-56

Mackay, LE, Morgan, AS, Bernstein, BA. (1999). Swallowing Disorders in Severe Brain Injury: Risk Factors Affecting Return to Oral Intake. Archives of Physical Medicine, 80: 365-371.

Mackay, LE, Morgan, AS, Bernstein, BA. (1999). Factors Affecting Oral Feeding with Severe Traumatic Brain Injury. Journal of Head Trauma Rehabilitation, 14:435-447.

Marion, DW (1998). Head and spinal cord injury. Neurology Clinics 16:485-502.

Markwalder, T (1981). Chronic subdural hematomas: a review. Journal of Neurosurgery 54:637-645.

Nemetz, PN, Leibson, C, Naessens, JM, Beard, M, Kokmen, E, Annegers, JF & Kurkland, LT (1999). Traumatic brain injury and time to onset of Alzheimer's Disease: A population-based study. American Journal of Epidemiology, 149(1):32-40.

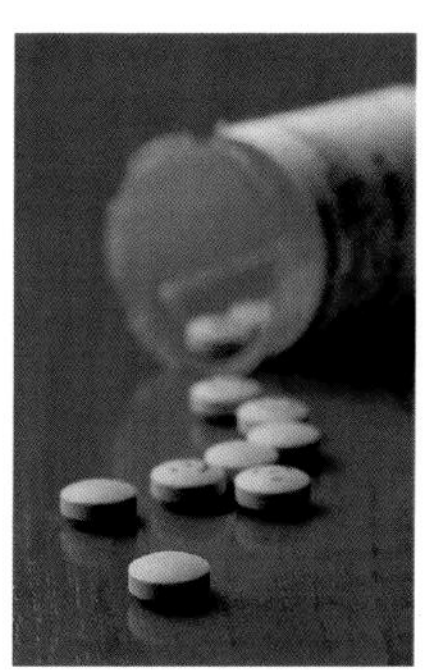

O'Donnell, ML, Creamer, M. Pattison, P, Atkin, C (2004). Psychiatric Morbidity Following Head Injury. American Journal of Psychiatry, 161, 507-514.

O'Neill, J, Hibbard, MR, Brown, M, Jaffe, M, Sliwinski, M, Vandergroot, D, & Weiss, MJ (1998). The effect of employment on quality of life and community integration after traumatic brain injury. Journal of Head Trauma Rehabilitation, 13(4):68-79.

Packard, RC & Ham LP (1994). Post-traumatic headache. Journal of Neuropsychiatry and Clinical Neurosciences, 6 (3), 229-36.

Rasmusson, DX, Brandt, J, Martin, DB, & Folstein, MF (1995). Head injury as a risk factor in Alzheimer's disease. Brain Injury, 9(3):213-219.
Rosenthal, J, Christensen, B, & Ross, TP (1988). Depression following traumatic brain injury. Archives of Physical Medicine and Rehabilitation, 79:90-103.

Rothweiler, B, Temkin, NR.. & Dikmen, S (1998). Aging effect on psychosocial outcome in traumatic brain injury. Archives of Physical Medicine and Rehabilitation, 79:881-887.

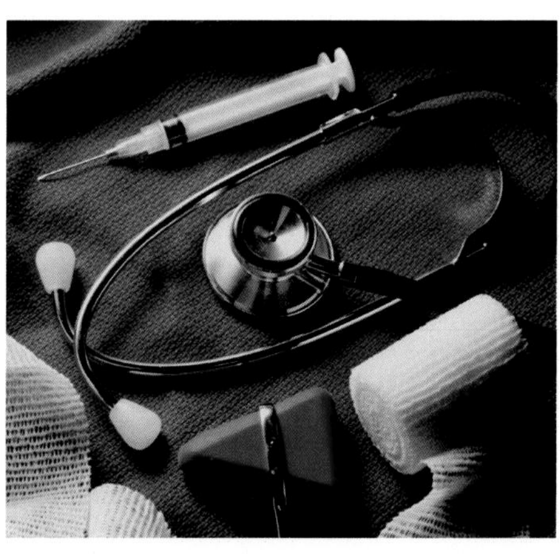

Schmitt, JA, Kruizinga, MJ, & Reidel, WJ (2001). Non-Serotonergic Pharmacological Profiles and Associated Cognitive Effects of Serotonin Reuptake Inhibitors. Journal of Psychopharmocology, 15: 173-179.

Sparadeo, FR, Strauss D & Barth, JT (1990). The incidence, impact and treatment of substance abuse in head trauma rehabilitation. Journal of Head Trauma Rehabilitation 5 (3),1-8.

Speed, WG (1991). Post traumatic Headache. Headache Review, 4 (3):1.

Sullivan, P., Petitti, D. & Barbaccia, J. Head trauma and age of onset of dementia of the Alzheimer's type. Journal of the American Medical Association, 257:2289-2290, 1987.

Tennant, A, MacDermott, N, & Neary, D (1995). The long term outcome of head injury: Implications for service planning. Brain Injury, 9(6):959-605.

Thomsen, IV (1984). Late outcome of very severe blunt head trauma: A 10-15 year second follow-up. Journal of Neurology, Neurosurgery, and Psychiatry, 47:260-268.

Trudel, TM, Tryon, WW & Purdum, CM (1998). Awareness of disability and long term outcome after traumatic brain injury. Rehabilitation Psychology, 43(4):267-281.

Trudel, TM. & Purdum, CM (1998). Aging with brain injury: Long term issues. The Rehabilitation Professional, 6:37-41.

Turner-Stokes, L, Hassan, N & Clegg, F (2002). Managing Depression in Brain Injury Rehabilitation: The Use of an Integrated Care Pathway and Preliminary Report of Response to Sertraline. Clinical Rehabilitation, 16: 261-268.

Van Reekum, R, Bolago, I, Finlayson, MAJ, Garner, S & Links, PS (1996). Psychiatric disorders after traumatic brain injury. Brain Injury, 10(5):319-327.

Varney, N, Martzke, J, Roberts, R (1987). Major Depression in Patients with Closed Head Injury. Neuropsychology, 1, 7-9.

Weinstein, CJ (1983). Neurogenic Dysphagia: Frequency, Progression, and Outcome in Adults Following Head Injury. Physical Ther., 63: 1992-1996.

Whyte, J (1992). Attention and Arousal: Basic science aspects. Archives of Physical Medicine and Rehabilitation 73:940-949.

Yablon SA (1993). Post-traumatic seizures. Archives Phys Med Rehabil 74; 983.

Yudovsky SC, Silver JM, Jackson W (1986). The Overt Aggression Scale for the objective rating of verbal and physical aggression. Am J Psychiatry 143:35-39.

Zafonte RD, Elovic E, Mysiw, WJ et al (1999). Pharmacology in traumatic brain injury: fundamentals and treatment strategies. In: Rosenthal, M., Griffith, E.R., Kreutzer, J.S. et al. eds. Rehabilitation of the adult and child with traumatic brain injury. Philadelphia, PA: F.A.Davis Company.

Chapter 5

Understanding and Treating Functional Impacts of Brain Injury

Learning Objectives

By the end of this chapter, you will be able to:

- Describe common cognitive, physical, emotional, behavioral, and social changes after brain injury.
- Describe how these changes affect the person's functioning.
- Describe the outcome-driven rehabilitation process.
- Describe and give examples of three environmental influences on behavior.
- Describe active treatment planning.

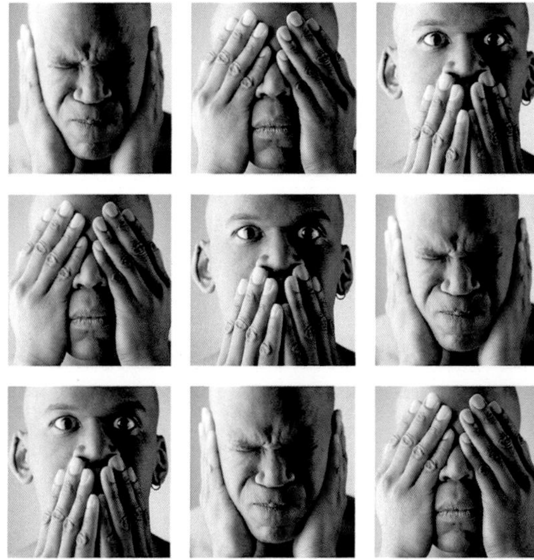

Introduction

There may be many changes in how a person thinks, feels, and acts after a brain injury. Cognitive, physical, behavioral and emotional changes can greatly affect a person's ability to live independently. These changes can affect virtually every aspect of a person's daily existence from routine activities of daily living, to interactions with loved ones, to being safe in the community.

Effective rehabilitation is based on:

- Knowledge of changes that occur after a brain injury.
- Environmental factors that influence people's behavior (wanted as well as unwanted).

Rehabilitation usually focuses on increasing adaptive behaviors that lead to more independent living. This involves helping individuals relearn lost skills and then using them in meaningful ways. For example, learning to manage one's finances and shop for necessary items are important to living independently in the community.

A Special Note about Chapter 5

Because effective treatment is based on the specific needs of the individual, great attention to detail is required. It is simply not possible to go into detail on the specifics of treatment design within the length of this chapter. Treatment design may vary from one setting to another. Thus, this chapter is an overview of general considerations for effective treatment planning in an active rehabilitation context.

Reducing certain unwanted behaviors is another fundamental focus of rehabilitation for some individuals. This involves helping a person learn alternative skills to replace existing unwanted behaviors. For example, learning alternative ways of expressing displeasure is preferable to loud, threatening behavior.

Functional Impact of Brain Injury

Functional changes following brain injury are different than a broken bone that heals over time. While broken bones eventually heal, cognitive, sensorimotor, and behavioral deficits can result in lifelong changes in how an individual functions in society. Any one of the functional changes discussed here can significantly affect every aspect of a person's life.

Brain injury can affect how a person feels, thinks, acts, and relates to others.

Most people who have survived brain injury have impairments in several areas, which complicate living independently, working, and relationships with others. Some people have physical changes, such as paralysis, or loss of a limb, that may alter their ability to move about. Many have emotional problems, such as depression or severe mood swings. Most often cognitive problems, such as memory loss, and difficulty with problem solving and decision-making are prominent. Changes in behavior after brain injury presents special difficulties. In some cases, behavioral changes such as aggression or property destruction can present additional challenges.

Memory Impairments

Are considered the most disabling consequence of brain injury.

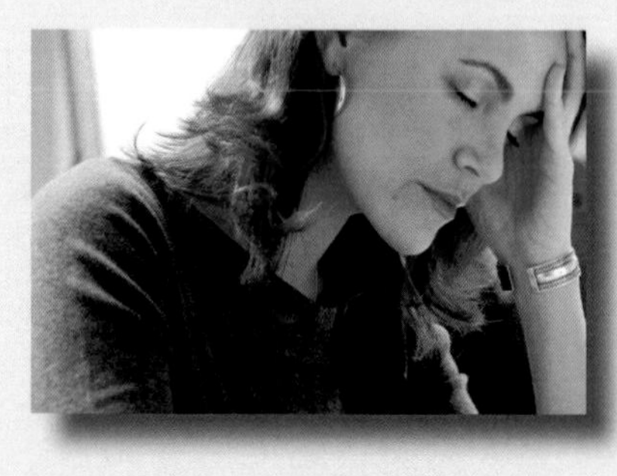

Cognitive Impairments

Cognitive impairments can affect activities of daily living, such as hygiene, eating, household management, community re-integration, and many other aspects of day-to-day living.

Memory Impairments

Memory problems are considered to be the most disabling consequence of brain injury. Impaired memory affects a person's ability to learn, retain, and use new information. In many cases, memory problems significantly affect a person's ability to live independently.

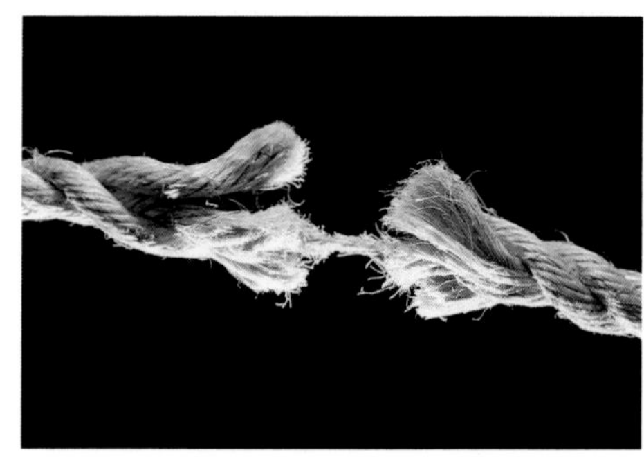

Executive Functioning Impairments

Executive functioning refers to the ability to plan, initiate, direct, and monitor one's activities, much like what an executive does to keep a business running. It involves organizing, planning, creating, evaluating, and initiating projects and activities. In many ways, executive functioning defines an individual, as it is the ability to engage in meaningful tasks, whether necessary or enjoyable, and evaluate performance. It is a large part of being able to understand oneself.

With impaired executive functioning, a person may not respond to stimulation from the environment in the same way as before a brain injury. For example, a common response to a difficult situation, or some type of overstimulation, may be yelling, throwing things, or being aggressive toward another person. These unwanted behaviors may be related to a person's inability to accurately recognize the problem, or poor judgment in arriving at a solution.

Initiation Impairments

Initiation problems may result in a person failing to engage in an important activity unless prompted. It is easy to see how failure to pursue interpersonal relationships, work, perform hygiene, or maintain a safe residence can affect a person's ability to live independently.

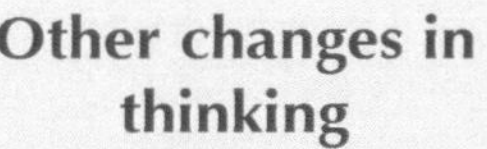

- Lack of awareness of deficits (anosognosia).
- Confusion about who one is, where one is, and the time (disorientation to person, place, and time).
- Distractibility.
- Reduced ability to pay attention.
- Difficulty with changes in routine.
- Difficulty with basic calculation.
- Difficulty sequencing.
- Lack of empathy.
- Impaired ability to evaluate what is important.
- Relating information or events believed to be true, that have not happened.
- Impaired ability to think abstractly.
- Perseverative verbal or motor behavior.
- Difficulty understanding cause and effect.
- Impaired safety awareness.
- Poor insight.

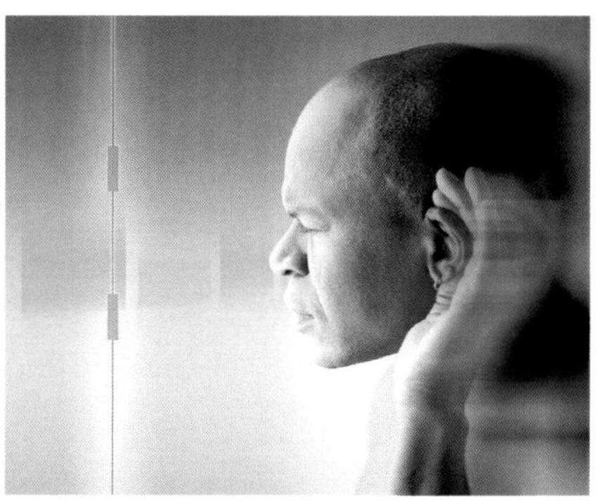

Speech and Language Impairments

Speech and language difficulties can take many different forms. Impaired word-finding abilities, repetition of words or phrases, disorganized spoken or written communication, and incomplete or incoherent expression of thoughts are common following brain injury. Speech and language problems can be either receptive (the ability to understand others), or expressive (the ability to express oneself to others).

Sensorimotor Impairments

Sensorimotor impairments vary, depending on the location and extent of injury to the brain. Sensorimotor impairments can be localized to one extremity or side of the body. In other cases, the effects can be generalized and affect most muscle groups and sensory modalities. When individuals have a combination of sensory deficits, it can have a major functional impact on the person's autonomy. For example, when impaired vision is combined with balance and coordination problems, it can affect the person's motor skills, hand-eye coordination, dexterity, spatial orientation, depth perception, and other areas of functioning.

Sensorimotor Impairments

- Variations in weight or body temperature.
- Variations in appetite.
- Constipation or incontinence.
- Headaches or seizures.
- Paralysis or paresis (weakness) of one or more limbs.
- Balance or coordination problems (ataxia).
- Difficulty planning muscle movements (apraxia).
- Increased muscle tone (spasticity) or deceased muscle tone (flaccidity).
- Decreased endurance.
- Swallowing difficulties (dysphagia).
- Vision problems or impaired depth perception.
- Involuntary eye movements (nystagmus).
- Increased sensitivity to light (photophobia) or sound (sonophobia).
- Hearing impairment or ringing in the ear (tinnitus).
- Impaired ability to smell (anosmia) or taste.
- Increased sensitivity to touch (tactile defensiveness).
- Chronic pain.

Behavioral and Emotional Changes

Behavioral and emotional changes are common following brain injury. It is easy to understand how the behavioral changes listed below may have a major impact on a person's ability to live independently.

In addition to the cognitive, sensorimotor, and behavioral and emotional changes already described, an individual may have medical issues. These medical issues may be temporary or ongoing. They can further affect any of these changes and complicate evaluation and treatment. Changes may include the following:

- Ability to respond to requests.
- Aggression or property destruction.
- Yelling and angry outbursts.
- Self-injury.
- Decreased frustration tolerance.
- Depression and emotional swings (lability).
- Impulsivity and hyperactivity.
- Inappropriate sexual behavior.
- Immature self-focused behavior.
- Hoarding.
- Decreased sensitivity to others.
- Paranoia.

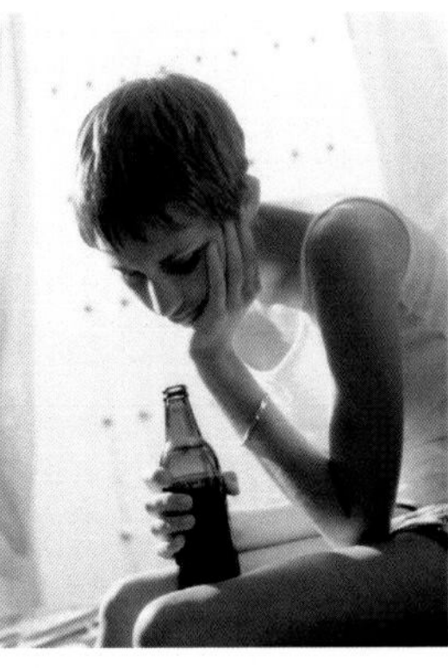

Substance Abuse

Substance abuse is another area of concern for rehabilitation professionals working with individuals with brain injury and their families. An individual with a pre-injury substance abuse history may not have difficulties right after an injury due to limited access to the substance. Physical and cognitive impairments may affect their ability to obtain drugs or alcohol. However, substance abuse difficulties can arise when an individual becomes able to gain access to drugs or alcohol. Substance abuse can be related to any of the following factors:

- Increased access.
- Depression.
- Isolation.
- Increased awareness of limitations.
- Re-involvement with friends who misuse substances.
- Denial that substance abuse is a problem.
- Poor coping strategies.
- Limited therapeutic recreation outlets.
- Limited vocational opportunities.
- Pre-injury pattern of use or abuse.

Treatment Planning

An individual may need varying degrees of support throughout life after a brain injury. This section refers primarily to persons in structured active rehabilitation programming. Certainly the concepts and strategies are also applicable for persons receiving any level of support.

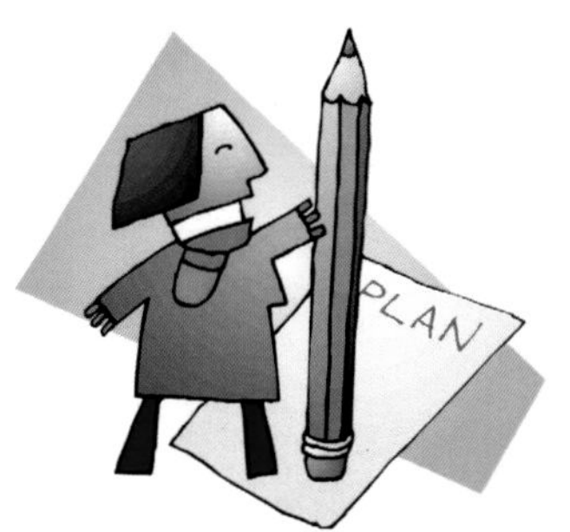

Treatment proceeds most effectively after systematic planning. This applies whether treatment is for teaching new skills or addressing unwanted behaviors. Depending upon the individual's time since injury or access to resources, a plan of treatment should be the product of a trans-disciplinary team of individuals. This team includes the person with a brain injury and family members, as well as professionals and brain injury specialists. Identifying realistic goals or outcomes is an important part of the planning process.

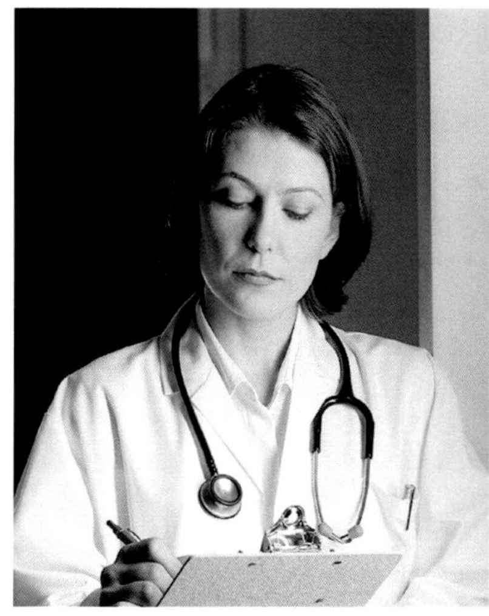

Steps to Effective Rehabilitation

Step 1	Identify important skills that an individual currently: a. can do independently, b. can do only with assistance, c. can not do.
Step 2	Help the individual develop a realistic long-term plan, including where and how to live.
Step 3	Determine what the individual needs to accomplish to achieve the plan.
Step 4	Identify long-term goals.
Step 5	Break long-term goals into specific short-term objectives.
Step 6	Design a plan for helping the individual meet the objectives.
Step 7	Evaluate progress on the basis of measurable outcome criteria.
Step 8	Based on regular reviews of outcome criteria, revise Steps 1-7, as necessary.

Outcome-Driven Rehabilitation

It is not enough to simply provide treatment and assume that the services are helpful. Treatment must be planned and provided within the framework of a systematic process. Results must be evaluated on the basis of specific outcome criteria. These outcome criteria are expressed in the form of therapeutic or life goals. They relate directly to functional improvements in the individual.

Identifying outcome criteria is a critical step. It is done not just by physicians and clinicians. It should also include the individual with a brain injury, brain injury specialists, significant family members, and funding representatives (such as a funding case manager). These people must all function as a team to identify realistic expectations. These expectations, or outcome criteria, are the basis for treatment planning.

When treatment planning is outcome-driven, the discharge site or the next setting is a primary focus for treatment planning. However, it is important not

When treatment planning is outcome-driven, the discharge site or the next setting is a primary focus for treatment planning.

to lose sight that the individual is the core element in the treatment plan. While the outcome may change, the individual is the constant element in the treatment plan.

The outcome or next environment varies among individuals. For example, primary discharge sites might be home to live with a spouse and children, and the job setting. For a teenager, discharge sites might be home to live with parents and school. For another individual, already living in the community, social and vocational integration may be key issues.

Not everyone may be able to return to independent community living and working. For example, it may be that someone with severe cognitive problems such as impaired memory, poor judgment, and impulsivity, along with high rates of aggression and property destruction, may need a structured environment with appropriate supports for the near future.

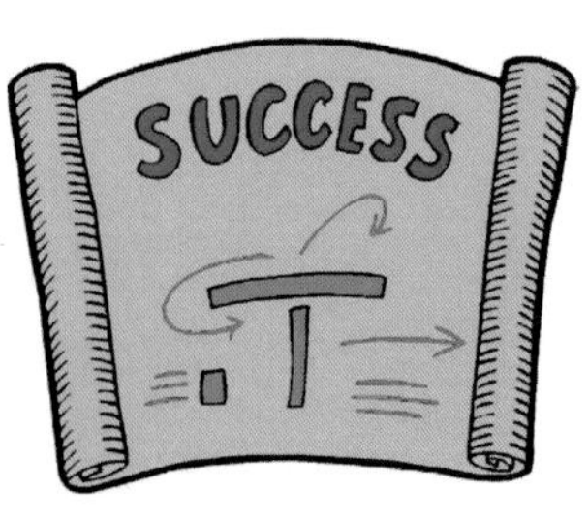

It is important to ensure that the individual's preferences are a primary driver in considering living options. The individual's choice is a fundamental element of the treatment plan.

Once a possible discharge environment is identified, the team can identify what skills are needed for the individual to live and adjust to that setting. The identified skills can be developed into treatment goals or outcomes of rehabilitation. All treatment is then directly related to the desired outcomes.

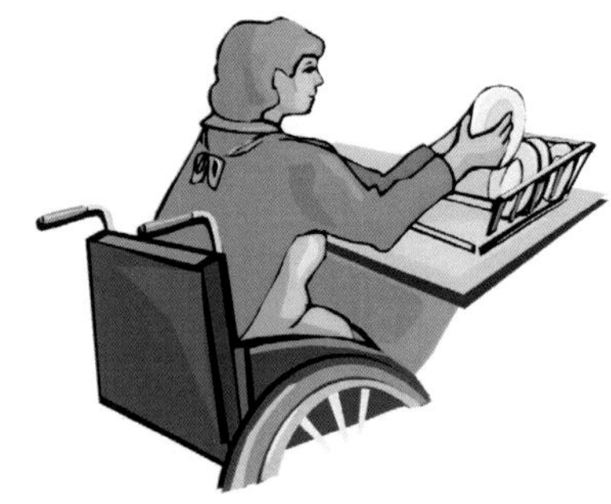

Domains of Functioning

Selecting relevant outcomes can be a complex process. Results of clinical assessment instruments are combined with the expectations and desires of the individual, family, and funder.

The process is complicated because there are many different skills related to successful long-term outcomes. Considering all the activities that go into being an independent person in society today, it would be difficult to get everyone to agree on which are most important to rehabilitation. As a result, different experts have different ways of looking at this issue.

The domains of functioning described below are presented as a guide. They are one possible way of considering outcomes:

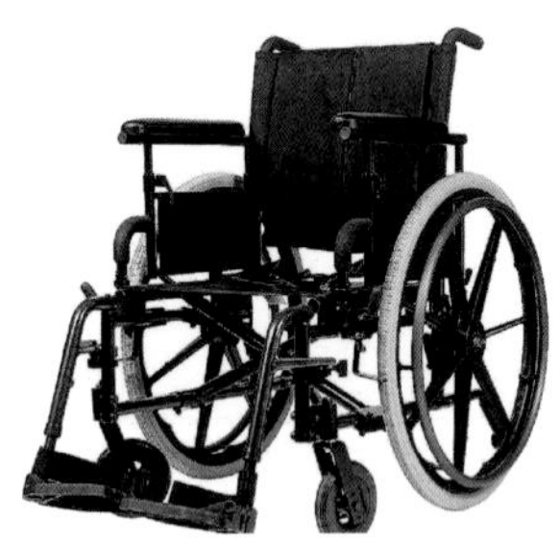

Mobility

Mobility is the ability to move about, either by walking, or with the aid of some form of assistive device such as a wheelchair, walker, or cane. A second aspect of mobility refers to the ability to transfer from one position to another. For example, transferring from a car to a wheelchair, or from standing with a walker to lying on a bed.

Cognition

Cognition refers to mental processes. This includes memory, attention, concentration, thinking, listening, judgment, decision-making, and awareness of the immediate environment including other people, places, and time.

Communication

Communication is broken down into two separate skills, receptive language, and expressive language.

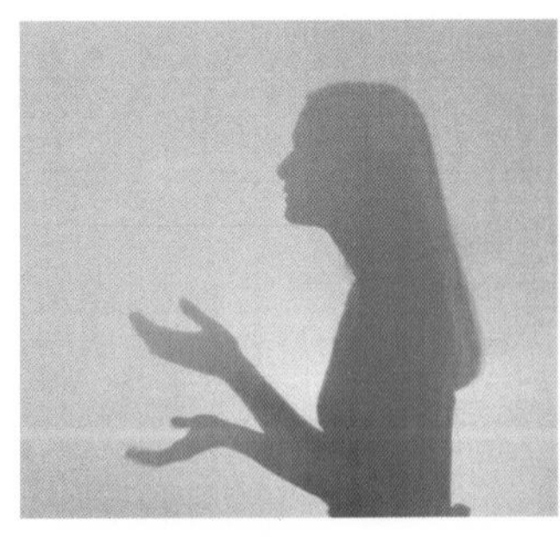

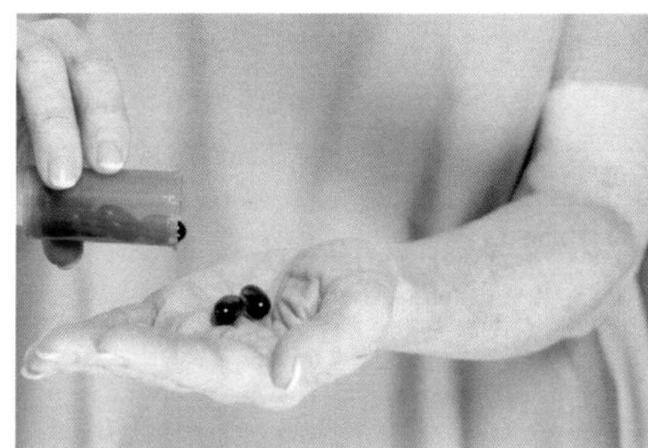

Health & Wellness

Health issues include any factor that affects a person's physical well-being. For a person with a brain injury, health issues may include a seizure disorder, respiratory problems, feeding difficulty, or bone or muscular complications. This domain also includes the ability to care for health and medical needs, such as first-aid, or taking medication.

Self Help Skills

Self-help skills include bathing, dressing, eating, grooming, and toileting. These are often referred to as activities of daily living (ADLs). They are central to reaching a basic level of independence.

Household Management

Household management includes meal preparation, housekeeping, money management, and other activities related to managing where one lives.

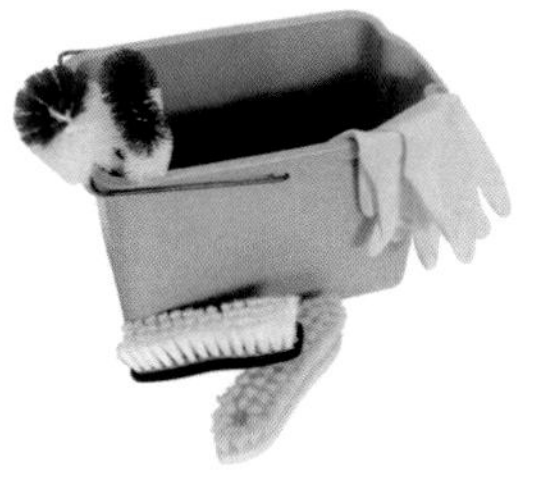

Community Skills

Community skills are what enable someone to live and function safely in the community. They include getting around, using public transportation, shopping, eating in restaurants, participating in recreational activities such as movies, concerts, or sporting events.

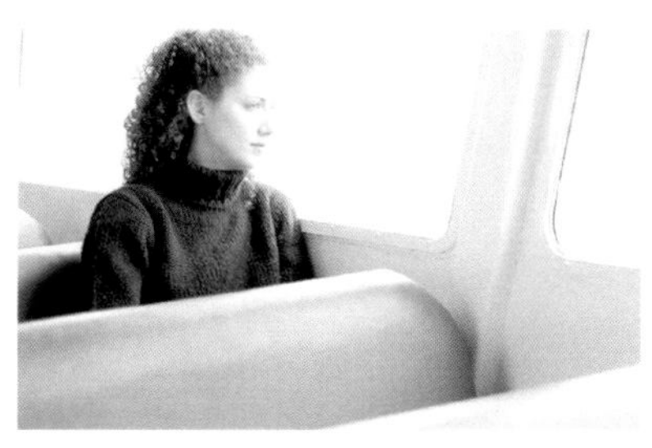

Leisure Skills

Leisure skills relate to the ability to use free time in ways that are not harmful (i.e., substance abuse, or other dangerous activities). In addition to the recreational activities listed under community skills, this category includes reading, television, music, and other activities done at home.

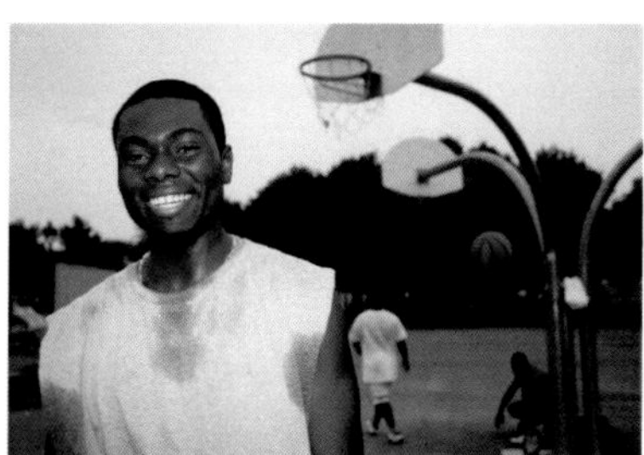

Vocational Skills

Vocational skills refer to behaviors needed to get and keep a job. This domain includes everything from simple on-task behavior in a structured workshop setting to higher-level cognitive functions in competitive employment.

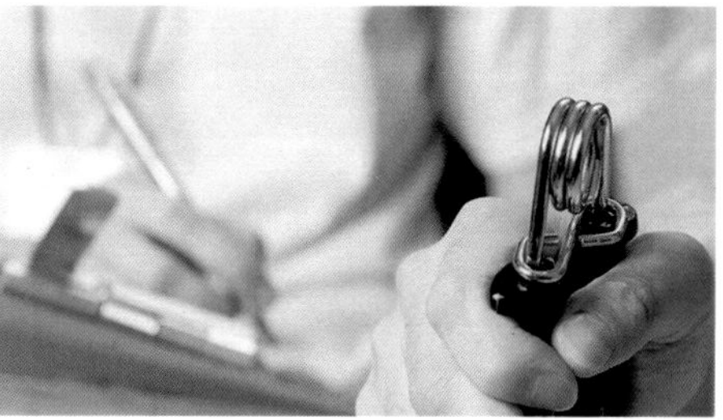

Assessment

Professionals from many disciplines are involved in the treatment of persons with brain injury. They include behavior analysts, cognitive therapists, neurologists, neuro-psychologists, nurses, occupational therapists, physiatrists, physical therapists, psychiatrists, psychologists, rehabilitation counselors, social workers, speech pathologists, vocational specialists, and others.

Each professional assesses an individual's performance in the domains of functioning. The primary focus of assessment is to identify precisely how an individual's strengths and weaknesses relate to the expected discharge environment. In most cases, professionals evaluate a person with a brain injury by using standard assessment strategies specific to their disciplines. Each discipline has specific assessment instruments.

Outcome Measures

Once the assessment is done, the next step is to identify exactly what skills are needed for each desired outcome. In general, each outcome will have one or more goals. Each goal has one or more behavioral objectives. They describe a logical path to reach the goal.

This process is illustrated below, first with the mobility domain, and then with community skills and mobility. As illustrated, outcomes progress to goals and then to objectives. Outcomes describe what performance is expected for success in the discharge site. Goals break the general outcome criterion down into more specific activities. Objectives further break down the goals into observable and measurable performance criteria that are taught in order.

Objectives must be written with a clear way to evaluate performance.

Outcome Measure Example

Outcome 1 Independent mobility in home with a walker.

Goal 1 Rhonda will ambulate safely in her apartment.

Objective 1: With stand-by assistance, Rhonda will ambulate from her bedroom to the kitchen within 5 minutes, with no more than two instances of losing her balance, for 10 consecutive days.

Objective 2: Rhonda will independently ambulate from her bedroom to the kitchen within 5 minutes, with no loss of balance, for 10 consecutive days.

Goal 2 Rhonda will engage in safe transfers in her apartment.

Objective 1: With hands-on assistance, Rhonda will successfully transfer from standing with walker, to a dining room chair within 30 seconds, for 10 consecutive days.

Objective 2: Rhonda will independently transfer from a standing position to a dining room chair within 30 seconds, for 10 consecutive days.

Outcome 2 Independent mobility in the community.

Goal 1 Rhonda will independently access public transportation.

Objective 1: With the assistance of a bus schedule, Rhonda will indicate the location and time of the bus she needs to catch to go to the mall, at 100% accuracy, for five consecutive days.

Objective 2: With the assistance of a bus schedule, Rhonda will indicate the location and time of the bus she needs to catch to return from the mall, at 100% accuracy, for five consecutive days.

Objective 3: Rhonda will independently negotiate the entrance to the bus with her walker, and sit down on the bus, within one minute of the bus stopping, for five consecutive days.

Goal 2 Rhonda will independently complete a shopping trip to the mall.

Objective 1: Rhonda will ambulate to the store of her choice within 15 minutes of arriving at the mall, with 90% accuracy, for five consecutive trips.

Objective 2: Rhonda will select an item from her shopping list within 20 minutes of entering the store, for five consecutive days.

Objective 3. Rhonda will accurately complete a purchase transaction, offering the correct dollar amount, and checking her change, with 100% accuracy, for five consecutive days.

Ideally, objectives are written with no ambiguity about whether the individual has achieved the goal. The objective must describe the behavior in terms that are observable and measurable.

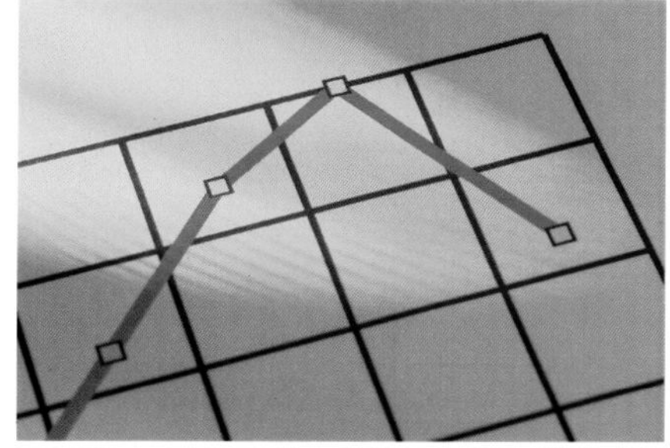

Evaluation of Outcomes

Evaluation of treatment effects is a critical aspect of outcome-driven rehabilitation. It is important to thoroughly evaluate whether treatment plans are preparing the person for the planned discharge environment.

There are many ways to collect outcome data on objectives, goals, and outcome criteria. Each method relies on counting or measuring some aspect of an individual's behavior. The brief overview below describes various dimensions of performance that are commonly assessed.

ABC Data

A-B-C data provide information on events in the environment. These correlate with under what conditions a behavior occurs. Knowing what factors contribute to a behavior's occurrence is critical for understanding and treating behaviors. Collecting data, not only on the behavior, but also what immediately precedes and follows the behavior is one method. This is accomplished with A-B-C data. "A" stands for antecedents to the behavior. "B" is for the behavior. "C" is for consequences to the behavior. Behavior change may then result from changing the antecedents or the consequences.

It is possible to analyze factors contributing to behaviors by analyzing data this way. In the example, both antecedents and consequences to targeted behaviors were preceded by increased expectations (laundry and meal preparation).

In both situations, the consequence to the target behavior was escaping the demanding situation. In particular, focusing on antecedents for persons with brain injury is critical. For example, a person with severe cognitive problems may become agitated when asked, "What do you want for dinner?" The person might respond

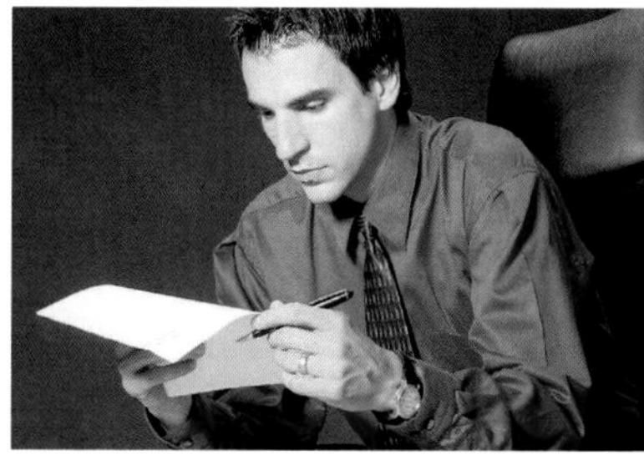

"yes" or "no" when asked if he would like "chicken." By focusing on the antecedents, one might be able to prevent an unwanted behavior from happening in the first place.

Frequency

Frequency is the number of times that a skill or behavior is observed to occur.

Examples are counting the number of independent social initiations, aggressions, or just about any other behavior of interest.

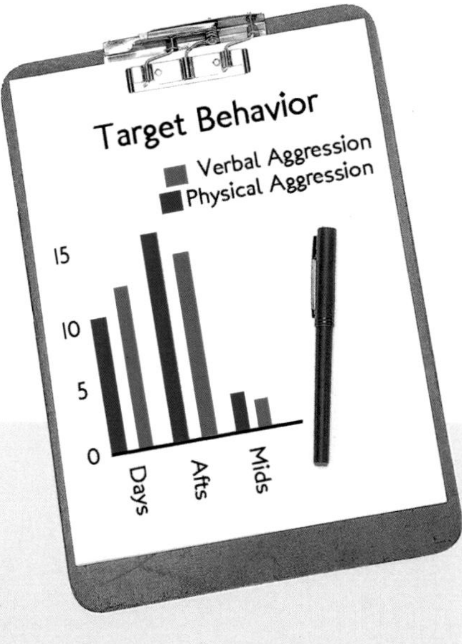

ABC Data Example

Date	Time	Antecedent	Behavior	Consequence
12/8	3:15p	Laundry task	Yelling, cursing	Sat on porch with staff
12/8	9:00p	TV time	Aggression to peer	Watched TV show of choice
12/9	9:20a	Meal prep	Throwing food	Went to bedroom until staff prepared meal

Rate

Rate is the number of times a behavior occurs in a specified time period.

Examples are the number of times per hour that independent ambulation occurs, or the number of cursing episodes per hour.

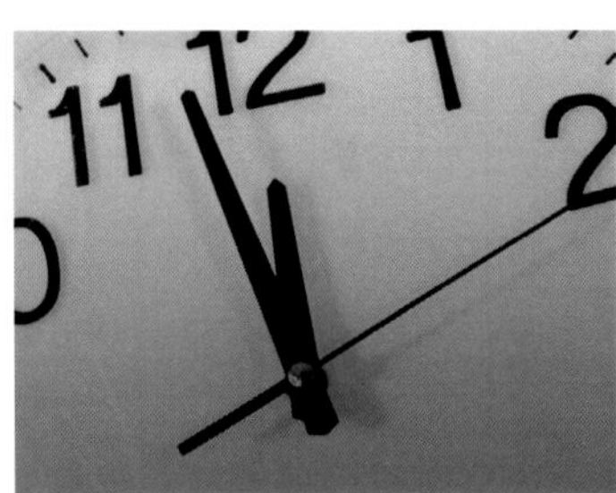

Duration

Duration is the length of time that a behavior occurs.

Examples are the length of time that a person walks without assistance, or the time someone continuously works at a task.

Latency

Latency is the length of time that it takes a person to initiate (or complete) a behavior.

Examples are measuring how long it takes a person to initiate a social interaction following a cue or measuring how long it takes to complete a transfer from wheelchair to car.

Magnitude

Magnitude or intensity is especially important for unwanted behaviors, such as aggression or self-injury. This measure is seldom used because it is difficult to objectively measure the intensity of an aggressive or self-injurious response.

An example is determining if an injury required on-site first aid or required an emergency room visit.

Percent of Opportunities

Percent of opportunities is a useful measure for knowing whether or not a behavior occurred when the opportunity was available. It makes little sense to record frequency, rate, or duration data on whether someone correctly dresses appropriately for the job site, arrives on time to scheduled appointments, or completes a grocery store purchase. These skills are best measured by recording the percentage of times that a behavior was performed correctly.

For example, when assessing punctuality, staff might keep track of the percentages of days in a month that the person arrived to work or appointments on time.

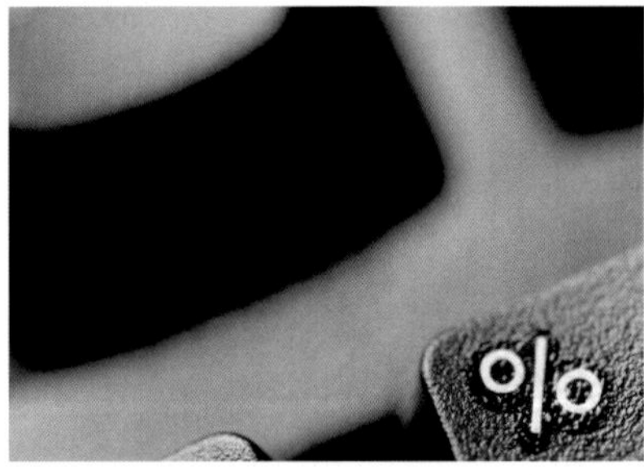

Differences between Rate and Duration

While rate may seem very similar to frequency, there is one critical difference. When frequency data are collected, the basic level of data typically is the daily total of a behavior's occurrence. However, the occurrence of observed behavior may vary dramatically from day to day if an individual is not in a setting for the same amount of time every day. The example below illustrates this problem.

Vocational staff reported 8 episodes of aggression for an individual on Monday. The person was in the vocational area all day. Tuesday, the daily total of aggression reported was 4. When data are analyzed at the monthly rehabilitation meeting, the fact that the individual spent the majority of Tuesday on an outing with family does not show up.

Using a rate measure shows that aggression occurred 8 times in 8 hours on Monday for a rate of 1 per hour. Because the individual was only in the vocational area for 2 hours on Tuesday, the rate for that day was 2 per hour.

Relying on frequency of behavior leads to the erroneous conclusion that the person was less aggressive in the vocational setting on Tuesday. Rate can be a better method of reporting outcome data.

Treatment Components

Each person in rehabilitation must be approached as an individual with unique backgrounds and current abilities and disabilities. The most effective treatment planning is tailored to the specific needs of the individual. The plan is developed based on the expected discharge site, the expectations of the individual and family, and knowledge about methods for changing behaviors to improve performance.

Steps to Treatment Planning

Treatment planning can vary dramatically from one setting to another. It may also vary on the basis of an individual's needs. However, effective treatment planning should generally include these components:

Assess Neuropsychological Factors

Because cognitive deficits may affect behavior, it is usually helpful to have a comprehensive neuropsychological assessment. This evaluation pinpoints specific strengths and weaknesses in areas such as attention, concentration, memory, language, spatial reasoning, general intelligence, abstract reasoning, conceptual thinking, judgment, and problem-solving, as well as sensory and motor skills. It also includes an analysis of a person's pre-injury personality, psychiatric disorders, and current patterns of emotional behavior.

Collect Baseline Data

Collecting outcome measures establishes at what frequency (or rate, duration, intensity or percentage of opportunities) the behavior occurs prior to treatment. This is important to evaluate treatment effects.

Assess Environmental Influences

As described earlier, a simple method for identifying environmental factors is to collect A-B-C data on the unwanted behavior. Whether the team collects A-B-C data, or merely draws conclusions about environmental factors, this is a critical step in understanding both adaptive and unwanted behaviors.

Identify Positive Reinforcers

Understanding what is rewarding to a person is an important step for effective rehabilitation. Some individuals seem self-motivated to work as hard as possible during rehabilitation. They never seem to need even a word of encouragement.

Unfortunately, this is not the case with many people. Brain injury rehabilitation can be a long, difficult, challenging, and sometimes painful process. Many people find aspects of rehabilitation confusing and frustrating. It sometimes seems as if the failures outnumber the successes. As a result, some individuals need help to be motivated to put up with the rigors of rehabilitation.

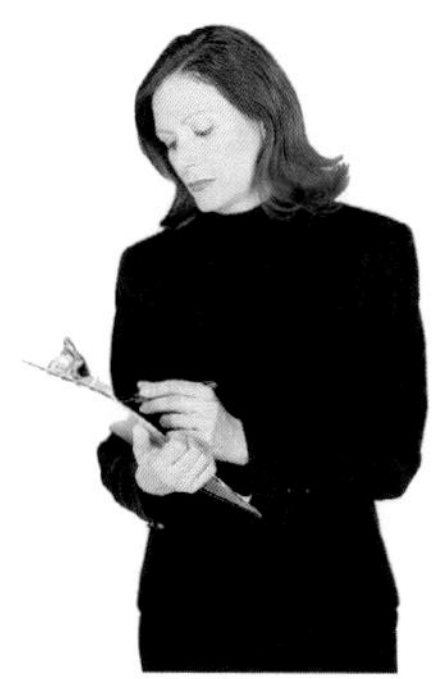

Identifying positive reinforcers is a critical step in motivating active participation in rehabilitation. It can be used to support positive behavior. This is such a critical step because everyone puts their own value on potential reinforcers. If 10 people from different walks of life listed the top 10 things they would do if they won the lottery, everybody's list would be different. The same principle applies to people in rehabilitation. Each person is an individual, whose unique value systems must be considered during treatment planning.

There are three basic methods for identifying positive reinforcers for individuals in rehabilitation:

1. The simplest method is to ask a person what kinds of things and activities are rewarding. In many cases, a person is willing to work for special time with a preferred staff member, sleeping an extra 30 minutes in the morning, having a way to track their accomplishments, or many other reinforcing activities.

Steps to Treatment Planning

1. Assess Neuropsychological Factors
2. Collect Baseline Data
3. Assess Environmental Influences
4. Identify Positive Reinforcers

The following list of potential reinforcers is a guide. Remember, everyone is different, and what works with one person may not work with another.

- Praise.
- Attention.
- Outings.
- Praise.
- Time with preferred staff.
- Favorite television shows.
- Buying new CDs.
- Snacks.
- Praise.
- Increased independence.
- Eye contact.
- A pat on the back.
- Smiles.
- Concerts.
- Sporting events.
- Praise.
- Trips to the mall.
- Being given choices.
- Being in charge of a particular situation.
- Praise.

2. If an individual is not able to provide meaningful information, family members may have insights or suggestions to identify effective reinforcers.

3. When no one can identify potential reinforcers, watch how a person spends free time or what makes them smile. With most people, highly preferred activities can be used as reinforcers for less preferred activities.

For example, wearing a Sony Walkman might be contingent on punctual attendance at all scheduled sessions. This principle is the Premack Principle, named after the man who first documented its effects.

Treatment plan

Generally, it is good practice to include the following sections in a treatment plan:

- Describe the desired behaviors, e.g. unassisted ambulation, that are related to outcomes in the same operational terms used in data collection.

This ensures that the individual and everyone working with the individual are clear on exactly what the target behaviors are.

- Identify the antecedent situations in which the behaviors occur or do not occur.

This is important for two reasons. In some cases, the actual treatment will consist entirely of rearranging the antecedent conditions that precede a behavior, e.g. a cue card in the bathroom listing the sequence of showering steps. The second reason is that identifying antecedent factors provides information about why a behavior occurs or does not occur, e.g. when the cue card is not in the bathroom, the person may not know the first step to initiating the shower routine.

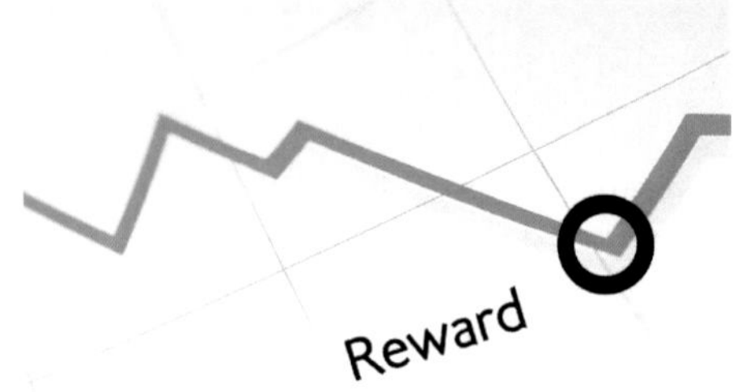

- Be absolutely clear on whether the plan involves staff providing consequences following the behavior. For example, a personal assistant may verbally praise use of the checklist.

All staff must be very clear, not only on what the target behavior is, but exactly what they are to do when the behavior occurs. The less clear this is, the more likely staff will do things differently. This sends mixed messages.

Treatment Evaluation

It is always important to evaluate the effectiveness of a treatment plan. This is done by comparing performance prior to the start of treatment (baseline data). Baseline data give a point of comparison. They make it possible to see whether treatment is having positive effects, negative effects, or no effect.

It is especially important to evaluate the effects of psychotropic and other medications. Many neuroleptic medications have potential harmful side effects. The specific behaviors that medication was prescribed for should be continually monitored to establish an ongoing need (e.g. seizures, blood pressure, aggression, depression). By doing this, medications can be reduced to the lowest necessary level and totally eliminated in some cases.

Revision

A treatment plan may need to be revised based upon the data collected if a person is not reaching their goals. This step may involve more frequent reinforcement, clearer cueing procedures, a reassessment of the potential antecedents, or lowered response expectations.

No treatment plan should ever be considered static. Even a very good plan that is working well should evolve over time to focus more attention on desirable behaviors that are replacing undesirable behaviors.

Treatment Methods

The following are demonstrated effective treatment strategies whether teaching an individual to self-feed, walk, use memory strategies, or to self-manage unwanted behaviors.

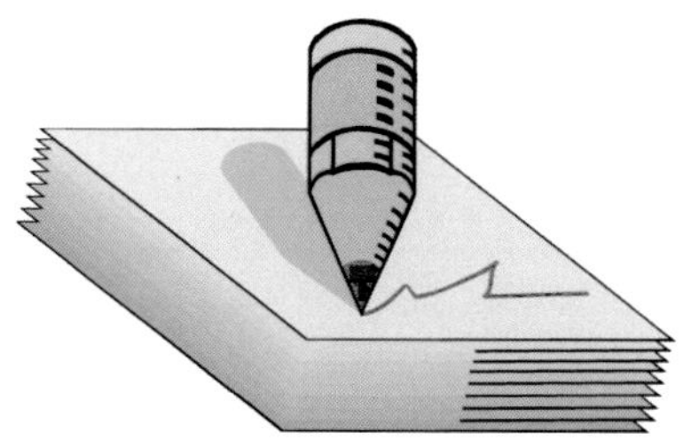

Task Analysis

Many of the skills taught to persons with brain injury involve sequences of smaller chunks of behavior. In conducting a task analysis , the overall skill is analyzed into components that can be taught and measured.

For example, brushing teeth involves getting a toothbrush, wetting it, applying toothpaste, moving the brush around the teeth, rinsing the mouth, rinsing the toothbrush, and putting away the toothbrush and toothpaste. It is much easier to help someone relearn tooth brushing by teaching one step at a time instead of trying to teach the entire sequence at once.

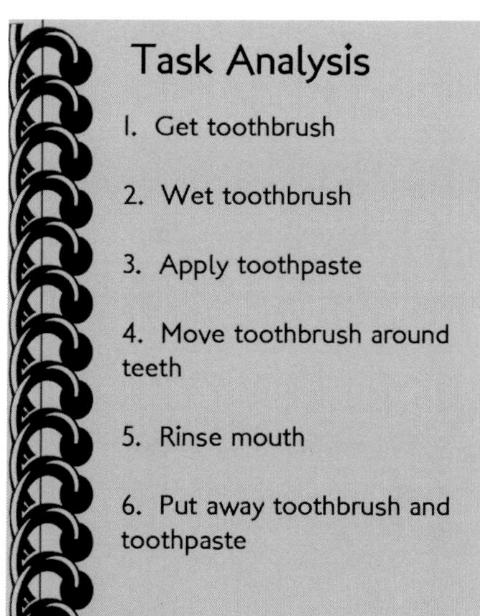

Task Analysis

1. Get toothbrush
2. Wet toothbrush
3. Apply toothpaste
4. Move toothbrush around teeth
5. Rinse mouth
6. Put away toothbrush and toothpaste

Just about any skill can be task analyzed into meaningful, teachable components. The process can be applied to skills in each of the domains discussed earlier. In fact, the process for breaking outcomes into goals, which are then broken down into objectives, is actually a form of task analysis. Once functional objectives are developed, behaviors that may have seemed complex and difficult to teach have been task analyzed into smaller teachable units.

Shaping

It is unrealistic to expect everyone to fully develop the target skill all at once. In shaping, reinforcement is provided only when a person gets progressively closer to the ultimate target behavior.

For example, a person with cognitive and neuro-muscular problems might find it hard to correctly make the bed. The sustained physical effort might be too much. This could be complicated by an inability to correctly sequence the steps involved in bed making.

Shaping relies on steps identified in a tasks analysis and only gradually requires more complete bed making. In the beginning, it might be enough that the person only pulls the sheets haphazardly across the bed. Although this is far from successful bed making, it is the first successful step that is reinforced. Over time, other aspects of bed making can then be added sequentially, while refining overall attention to detail. This example shows that it is possible to teach a skill through shaping that the person might otherwise not be capable of learning.

Fading

A person's current skills may not enable them to respond to environmental cues as effectively as before the brain injury. Fading uses a gradual change from artificial to more natural cueing stimuli.

For example, someone relearning how to set the table might not respond correctly to the natural cues of a place mat on the table, and plates and tableware in the adjoining kitchen. The person may have no idea of where to put the various items in relation to each other. In a fading procedure, a place mat is used with outlines of the plate, knife, spoon, fork, and glass clearly marked. If this cueing produces the desired effect, the artificial cues are slowly faded away over time. As the outlines on the place mat become progressively fainter, the person's behavior gradually comes under the control of the natural cues that control table setting.

Incidental Teaching

Many of the interactions between staff and individuals with brain injuries occur outside the structured program. This is particularly so in residential programs or when one spends a lot of time with the person, such as family.

For example, a structured therapeutic context is a session with an OT, working on cooking skills. The brain injury specialist or family later works with the person to incorporate the OT's recommendations into the residential environment.

Even though the OT has developed a prescriptive program for cooking, there will still be incidents that are not explicitly covered in the OT program. When unprogrammed situations arise, they present opportunities for teaching and sometimes provide the best opportunity to teach carryover or generalization of skills to other settings or other persons.

For example, a person accidentally burns the toast while making breakfast. This is not mentioned in the OT protocol. The staff member has several options at this point:

1. *Ignore the problem, and let the person eat the burned toast.*

2. *Demonstrate displeasure at the person's mistakes.*

3. *Take over the situation, and quickly make new toast so the person can eat the breakfast.*

4. *Turn the situation into a learning opportunity by helping the person troubleshoot why the toast was burned and what could be done to prevent it from happening again.*

As the primary support person, it is important that the brain injury specialist choose the fourth option. Although this is the obvious answer in this example, many staff unknowingly choose one of the first three options. Similar scenarios occur dozens of times a day with many important skills, from social interactions, to self-care, to anger control, to any other situation related to a person's rehabilitation. As an exercise, try to identify an opportunity for incidental teaching for each domain of functioning.

Decreasing Unwanted Behavior

Aggression toward others, self-injury, property destruction, tantrums, yelling, cursing, and failure to respond to requests are unwanted and counterproductive behaviors. Unwanted behaviors can seriously concern families, friends, teachers, co-workers, and others. At the very least, these behaviors are annoying and troubling. At worst, such behaviors cause serious injury or property damage. Perhaps most important, such behaviors may interfere with a person achieving rehabilitation goals and are an obstacle to community reintegration.

Fading Example

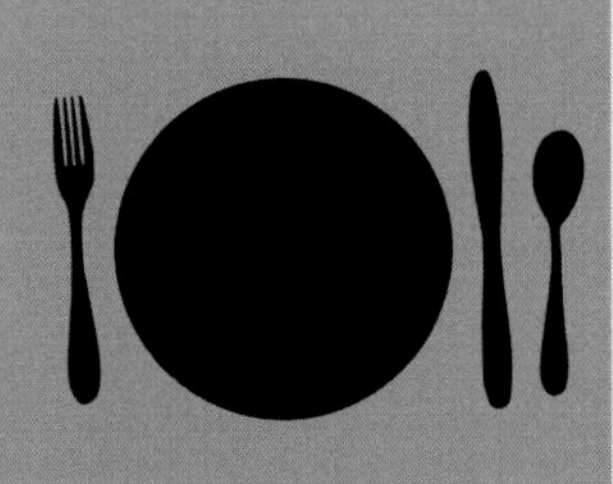

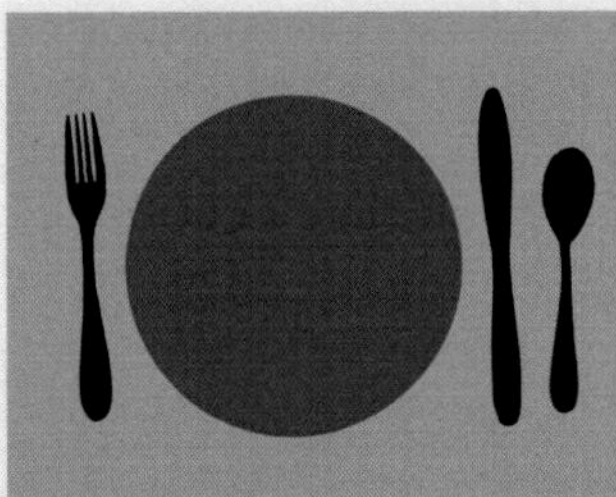

As the individual learns to place the plate in the correct location, the artificial cue (the plate outline), becomes more and more faded. This continues until the individual no longer requires the artificial cue to correctly place the plate.

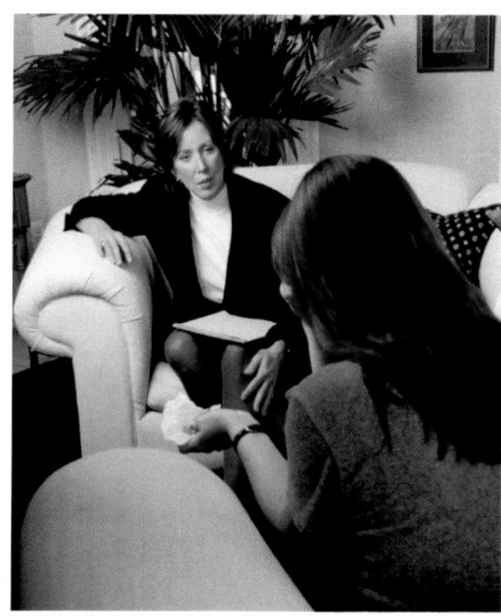

Role of the Brain Injury Specialist in Treatment Planning

The brain injury specialist plays a critical role in evaluating therapeutic effects, implementing treatment plans, interacting with professionals outside the facility such as physicians, meeting with family members, and many other aspects of rehabilitation. In many ways, brain injury specialists are the most important part of the treatment team because they spend so much more time with individuals than do other members of the team.

In addition, brain injury specialists spend time with individuals under the more natural conditions than other team members. In some cases, physicians, psychologists, or any other professional team members may see an individual who is interested in impressing the professional. Seldom does this effort to be on one's best behavior extend into the many hours in the living (or vocational) environment. Brain injury specialists are more likely to see individuals' daily difficulties and frustrations as they undergo rehabilitation.

General Guidelines for Treatment Planning

Person-Centered

Include the individual as much as possible, in the development and design of the treatment plan. Discuss the treatment plan with the individual, in terms of expected discharge site, outcome criteria, goals, objectives, and treatment methods. Involving the individual usually increases the chances for a positive outcome. It is also appropriate from an ethical point of view.

Supportive

Design a plan that makes it very likely the individual will succeed, especially in the early stages. This is done by using shaping procedures.

For example, a person who is anxious about ambulating in the community may feel more comfortable ambulating to a preferred site (mall, clothes store, movie theater) than some site chosen at random. Once a certain comfort level is established, additional sites can be added with input from the individual.

Simplicity

Make the plan easy for staff and the individual to understand. Complicated plans that try to do too much at once can be confusing. They make it less likely the individual will comply with requests.

Consistency

Implement the plan consistently. Everyone who implements the plan, whether residential staff, vocational specialist, occupational therapist, or whoever, must have the same expectations and be consistent when interacting with the individual. Anyone who implements a plan must do it the same way every time. Abrupt changes in a plan send mixed messages. This can reinforce inappropriate behavior.

Flexibility

Make the plan flexible enough to adapt to changes in the individual. Although spur-of-the moment changes are not good, there is nothing wrong with thoughtful changes on the basis of progress or lack of progress.

Avoid making changes while the activity or interaction is occurring. For example, don't critique social skills and suggest changes while the person is in the midst of a conversation or discussion. Talk about changes before the next interaction.

Positive

Only discuss the person's successes when the person is nearby. It's very helpful if a person overhears others talking about something positive, no matter how minor. Conversely, overhearing people discuss some shortcoming, or behavioral outburst can have very negative effects.

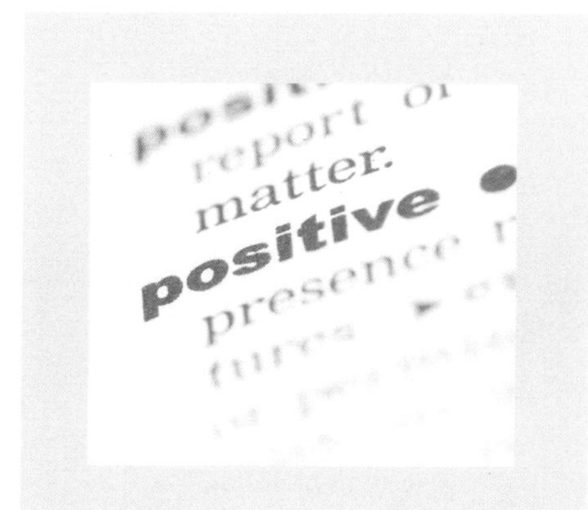

Treat Everyone with Dignity and Respect

Treat individuals in rehabilitation with dignity and respect. Although this may seem obvious, it does not always happen. Staff sometimes start to look down on persons they are treating. Being a specialist in brain injury does not make any staff better than the person in rehabilitation who is a "client."

Demonstrate an honest interest in individuals. For example, comment on some topic of interest to the individual. The most effective staff are those who treat people as unique individuals with dignity and respect.

Don't Talk Down to People

Persons in rehabilitation are people like you and I, autonomous individuals prior to the brain injury. The person may have had an active dating life, a family, career aspirations, and a network of friends. The person was living a life not much different than that of a staff member.

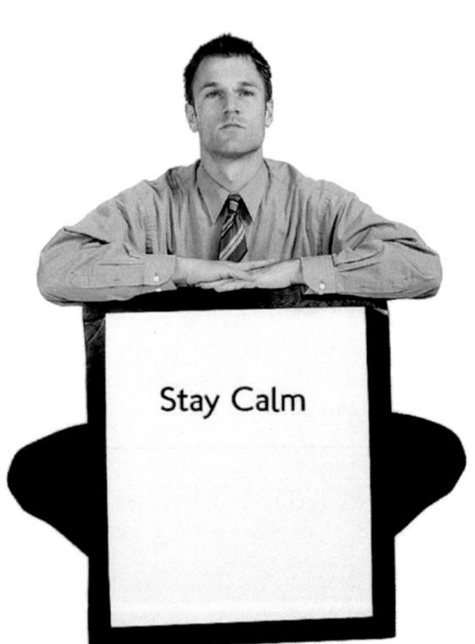

Most individuals recall their former lives quite clearly. It is critical to keep this in mind and show the same respect that would be offered to friends or fellow employees.

Stay Calm

Staff who are most effective working with individuals with brain injury stay calm in the midst of crisis situations. When an individual is confused, frustrated, depressed, or even actively agitated, the last thing needed is a staff member who exacerbates the situation by failing to stay calm.

Don't Take Things Personally

There is never a good reason to take it personally when things don't go as planned. It is human nature to be personally offended when assaulted, or verbally attacked or ethnically slurred. Don't reveal personal reactions to such actions to the individual.

Unwanted behavior occurs for very specific reasons. The individual may not have control over them so there is no reason to take things personally. If someone hits or insults a staff person, it is because of premorbid history, brain injury, environmental influences, or a combination. The unwanted behavior occurred for reasons, none of which have anything to do with a staff member personally.

Staff sometimes take things personally when a person fails to achieve some outcome. In most cases, the fault lies with the team's assessment or treatment plan, not the individual. Whether a person in rehabilitation is motivated and prepared to achieve outcomes is determined by the ability of the team to provide effective programming.

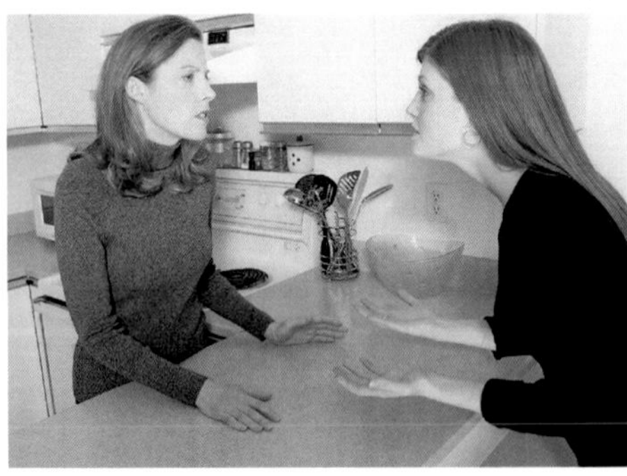

Avoid Arguments

Little good comes from arguments. Even if the staff member is right, it is often impossible to "win" the argument in light of the individual's cognitive deficits in reasoning, judgment or impulsive decision making. It is better to avoid arguments completely by declining to discuss an issue and redirecting the person to another topic.

Maintain a Sense of Humor

Interacting with individuals humorously is part of treating them with respect. It sends a message that a staff is comfortable with a person as an individual, and not just as a client or patient. In many cases, a little humor is an antecedent to more relaxed, comfortable and effective performance by the individual.

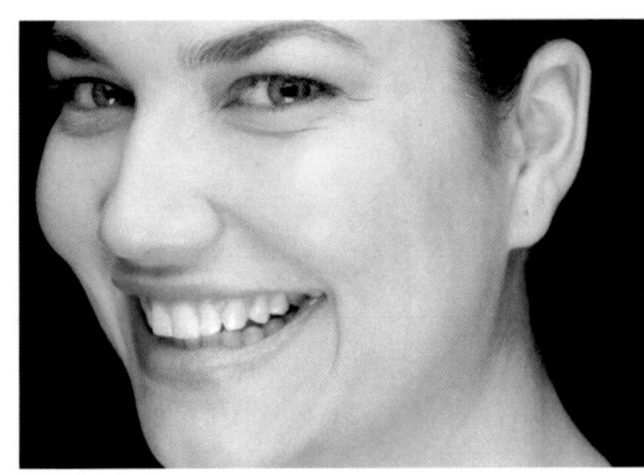

Understanding Behavior

Measurability and objectivity are essential for understanding behavior so consistent observations can be made. It is important that the reader understand that "behavior" is everything and anything we do. Treatment planning for unwanted behaviors is discussed in a separate section in this chapter.

Human behavior is very complex. What we do, why we do it, and how we do it have been the subject of scientific study for centuries.

The factors that influence all people's behavior are the same factors that influence the behavior, both good and bad, of persons with brain injury or another disability. This important point is overlooked sometimes by specialists in brain injury rehabilitation.

Human Behavior & Brain Injury

Human behavior is very complex.

All behavior is lawful and occurs for specific reasons.

Behavior is controlled by the human nervous system and the environment.

Behavioral excesses (e.g., aggression) and weaknesses (e.g., lack of initiation) are not the fault of the person with a brain injury.

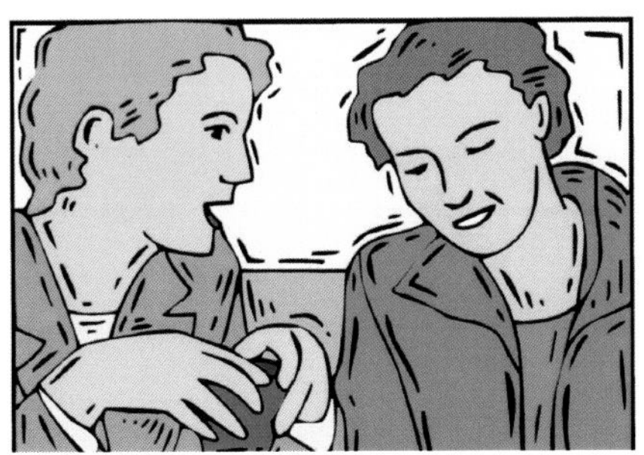

Regardless of an individual's disabilities, it is important to remember two facts when planning and implementing treatment.

The first is that every person with a brain injury is an individual.

Each one of us, whether or not we have experienced a brain injury, behaves the way we do because of how our brain functions and our unique life experiences. It is important to approach each person in rehabilitation as an individual. Do not assume that what works with one person will automatically work with another.

The second fact is that all behavior is lawful and occurs for specific reasons. Behavior is controlled by the human nervous system and the environment.

When brain functioning is altered by an injury, behavior can change. Unfortunately, some changes to the brain and the environment decrease adaptive behaviors and/or strengthen unwanted behaviors. As highlighted in Chapter 2, both behavioral excesses (e.g., aggression) and weaknesses (e.g., lack of initiation) are not the fault of the person with a brain injury.

Altered behavior occurs as a result of brain injury and environmental influences.

Neurologic Influences

The brain controls a person's thought processes and all bodily functions. In short, it controls behavior. When the brain is injured, the ability to perform certain tasks can be affected as can the ability to control unwanted behaviors.

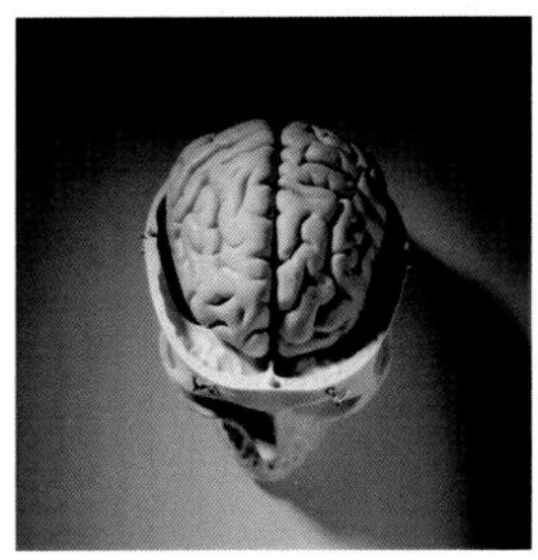

Environmental Influences

The environment consists of everyone a person has contact with and everything that happens to an individual. It also includes a person's history with the environment and what is learned from that history. The environment's responses to behaviors greatly affects how a person acts. There are four primary ways that the environment affects behavior.

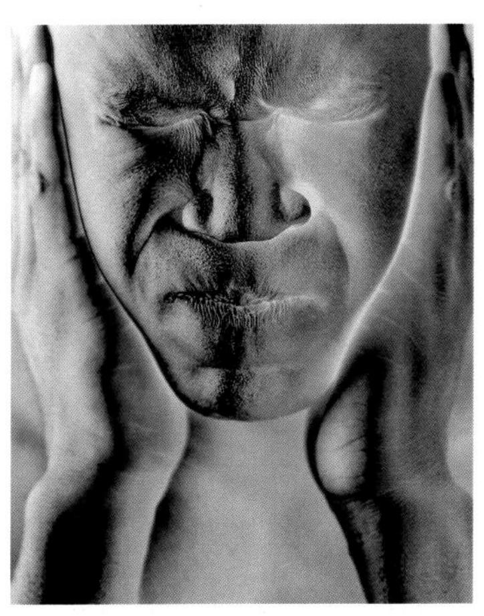

Likelihood of Behaviors Increasing

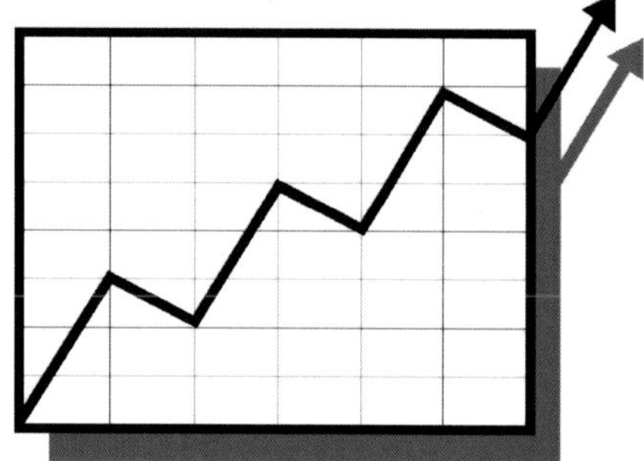

Likelihood of Behaviors Decreasing

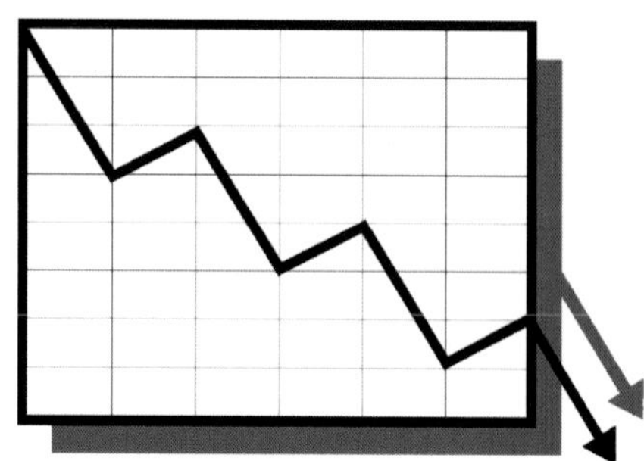

Rewards

When good things happen after a behavior, that behavior is more likely to be repeated in the future. The behavior has been strengthened or reinforced.

For example, if people always laugh when a person tells a particular joke, chances are that the joke will be repeated to others. But if the same behavior of telling a joke prompted frowns or criticism, most likely the person would stop telling that particular joke.

The same principle applies to all behavior. Things that are followed by something enjoyable (rewards) are more likely to occur than actions followed by non-enjoyable things. This is positive reinforcement.

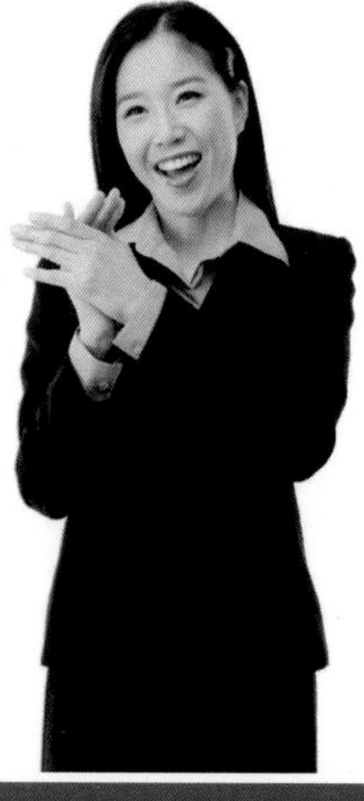

Escape and Avoidance

When behavior gets someone out of an unpleasant situation, or removes the threat of one, that behavior may be strengthened. It is more likely to occur again in the future.

For example, a person is at a store with a young child who asks for candy. The child is told that she can't have candy because it's almost time for dinner. She begins to cry and scream. This causes everyone in the store to look at the adult who is with her. This is very uncomfortable for the adult, who gives in, and buys the candy. The crying and screaming stops and everyone stops looking.

The adult's behavior of buying the candy to <u>escape</u> from the crying and unwanted attention has just been strengthened. The adult's action was negatively reinforced by removal of the unpleasant situation. As with positive reinforcement, negative reinforcement strengthens many behaviors that allow someone to escape or avoid unpleasant situations.

Punishment

When behavior leads to a negative consequence (punishment), it is less likely to happen again.

For example, most people decrease their driving speed after receiving a traffic ticket, or they stop being late to work after being reprimanded.

Extinction

When a behavior that has been previously reinforced is now <u>not</u> followed by a positive reinforcer, the behavior is weakened.

For example, the family has been responding to John's requests when he shouts to them from his bedroom. It is likely that if they did not respond, the future of this shouting would decrease. In this example, it is also important to reinforce an alternative such as coming out of his bedroom to make a request in a normal tone of voice. It is also important to note that often with extinction, the behavior usually goes up, before it goes down or decreases.

In these four ways, environment affects the development and maintenance of

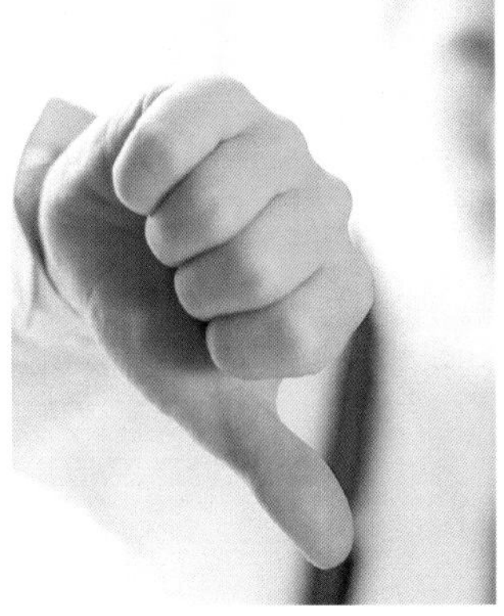

behaviors -- those that are acceptable as well as unwanted. People are sometimes skeptical about how much of their behavior is controlled by the environment. They object that relying on positive and negative reinforcement and punishment is overly simplistic.

In most cases, people - brain injury specialists, as well as persons with brain injury - are unaware of the many influences on their behavior.

There are thousands of examples of dramatically altered behavior without the person's knowledge. This is important to remember when working with individuals with brain injury, whether the intent is to increase adaptive skills or decrease unwanted behaviors. An individual usually is unaware of the factors influencing adaptive or unwanted behaviors.

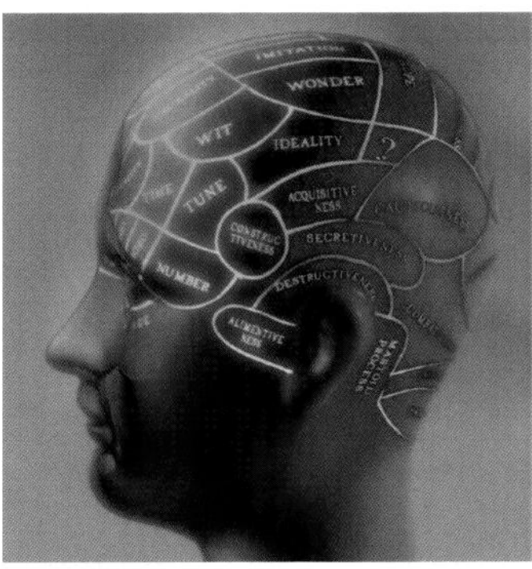

Example of the Influence of the Environment on Behavior

A college professor had just taught students about the power of positive reinforcement. He urged the class to use positive reinforcement and report on it. Several members decided to conduct an experiment using the professor as the subject. They convinced all the students to use a positive reinforcement procedure when the professor was lecturing.

The professor walked back and forth at the front of the room during the entire class. When he was on the left side of the room, all the students looked interested, wrote down notes, and asked questions. When he was on the right side of the room, the students yawned, looked out the window, and generally looked disinterested. After a couple of classes, the professor (who knew nothing about the experiment) was spending the entire class period on the left side of the room.

The students' attention was a powerful positive reinforcer and had a dramatic effect on the professor's behavior. He did not even realize that he was spending the entire class on the left side of the room.

General Behavioral Principles

Behavior will Increase	Behavior will Decrease
Reward	**Extinction**
Escape & Avoidance	**Punishment**

Understanding Unwanted Behavior

There are no simple universal solutions to treating unwanted behavior problems. Every person with behavior problems is an individual whose situation is unique. Still, certain approaches to treatment have proven effective. They should be included in most treatment approaches.

> *The general, but most effective, approach understands unwanted behavior is the product of brain dysfunction and environmental influences.*

As discussed in the section on understanding behavior, everything a person does occurs as a result of interactions between the brain and the environment. Chapter 3 described some ways that specific brain injuries can lead to unwanted behavior. Environmental factors discussed earlier in this chapter also play a key role in the development and maintenance of unwanted behavior.

Neurologic Influences

At the most basic level, damage to the brain can directly lead to changes in behavior. Damage to the limbic system, or temporal lobes, is often associated with aggression and other emotional responses. Damage to the frontal lobe can also result in inappropriate and emotional responses, as well as disinhibition. Problems with arousal and lethargy can be related to injury to the brain stem.

As a typical example, remember that problems associated with frontal lobe injury can be distractibility, inflexible thinking, poor judgment, and impulsive behavior. Many individuals have some combination of these problems, but are able to control their behavior in most situations. However, sometimes agitation leads to impulsive behaviors in a challenging or confusing situation. The unwanted behaviors can be as minor as lack of response to requests or yelling. They can be as severe as aggression, property destruction, or self-injury.

Positive Reinforcement

Scientific studies show that unwanted behaviors are sometimes maintained because they produce positive reinforcement. Sometimes unwanted behaviors are followed by attention from other people, such as staff, other individuals in the rehabilitation setting, staff, family, and even strangers in the community. Aggression, and other threatening behaviors, can result in a payoff to an individual. This can be access to preferred objects or getting one's way in personal choices by demonstrating the unwanted behavior.

Consider someone who has episodes of agitation accompanied by aggression and property destruction. During the outbursts, the individual becomes the center of attention. Following the outbursts, there may be individual meetings with a variety of people.

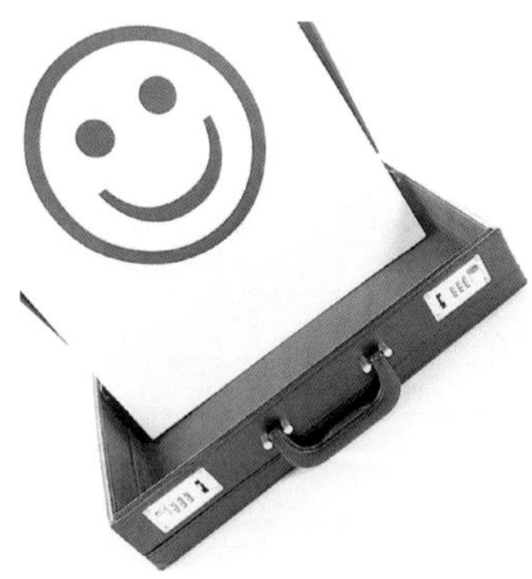

The attention from other people is comforting. It lets this person know that others care. Meeting with staff on a one-on-one basis is helpful and reassuring. This positive attention may inadvertently strengthen the unwanted behavior that preceded it.

In many cases, the response to unwanted behavior can include an element of counseling, or even reprimanding. Still, research has shown that even severe unwanted behaviors, such as aggression and life-threatening self-injury, can be maintained by positive reinforcement of another person's response. In many cases, a staff member thinks that effective counseling is given after a behavioral outburst, but what may actually be provided is positive reinforcement.

Negative Reinforcement

Despite the best intentions of skilled and caring rehabilitation professionals, the recovery process can be very unpleasant for individuals. Physical activities can be painful. Seemingly simple cognitive activities can be confusing and difficult to perform. Speech problems may make it difficult to speak or be understood. Many activities may seem childlike and are demeaning or embarrassing.

Individuals going through rehabilitation or community reintegration often face situations that are unpleasant.

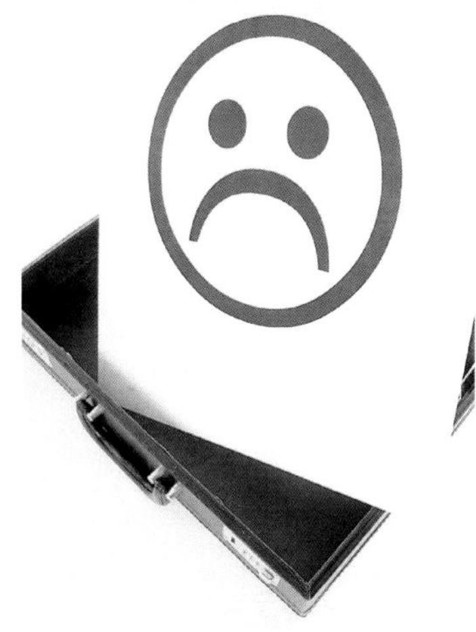

Sometimes, individuals learn to use unwanted behavior to avoid them. Consider someone who finds physical therapy painful and frustrating. Being aggressive toward the physical therapist or transporting staff member results in being rescheduled for easier therapy or being allowed to read or watch TV. When this happens, the unwanted behavior is strengthened by avoiding the unpleasant situation.

Similarly, a person may not like occupational therapy because the cognitive exercises aren't understood. Or the person may not like the therapist or other group members. This person may learn that an outburst that disrupts the session or scares others results in being excused from therapy. The outburst is reinforced by the escape from therapy. This makes it more likely to occur in the future.

Punishment

Behaviors that are followed by unpleasant consequences are less likely to occur again. Unfortunately, this can complicate the rehabilitation process when necessary measures result in unpleasant consequences, such as pain, confusion, embarrassment, or failure. A person's efforts to participate in rehabilitation can be discouraged in this way.

Most people learn what things they do well, and what they have trouble with. The same is true for the person in rehabilitation or returning to the community. When the skills that are most important to a person's recovery are followed by some type of punishment, those behaviors are weakened. This results in limiting a person's ability to obtain positive reinforcement. For example, a person may find using mass transit too confusing or has gotten lost. The person might choose not to go out alone to avoid this unpleasant outcome. The individual is then likely to find other behaviors that are effective, even if those behaviors are inappropriate sometimes. An example is making too many demands or requests for a neighbor to run errands. Other individuals withdraw into depression and social isolation as they experience more and more failure.

Multiple Causes

The unwanted behavior of most people with brain injury is the result of a combination of neurologic and environmental causes. In some cases, the initial occurrence of behavior problems is due solely to neurologic damage. Individuals who did not have significant unwanted behaviors previously may become aggressive, disruptive, and difficult to get along with. Clearly, the brain injury caused these problems.

But the environment plays a part in determining the future likelihood of behavior. So even in cases where the brain injury is the primary cause for the unwanted behavior, the reaction of the people in the environment affects how often the behavior will occur in the future.

For example, an individual with frontal lobe damage becomes easily frustrated. This leads to agitation and aggression. This aggression can be strengthened by positive reinforcement -attention - or negative reinforcement by escaping from un-

Unwanted Behavior

Unwanted behavior due to environmental factors is not the fault of the individual with the brain injury. The fault lies in the environment accidentally strengthening unwanted behaviors instead of wanted responses. It is very likely that the individual is not aware of why the behavior problems occur, and probably wishes to have more acceptable behavior.

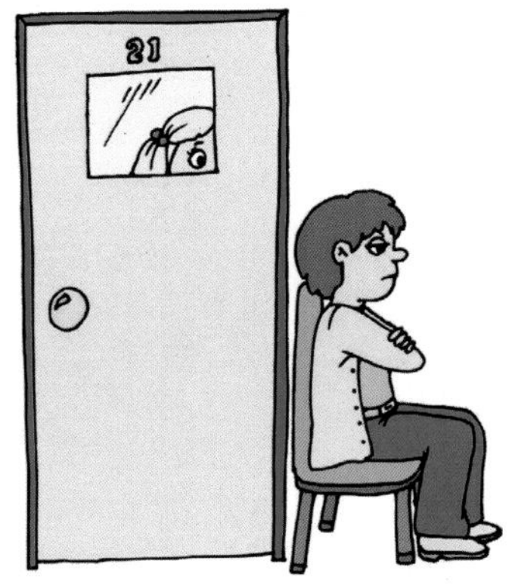

pleasant tasks. While the origin of the behavior is neurologic, the behavior continues to occur partly because of environmental influences.

Alternately, if the same individual becomes aggressive but the behavior is not reinforced, then the behavior is less likely to occur. The behavior is even less likely if the individual learns more adaptive strategies to get attention or escape unpleasant situations.

Treatment Planning for Unwanted Behavior

The steps are the same as those described earlier for general treatment planning. Identifying outcome criteria, goals, and objectives proceeds from understanding the discharge environment. Planning for treatment of unwanted behaviors is part of the process described earlier in Steps to Treatment Planning. Put most simply, treatment of unwanted behaviors involves the following:

- Define the behavior specifically in objective and measurable terms and give examples.
- Establish a baseline level of the behavior.
- Identify specific methods for discouraging occurrence of the behavior.
- Reinforce desirable behaviors that can replace the unwanted behavior.
- Continue to evaluate the behavior's occurrence.
- Revise the plan as necessary.

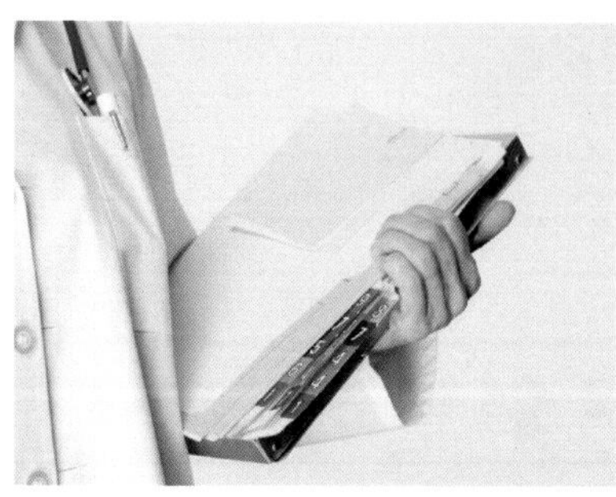

General Guidelines

- Emphasize strategies which focus on teaching the individual to self-manage unwanted behaviors instead of reliance on others to intervene. This insures maximum inclusion and control by the individual and has the greatest likelihood of maintaining and generalizing to other settings and persons.

The treatment plan should be discussed with the individual, in terms of what the problem is, why it is a problem, and what will be done to address it. As with all treatment planning, this usually increases the chances for positive outcome because the individual is involved in the process.

- Ensure programming is least restrictive and that more restrictive measures are used only after lesser measures have proved ineffective.

For example, if a person is demonstrating loud vulgar language, it may be more appropriate to walk away or put that person on extinction as opposed to restricting community access for the next 48 hours.

Even some professionals assume that the only effective means of decreasing unwanted behavior is through punishment or loss of privileges. While mild forms of punishment may sometimes be necessary, many behavior problems can be eliminated through strictly positive means. There should be many more rewards for wanted behavior than loss of reinforcers or other punishments for unwanted behavior.

- Use the plan to teach adaptive behaviors that replace unwanted behaviors.

If someone physically aggresses to escape from a task, part of the treatment is to prevent the escape. But it's just as important to teach the person acceptable ways of having more control over the task.

For example, give the person options of choosing what time tasks are done, the order of tasks, or what the consequence are for doing, or not doing, the tasks. Consider teaching how to request a short break, or ask for help or directions.

- Carry out treatment for behavioral issues in all therapeutic contexts.

Behavior problems do not occur in a vacuum. They occur in therapy rooms, the dining room, the residence, the grocery store, and many other places. Effective assessment and treatment require that unwanted behaviors be treated in all situations.

- Always attempt to be pleasant and positive in interactions.

Staff should interact in a manner that shows respect, caring, and positive concern for the person's well-being. For example, greet program participants by name and ask how they are

Chapter Note

It is important to note that this chapter does not address hands-on procedures to contain or restrain individuals during time of crisis. Each state and often licensing and accrediting agencies specify strict guidelines which must be followed to reduce risk of harm to the individual and others and ensure thorough documentation of the incident.

doing. When staff show an honest interest in individuals by commenting on some topic of interest to the individual, it is less likely that behavior problems occur to gain attention.

- People with behavior problems need a lot of encouragement that they can learn to control their behavior more effectively. Don't focus just on the problems.

A very common mistake by staff is discussing a recent behavior outburst in the person's presence. Nothing positive comes from this. There may be severe negative effects by further discouraging someone who already feels bad about their behavior. There is also the risk that overhearing two staff, or staff and family, discuss a recent behavioral outburst may be positively reinforcing for the individual.

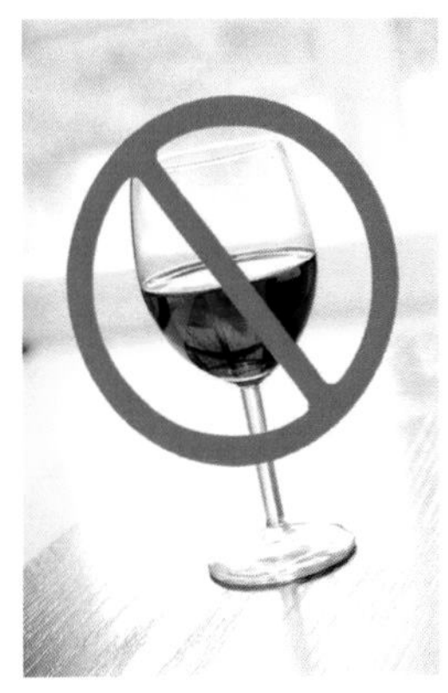

Treating Substance Abuse

Traditional substance abuse treatment strategies often do not work with people with cognitive impairments after brain injury. Concepts such as sobriety and commitment can be difficult to understand and integrate into daily life following brain injury. As a result, programs like Alcoholics Anonymous rarely work without additional education, professional support, and clearly defined strategies for recovery and staying sober.

Recent research has identified critical elements for effectively treating substance abuse after brain injury. They are:

1. Trained substance abuse counselors as part of the trans-disciplinary team.
2. Comprehensive assessment of substance abuse upon entry to a program.
3. Recognition of stages of readiness and willingness to commit to a sober lifestyle.
4. Group therapy approaches to build a person's ability to receive feedback and appreciate different points of view.
5. Family involvement.
6. Relapse is part of the recovery process, not failure.

General Components of Effective Programming

Whether treatment planning is aimed at increasing desirable skills, decreasing unwanted behavior, or both, deficits in cognitive functioning must be considered. Memory, attention, language, reasoning, and executive function are commonly affected areas. They are the areas most likely to affect the success of treatment planning. Below are general guidelines that may apply to individual plans.

Daily planner

Treatment plans should include using a daily planner. These are also referred to as organizers or memory journals, but the term planner is more common. The plan should describe specific ways to give assistance. If the individual resists using a planner, encourage carrying lists of cues.

For example, a person who speaks with great difficulty carries a laminated card. It lists 4-5 strategies that are helpful for clearer articulation.

A person prone to impulsive, explosive behavior carries a card with 3-4 de-escalation steps. The card is read at the first feeling of anger.

General Components of Effective Programming

Problem	Functional impact	Treatment strategies
Memory	Forgetting critical events	Review written diary of events in daily planner
	Forgetting appointments	Detailed schedule in daily planner, with prompts to check journal as needed
	Forgetting to take medication	Alarm on watch pre-programmed to provide cues
Executive Functioning	Poor planning	Use written task analysis to break task into smaller steps
	Trouble initiating activities	External prompts and fade out when no longer needed
	Difficulty paying attention	Require small amounts of attention to tasks initially Slowly require more attention
Language	Difficulty articulating words	Carry card with 4-5 steps to facilitate effective speaking
	Poor expressive speech	Cues to slow down
	Poor receptive speech	Ask speaker to slow down
Aggression	Limits opportunities for independence	Determine why aggression occurs. Reinforce appropriate means of obtaining same result
Verbal Outbursts	Limit opportunities for socialization	Carry card with 4-5 de-escalation steps to be read at first feeling of anger
Social skills	Inappropriate interactions	Task analyze appropriate interactions. Teach through modeling, role-playing, and praise
Employment	Difficulty recalling job	Task analysis to break task into simpler steps
	Anxiety	Relaxation strategies
Activities of daily living	Unclean, unhealthy	Task analysis with written, visual, or verbal cueing, as needed

Redirection

Many individuals in rehabilitation are easily confused, overstimulated, impulsive, and have other problems discussed earlier. It is not always therapeutic to directly confront a person exhibiting unwanted behaviors. In most cases, trying to resolve an active situation only leads to further escalation when a person is in the middle of an agitated outburst, whether it be yelling, aggression, property destruction, self-injury, or whatever. This applies regardless of what caused the behavior. It is sometimes more effective to redirect the person away from whatever is causing the unwanted behavior.

For example, if a person is perseverating or "stuck on" some perceived mistreatment by staff or a peer, there is little therapeutic value in trying to reason that the perceived mistreatment is just a misunderstanding. Redirection tries to get the person to interact on a preferred topic and completely avoids any mention of the original problem. Examples are redirecting a person to discuss a recent movie, TV show, sporting event, or an upcoming event.

> *Changing the focus from the cause of agitation usually results in reducing agitated behavior. Depending on the individual, it is often therapeutic to discuss the origin of an agitated episode after the person has calmed down.*

Summary

People with brain injury face difficult challenges. Each individual has a myriad of problems and challenges to overcome. The good news is that no matter what the problem, there is always something that can be done to improve a person's ability to function more independently.

Treatment planning to maximize gains must proceed from an identification of the discharge site. Whether the individual eventually returns to independence in the community, or needs ongoing assistance, the treatment team must know this to be aware of skills needed for maximal functioning. All treatment planning is oriented toward achieving objectives and goals for what will be needed upon discharge. These outcome criteria are the ultimate basis for evaluating whether a person's rehabilitation has been successful.

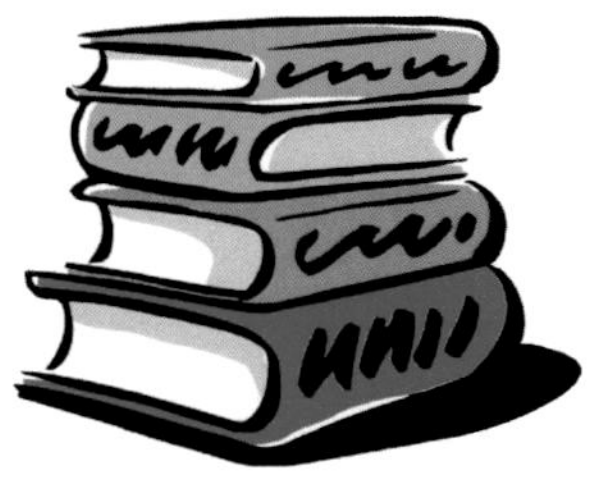

References

Bellack, AS, Hersen, M, & Kazdin, AE (Eds) (1990). International handbook of behavior modification and therapy. New York: Plenum Press.

Bombardier, CH & Heinemann, AW (2000). The construct validity of the Readiness to Change Questionnaire for persons with TBI. Journal of Head Trauma Rehabilitation, 15, 696-709.

Braunling-McMorrow, D (1988). Behavioral rehabilitation. In: P Deutsch, & K Fralish (Eds), Innovations in head injury rehabilitation. New York, NY: Matthew Bender and Company.

Delmonico, RL, Hanley-Peterson, P, & Englander, J (1998). Group therapy for persons with traumatic brain injury: management of frustration and substance abuse. Journal of Head Trauma Rehabilitation, 13,10-22.

DiLima, SN & Eutsey, DE (Eds) (1996). Brain Injury Survivor and Caregiver Education Manual. Gaithersburg, MD: Aspen Publishers.

Fralish, KB (1994). Functional rehabilitation: An outcomes oriented therapeutic approach to traumatic brain. Carbondale, IL: Center for Comprehensive Services Monograph.

Jacobs, H (1993). Behavior analysis guidelines and brain injury rehabilitation: People, principles, and programs. Gaithersburg, MD: Aspen.

Levin, HS, Benton, AL & Grossman, RG (1982). Neurobehavioral consequences of closed head injury. New York: Oxford University Press.

Pace, GM, Ivancic, MT, and Jefferson, G (1994). Stimulus fading as treatment for obscenity in a brain-injured adult. Journal of applied Behavior Analysis, 27, 301-305.

Page, TJ (1996). Navigating the curves: Behavior changes and brain injury. Washington, D.C.: Brain Injury Association.

Schmidt, ND (1997). Outcome-oriented rehabilitation: A response to managed care. Journal of Head Trauma Rehabilitation, 12, 44-50.

Treadwell, K, & Page, TJ (1996). Functional analysis: Identifying the environmental determinants of severe behavior disorders. Journal of Head trauma Rehabilitation, 11, 62-74.

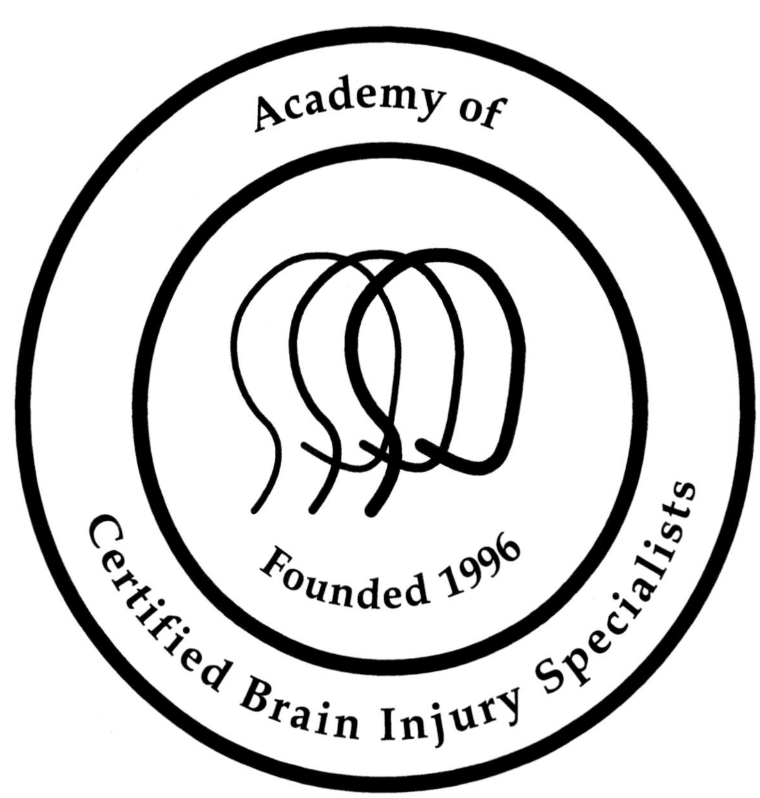
Academy of
Certified Brain Injury Specialists
Founded 1996

Chapter 6

Children and Adolescents with Brain Injuries

Learning Objectives

By the end of this chapter, you will be able to:

- Recognize developmental issues for children and adolescents after brain injury.
- Understand the public special education laws for children and adolescents with brain injuries.
- Understand the practice of individualized educational planning for children and adolescents.

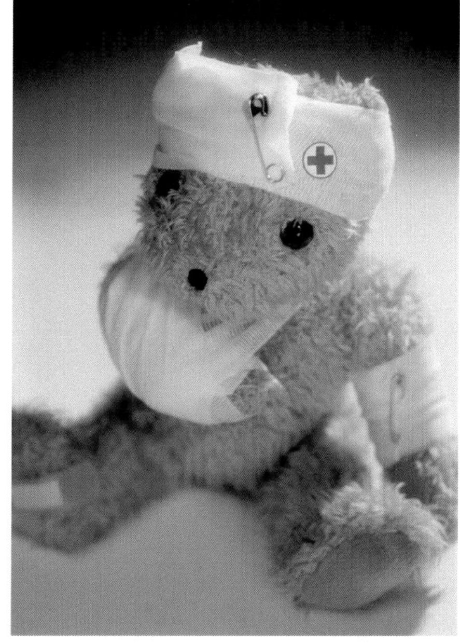

Introduction

In Chapter 1, incidence and prevalance data in children was presented. The 2006 CDC Report data show clearly that incidence rates of TBI for children are different than that of other age groups. For overall rates of TBI (including ED Visits, Hospitalizations, and Deaths) three of the top four incidence rates were in the age groups of children; **0-4** (1121 per 100,000), **15-19** (814 per 100,000), and **5-9** (659 per 100,000). Overall, children aged **0-4** had the highest rate of overall incidence of TBI (1121 per 100,000), the highest ED visit rate (1035 per 100,000), and had the highest ED Visit rates for males, females, Whites and Blacks. Thus children disproportionately incur TBI, and this chapter focuses on the effects of brain injury for the youngest of survivors.

Age Effects

It was formerly believed that children were wonderfully resilient little beings who could "bounce back" after even severe trauma. Now it is understood that children are just as vulnerable as adults. Sometimes it takes much longer for the effects of trauma to be seen in children, since their brains are still developing.

Preschoolers with injuries to their frontal lobes often look fine within a few weeks or months after an injury. However, as they get older and their brains mature, that part of the brain previously damaged may not work as well as it should. When a child's brain is injured, it can have long-term devastating effects on the child and family. Too often, children who sustain a brain injury early in life may look "well" at that moment in time, but more serious cognitive and behavioral problems may emerge as the child grows.

Brain Maturation - Age and Percent Maturation

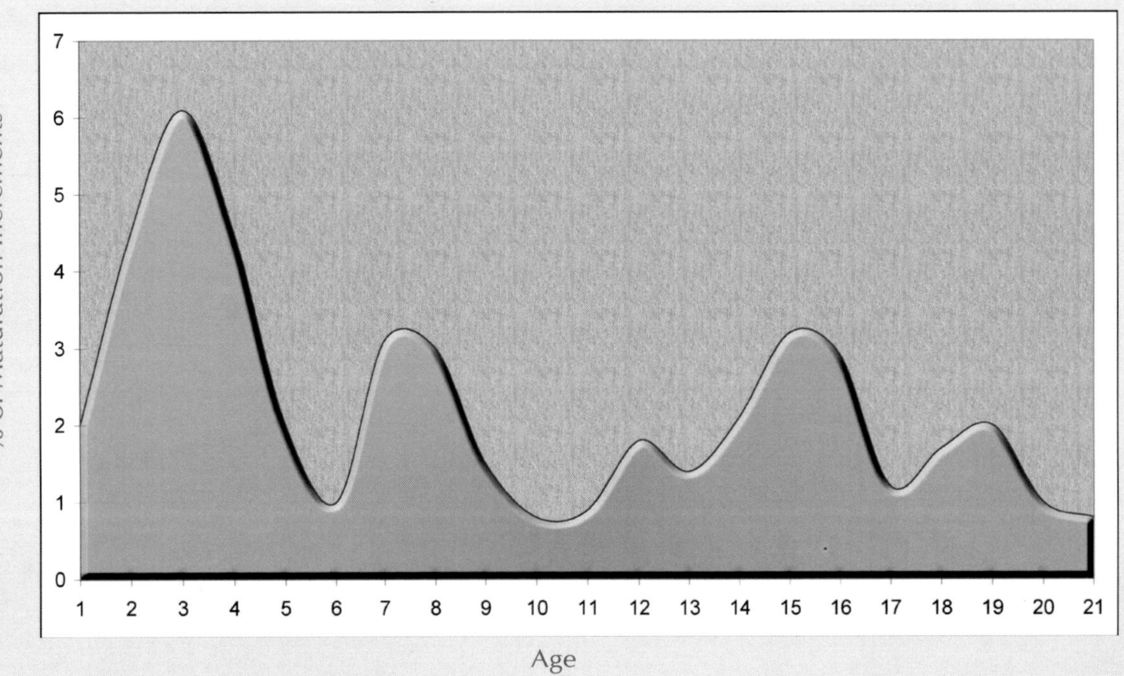

Maturation occurs in immediate and abrupt changes during childhood. Thus, depending on the age of the child when the brain injury occurred, one may be able to predict the kinds of cognitive and learning challenges that the child may experience now and in the future. This knowledge allows professionals working with the child to predict the resources that may be needed to better support the child in school.

New research using advanced scanning technology is identifying how a child's brain grows and matures from birth through adolescence. Five peak maturation periods have been identified in normally developing children. These may be significantly affected depending on the age of the child, the type of brain injury, and the region of the brain that is injured. The five peak maturation mileposts are ages:

1-6

7-10

11-13

14-17

18-21

Through developmental studies and techniques such as neuropsychological testing, magnetic resonance imaging (MRI), and special uses of electroencephalography (EEG), critical discoveries are being made about how the brain grows and matures throughout childhood. New research utilizing advanced scanning technology and statistical analysis of EEGs have better identified how a child's brain matures from birth through adolescence. The developmental stages of the 5 peak maturation mileposts are listed on pages 109 and 110.

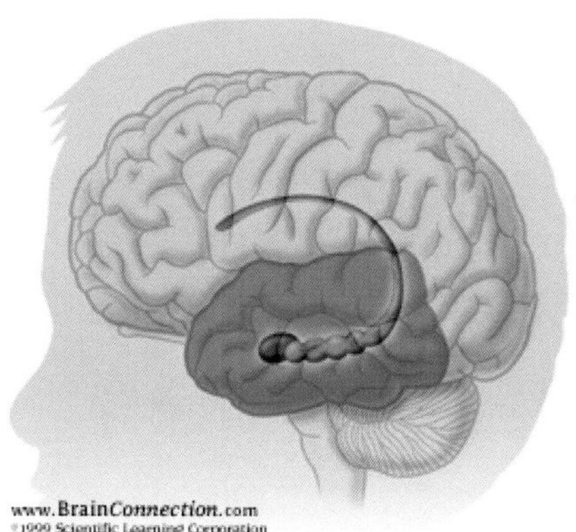

Maturation Mileposts

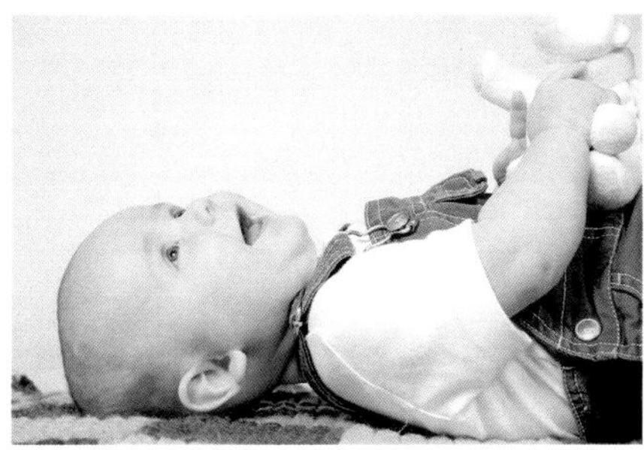

Ages 1-6

During this period of overall rapid brain growth, all regions of the brain – those governing frontal executive, visuo-spatial, somatic, and visuo-auditory functions – show signs of synchronous development until about the age of 6. Children are perfecting such skills as their ability to form images, use words, and place things in serial order. They also begin to develop tactics for solving problems.

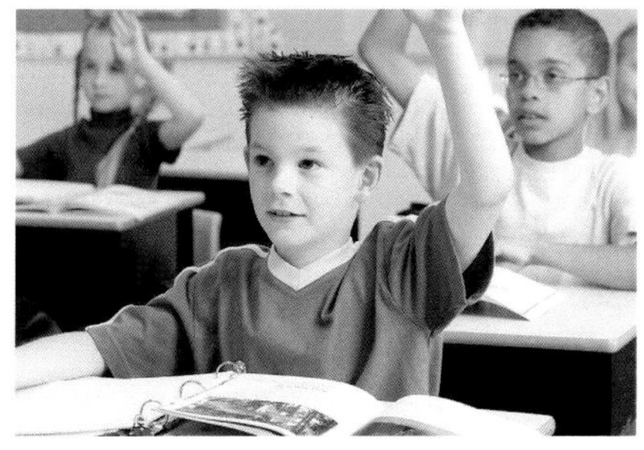

Ages 7-10

At this point, only the sensory and motor systems continue to mature in tandem up to about age 7 1/2, when the frontal executive system begins accelerated development. Beginning at about age 6, the maturation of the sensory motor regions of the brain peak. This occurs just as children begin to perform simple operational functions, such as determining weight and logical-mathematical reasoning.

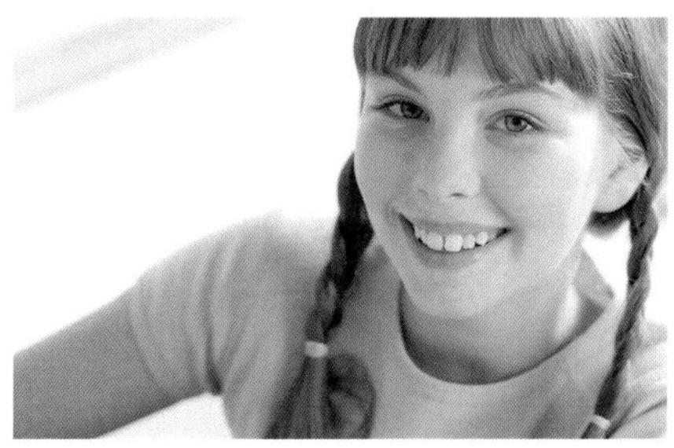

Ages 11-13

This stage primarily involves the elaboration of the visuospatial functions, but also includes maturation of the visuo-auditory regions. By the age of 10, while visual and auditory regions of the brain mature, children are able to perform formal operations, such as calculations, and perceive new meaning in familiar objects.

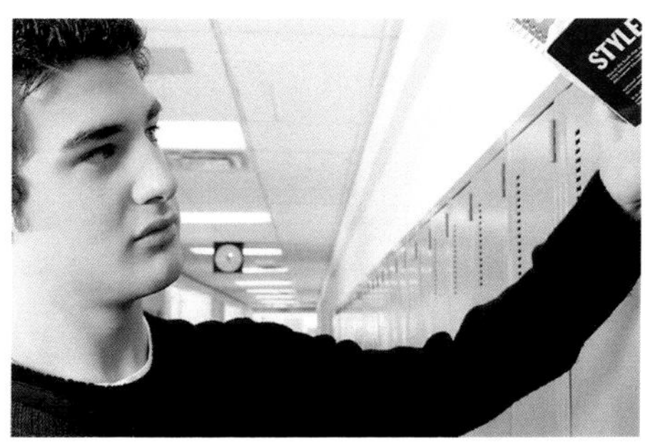

Ages 14-17

During these years, successive maturation of the visuo-auditory, visuospatial, and somatic systems reach their maturational peak within one-year intervals of each other. In their early years, young people enter the stage of dialectic ability. They are able to review formal operations, find flaws with them, and create new ones. Meanwhile, the visuo-auditory, visuospatial, and somatic systems of the brain are developing.

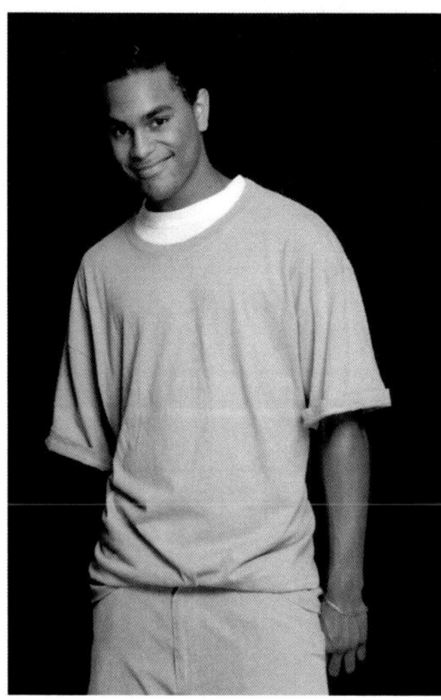

Ages 18-21

The final stage begins around 17-18 years as the region governing the frontal executive functions matures on its own. Young people begin to question information they are given, reconsider it, and form new hypotheses incorporating their own ideas. This development occurs in conjunction with rapid maturation of the frontal executive region of the brain.

Brain Growth

The greatest percent of brain maturation occurs in the early years, birth through age 5. Thus, injury to a child's brain before age 5 may be the most devastating time to sustain an injury. This may be why infants and toddlers who have had severe head trauma from being "shaken and impacted" have such poor outcomes. In addition, children with frontal lobe injuries early in life tend to develop long term psychosocial and behavioral problems.

Collaborating with Medical and Rehabilitation Systems

Medical and rehabilitation systems care for children who sustain brain injuries. However, their much needed services are short in comparison with the long term needs of these children and their families. Medical systems, involving emergency departments, acute care hospitals and rehabilitation facilities that do not communicate with each other, create referral gaps when children are discharged home and enter or return to school (Christensen, 1997; Savage, 1997).

Some children seen in emergency departments for mild brain injuries may not be referred to the school or to the child's primary care physician for follow-up. Other children, who are admitted to acute care services for more serious injuries, may not be referred to rehabilitation services, especially if those services do not exist in that hospital (Discala, Osborn, Savage, 1998). Children who do receive rehabilitation services may not be referred to their local school's special education department for educational services and educationally relevant rehabilitation services, e.g., physical, occupational, speech/ language therapy (Discala, Osborn, Savage, 1998; Janus et al., 1997).

Medical services are the "beginning" of the continuum of services necessary to support the long term needs of these children. Therefore, it is important for local hospitals and area schools to develop policies and procedures that promote effective communication and discharge planning. By developing referral systems that facilitate communication between hospitals, schools and families, children are more likely to receive appropriate services. Thus, those children who are properly referred will be better managed both from a medical as well as an educational perspective.

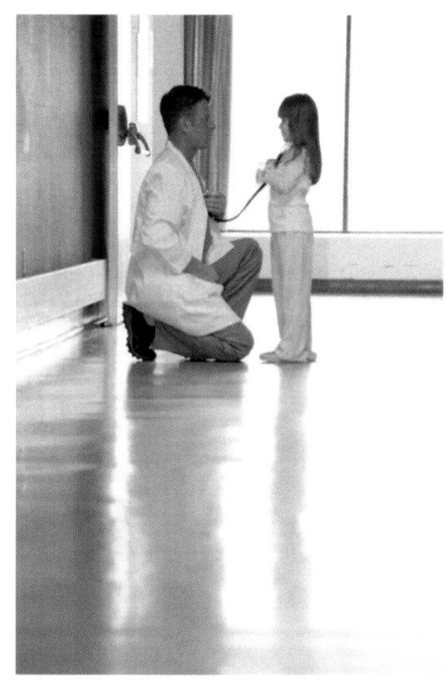

Collaboration

It is important to develop good systems of communication between Medical Service Providers, families and School Systems. This will help to ensure that children with brain injuries will be well served both medically and educationally

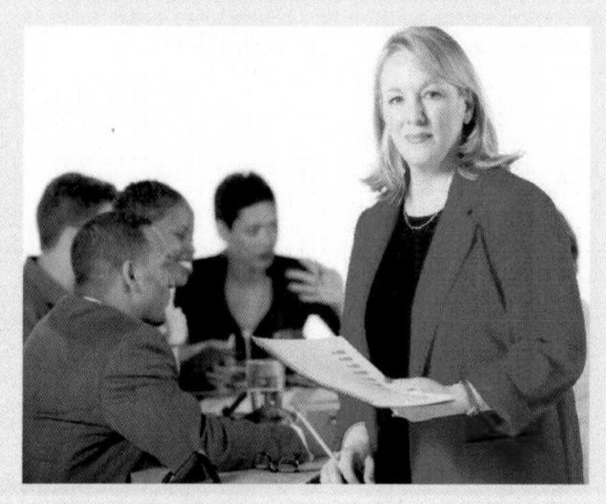

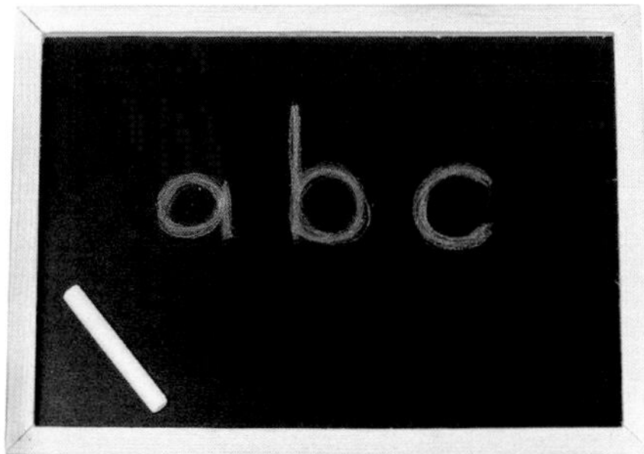

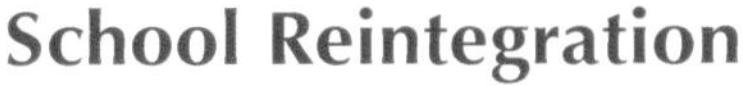

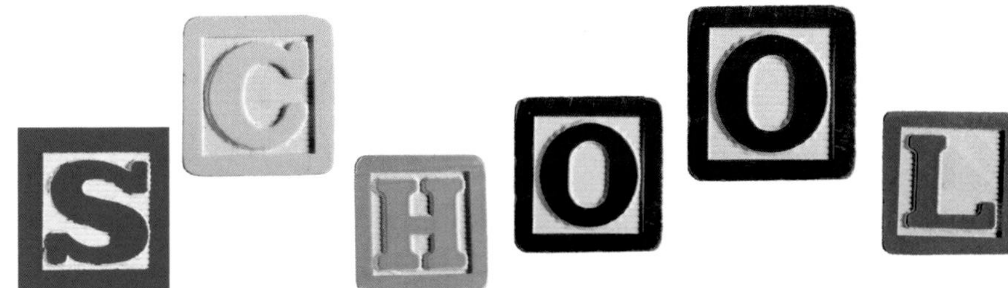

School Reintegration

Educating teachers and peers about the student who is returning to school is critical. Students with brain injuries need to be carefully transitioned into schools with support plans already in place (Blosser & Pearson, 1997; DePompei & Blosser, 1994; Savage & Wolcott, 1994; Tyler and Wilkerson, 1999; Ylvisaker, 1999). Students may need to reintegrate into school on a part-time basis or they may need in-home instruction for a period of time. Families can help schools by bringing copies of medical records, such as discharge summaries and evaluations by specialists. Families can also help educate school staff by requesting training for all school staff who will be working with their children; alerting teachers to information about students with brain injuries; or preparing classmates about their children (Glang et al., 1999; Glang et al., 1997). Families are a natural link between hospital, home and school; however, they need the full support of professionals to plan for the child's successful reintegration to school.

Persisting Effects of Brain Injury

A complete listing of common deficits following brain injury has been provided already in Chapter 5. These deficits can not only affect daily functioning among children, but may also have a major impact on their education. Following are a few examples of how common, long-term effects of brain injury can show up in the classroom and affect a child's learning.

Cognitive Effects

<u>Memory</u>

The student...

- Is unable to recall previously learned information that serves as the foundation for new learning.
- Can not remember a series of two to three step directions.
- Is unable to grasp new concepts without repeated exposures.
- Has difficulty recalling the day's schedule, what was assigned for homework, or what materials to bring to class.

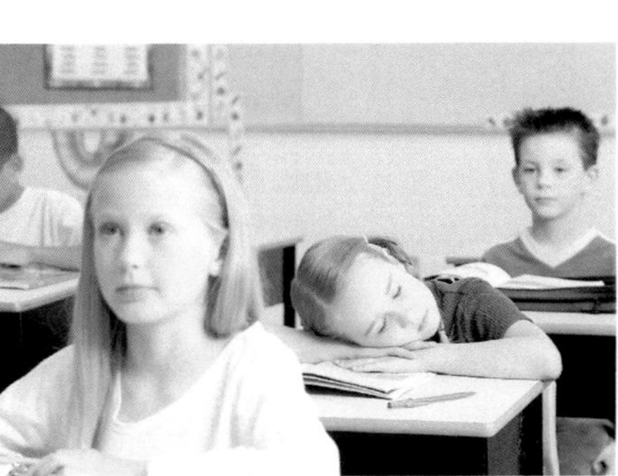

<u>Attention and Concentration</u>

The student...

- Is distracted by normal classroom activity.
- Has difficulty staying on topic during a class discussion.
- Is unable to complete a task without prompting.
- Blurts out answers in the middle of a class session.
- Becomes fatigued by mid-afternoon and appears uninterested in activities.

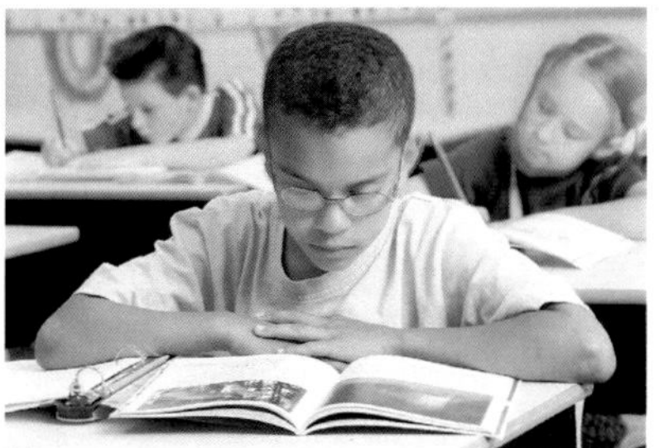

<u>Higher Level Problem Solving</u>

The student...

- Has difficulty organizing and completing long-term projects.
- Lacks ability to sequence steps necessary to plan an activity

- Is unable to come up with solutions to problem situations (e.g., lost lunch money).
- Has difficulty drawing conclusions from facts presented.

Language Skills

The student...

- Has difficulty taking turns in a conversation.
- Is unable to summarize and articulate thoughts.
- Talks around a subject or uses indefinite words.
- Does not understand the meaning of a conversation when figures of speech or metaphors are used.

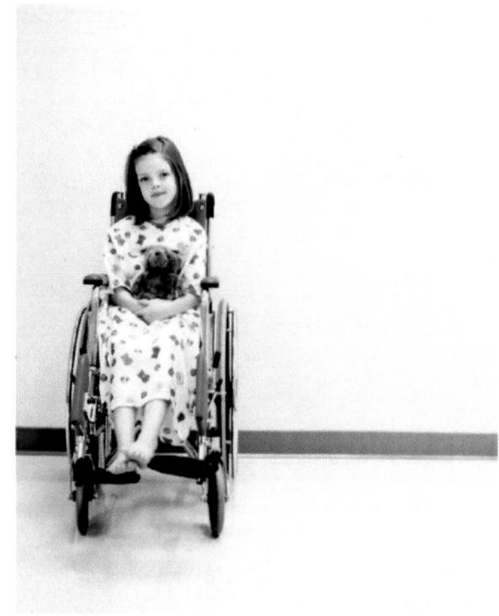

Sensorimotor Effects

The student...

- Takes an inordinate amount of time to produce written material.
- Is unable to take notes while listening to the class lecture.
- Has difficulty copying information from the board or overhead projector.
- Has difficulty completing simple math problems when presented with a worksheet full of problems.
- Completes only problems on one-half of the paper because of difficulty seeing objects in part of the visual field.
- Becomes disoriented in the hallway and has difficulty finding the classroom.

Behavioral & Emotional Effects

The student...

- Says or does socially inappropriate things.
- Has difficulty fitting in with peers.
- Is easily mislead by peers into making poor choices.
- Is unable to start or stop an activity without assistance.
- Impulsively leaves the seat or classroom.
- Becomes easily frustrated.
- Is unaware of and denies any impairments resulting from the injury.

The child also may have physical changes from the brain injury which affect daily functioning and

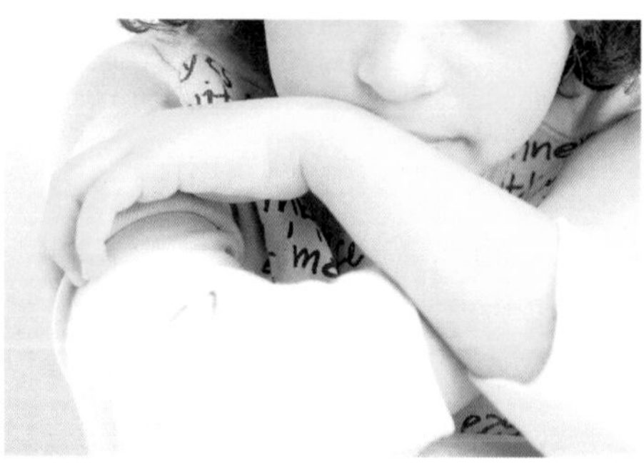

educational performance. Common physical effects include seizures, headaches, and lack of endurance. Motor problems may include rigidity, tremors, spasticity, ataxia (loss of ability to coordinate smooth movements), or apraxia (inability to plan and carry out movements purposefully on command). Less common, but very significant physical effects include disruption in growth, eating disorders, development of diabetes, and thermoregulation difficulties (e.g., spikes in body temperature). Educators need to have a clear understanding of the child's physical problems so they can evaluate their implications and modify the student's educational program accordingly (Tyler & Mira, 1999).

Many children, particularly those with severe deficits after a brain injury, will not be able to succeed in school without specialized programming and services. To obtain appropriate services for such students requires coordinated, interdisciplinary planning. This must involve all parties, including health care providers, educators, the family, child, and community.

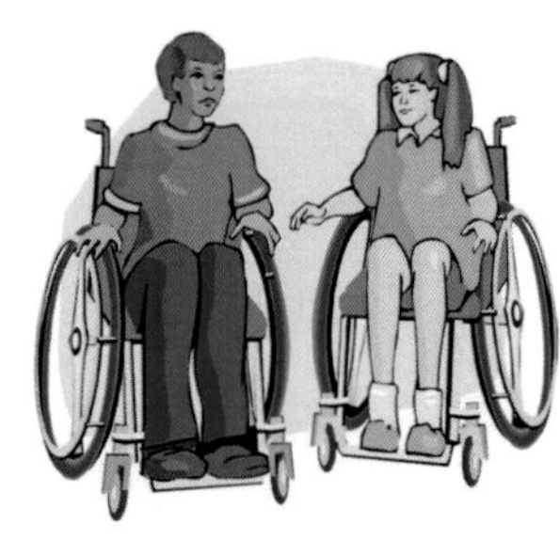

Qualifying for Special School Services

Ultimately, schools end up being the largest provider of services to children with brain injuries (Savage, 1997). Because of the unique needs of these students, many require specialized school services. These services may be provided under the Individuals with Disabilities Education Act (IDEA) or Section 504 of the Rehabilitation Act of 1973.

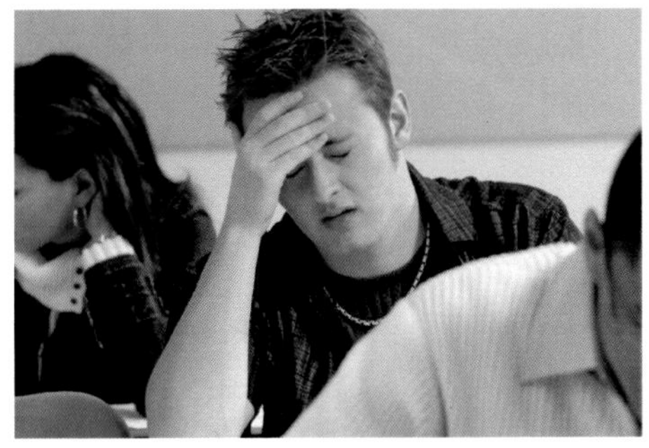

Individuals with Disabilities Education Act (IDEA)

In October 1990, a category of "traumatic brain injury" for students requiring special education services was authorized under IDEA (Public Law 101-476). IDEA enables school systems to better identify the students with traumatic brain injuries as well as their special needs. It helps avoid mis-classifying them as mentally retarded, learning disabled, behaviorally disturbed, or any other special education category. Traumatic brain injury is defined under IDEA as follows:

> *"Traumatic brain injury" means an acquired injury to the brain caused by an external physical force, resulting in total or partial functional disability or psychosocial impairment, or both, that adversely affects a child's educational performance. The term applies to open or closed head injuries resulting in impairments in one or more areas, such as cognition; language; memory; attention; reasoning; abstract thinking; problem–solving; sensory, perceptual and motor abilities; psychosocial behavior; physical functions; information processing; and speech. The term does not apply to brain injuries that are congenital or degenerative, or brain injuries induced by birth trauma. (Section 300.7b[12] 1999)*

While some states have expanded IDEA's definition to include all acquired brain injuries, most states follow this federal definition. Therefore, in several states, students with brain injuries from "internal" occurrences such as brain infections, strokes, anoxia, brain tumors, neurotoxic poisonings, or metabolic disorders do not qualify for special services under the educational definition of TBI since their injuries were not the result of an "external physical force." If these children are having educational difficulties as a result of their injury, they may qualify for special education services under the category of Other Health Impaired. Because state definitions vary, hospital and rehabilitation staff should be familiar with the definition used in the state where the child is returning to school.

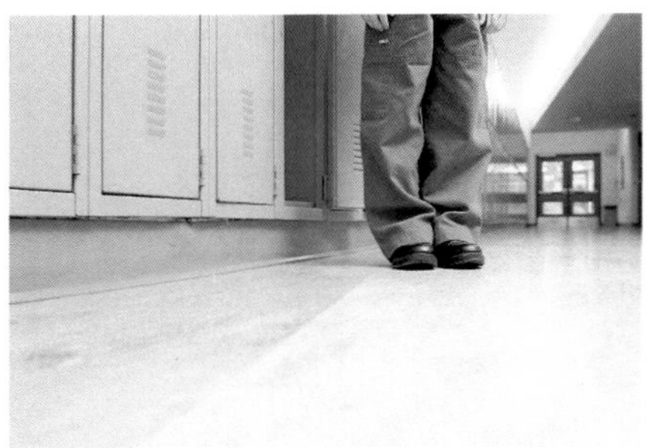

Some states have expanded the TBI definition to include acquired brain injuries, because the learning needs of students with brain injuries from external physical force and brain injuries from internal occurrences are similar, even though their course of recoveries may differ. Perhaps the most profound similarity is the sudden onset of disability. Prior to the injury, the majority of these students had a history of normal development.

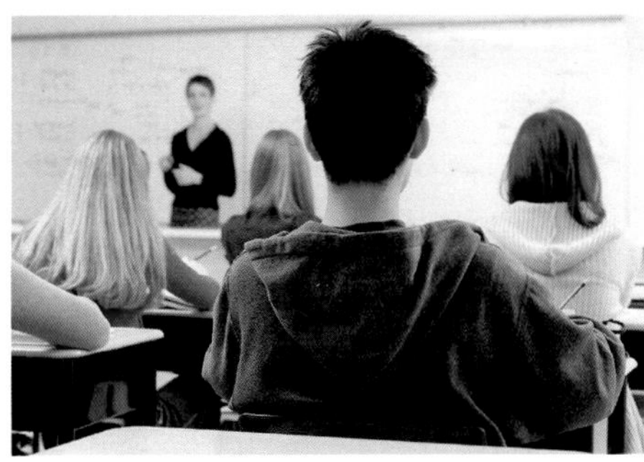

504 Plan

Another means of accessing educational services through the school system is a 504 Plan (sometimes referred to as a 504 Accommodation Plan).

> *Section 504 of the Rehabilitation act of 1973 requires schools receiving federal funding to provide reasonable accommodations to allow an individual with a disability to participate.*

To qualify for a 504 Plan, a student is only required to have a "presumed disability".

> The term disability means that an individual has a physical or mental impairment that substantially limits one or more major activities; has a record of the impairment; or is regarded as having an impairment.

Examples of academic accommodations that may be written into a 504 Plan include:

- Extended time on tests/assignments.
- Alternate formats for exams (e.g., oral vs. written, a scribe for writing answers).
- Note takers for lectures.
- Preferential seating.
- Assistance with project planning.
- Provision of audio-taped books.

In the elementary and secondary schools, a 504 Plan is generally reserved for students who:

- Do not require direct special education instruction or services.
- Can participate in the general education setting if accommodations are provided.

Schools and teachers across the country have been, and are still, receiving training about TBI. This training will lead to providing improved special education services for these students. Many states have set up interdisciplinary teams to develop programs to coordinate school re-entry and help students with TBI in their ongoing recovery.

Preparing for School Re-Entry

Returning to school can be devastating if the health care facility (hospital or rehabilitation center) and the student's home school do not interact as soon and as frequently as possible after the injury. This communication is important throughout the child's rehabilitation. As soon as a student is admitted to a health care facility, the school reintegration and transition process should begin. Hospital and/or rehabilitation professionals need to immediately inform the school that they are presently caring for one of their students. The family and/or attending physician should formally request that the school begin the evaluation process.

This evaluation is the important first step in initiating the special education process for identification and classification purposes. Unfortunately, many students are not referred to the school system for special education evaluation and are merely discharged back to school with little, if any, support services in place (DiScala, Osberg, & Savage, 1997). To insure that the student receives appropriate services after discharge, a referral for evaluation must be made while the child is still hospitalized. With this referral, school–based special educators or psychologists can then visit the student in the health care facility and begin the process to determine if the child will require special education services (Savage, 1991; Ylvisaker, Hartwick, & Stevens, 1991; Savage & Wolcott, 1995; Blosser & DePompei, 1994).

Hospital/rehabilitation staff can provide a great deal of information that will assist the school staff in evaluating a student. For example, DePompei, Blosser, Savage, and Lash (1999a) suggest the following information that hospitals can share with the schools:

Sharing Information with the School

Let the school staff know:

- When the child was injured.
- How the child was injured.
- How long the child was in the hospital or rehabilitation center.
- When the child will return to school.
- How the brain injury has affected the child.
- How the child best learns.
- What medications the child is taking.
- What special equipment may be needed in the school.
- What environmental accommodations the child will need.

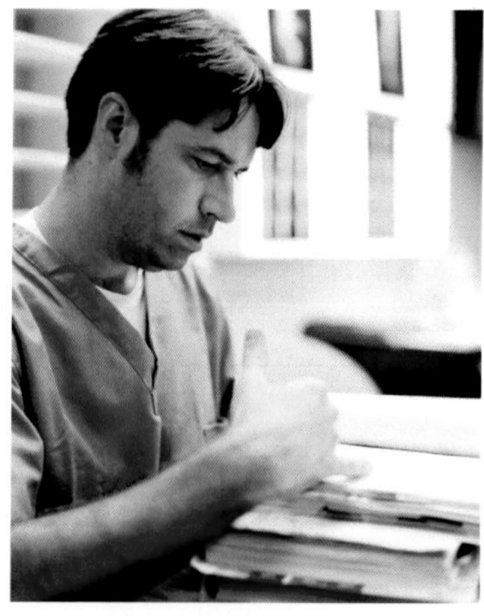

Hospital & Rehabilitation Staff Responsibilities

- Identify someone responsible to coordinate planning with the school.
- Determine with the school if the child needs to be referred for a special education evaluation.
- Meet with the child's teacher, school nurse, and special education director.
- Visit the child's school and complete an environmental assessment.
- Keep in contact with school staff by phone for updates.
- Conduct an in-service training for school staff.
- Be available for follow-up planning and consultation.

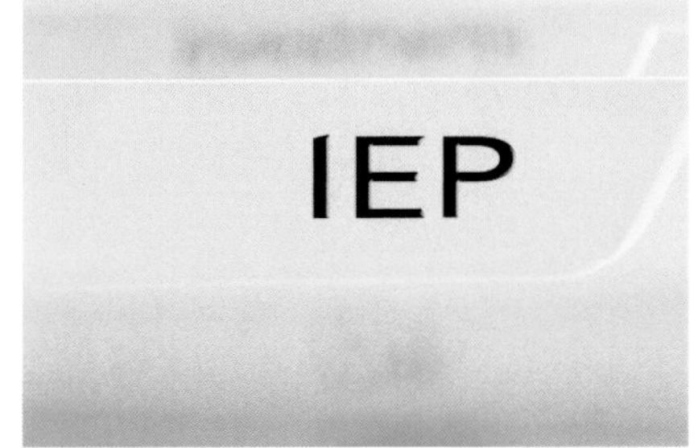

Developing the Individualized Education Plan (IEP)

Once the school has determined that the student needs special education services and has appropriately identified the student as having a TBI or Other Health Impairment, the school can begin to develop the Individualized Education Plan.

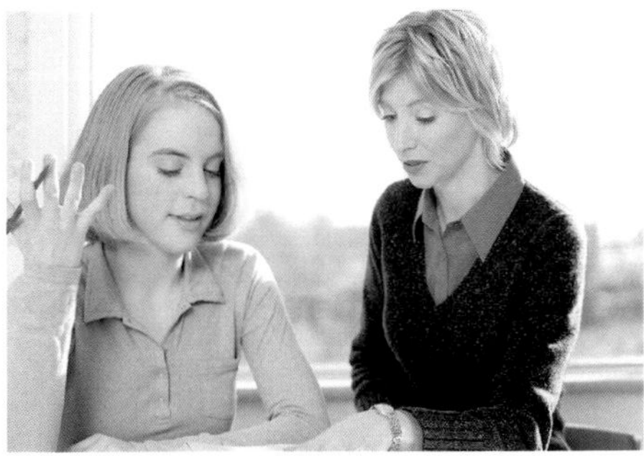

The IEP is essentially a contract between the student's family and the school system designating the kinds and extent of services that the student needs.

For those students whose brain injuries are mild, full–fledged special education programming may not be immediately necessary. Those students may only need to be monitored or have their schedules modified for a period of time to insure that any neurologic sequelae or changes have resolved. However, it is important to note that current medical definitions of mild, moderate and severe brain injury may not be the best indicators of outcome or potential for school related problems.

Some students with mild traumatic brain injuries, for example, may have problems months or even years later that may be just as disabling as those experienced by a student with more severe injuries (Savage & Wolcott, 1995). Therefore, it is crucial that the school nurse, classroom teachers, and family closely monitor the child's performance and alert the child's physician and/or neuropsychologist, of any persistent problems.

For students with more severe injuries, coordinated systems of care are necessary for the student's return to school. Merely passing the child from the medical to the educational system is not effective. It results in many students and their families falling into the "cracks" between the two systems. Developing communication protocols between health care facilities, school systems, and families is essential to avoid this breakdown in communication and services.

Thus, the initial IEP should be a "joint venture" among the health care facility, the school, and the family. It can reflect the cognitive, psychosocial, and neuro-motor needs of the student. By using a functionally–based and holistic approach, the student can become increasingly more involved at school, with the family, and community during recovery. A student's IEP can even involve vocational rehabilitation and community transition services by state and local agencies. This is important to ensure continuity of services for the adolescent before and after graduation from high school.

The IEP is a tool that describes what help the student will be given. The IEP should identify the skills, strategies, and behaviors that the student needs to learn and function at school.

DePompei, Blosser, Savage, and Lash (1999b) recommend that the team ask the following questions when developing the IEP:

The IEP

The IEP is a tool that describes what help the student will be given. The IEP should identify the skills, strategies, and behaviors that the student needs to learn and function at school.

Does the *IEP* help the student think and communicate by improving the student's ability to:

- Pay attention and concentrate?
- Get started in activities and work?
- Become organized and plan ahead?
- Reason and problem solve?
- Learn new information?
- Recall previously learned information?
- Communicate clearly and effectively in speech and writing?
- Make good and safe decisions?
- Be flexible and adjust to change?

Does the *IEP* help the student with feelings and behaviors by improving:

- Self esteem and self control?
- Awareness of how feelings effect others?
- Knowledge of expectations in social situations?

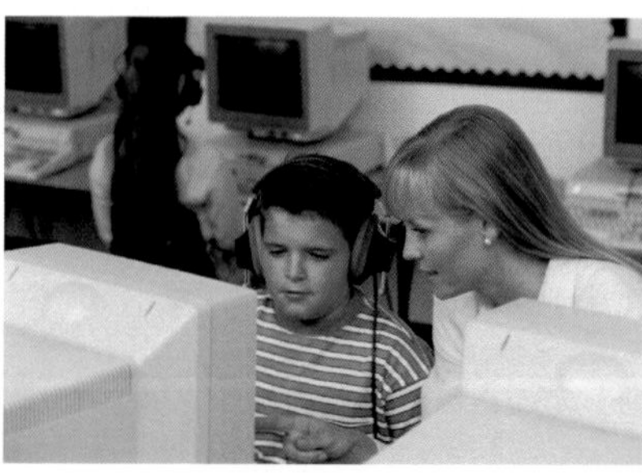

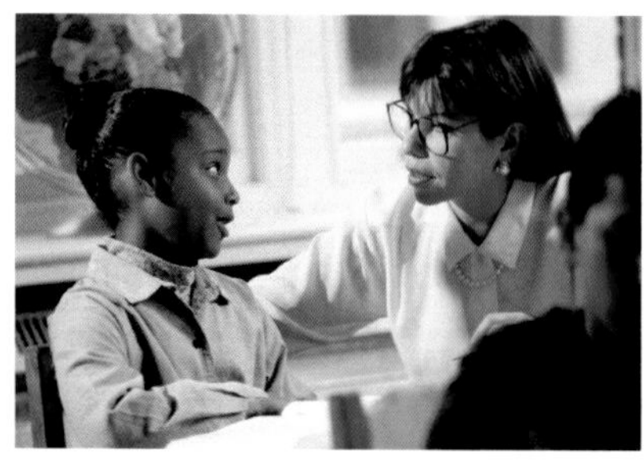

- Awareness of appropriate dressing and grooming?
- Ability to control sexual comments, gestures and actions?
- Ability to handle frustration and control anger?

Does the *IEP* help the student with physical and sensory issues by describing what the student needs to do to:

- Compensate for changes in vision and hearing?
- Detect changes in sound, height, distance, and touch?
- Adjust to changes in body coordination?
- Slow down or speed up movements?
- Improve balance & steadiness?
- Recognize and handle fatigue?
- Improve eye & hand coordination?

Generally, an IEP is written for a twelve-month period. However, the IEP for a student with a brain injury should be reviewed more frequently (every 2-4 months) with changes made as needed. This is because of the dramatically changing needs of students with brain injury, especially in the early months of recovery.

Planning the Academic Program

Teaching Strategies

While planning for school re-entry, educators need to develop programming strategies to meet the specialized needs of each child with a brain injury. Unfortunately, there is no standard procedures or curricula specifically for students with TBI and this is further complicated by the diversity of students (Ylvisaker et al., 2001). Instead, teaching methods are developed based on information obtained from hospital/rehabilitation staff and school personnel during the assessment process. Consideration of the functional needs of the student will also assist in the determination of the most effective teaching strategies (Ylvisaker et al., 2001).

These assessments may reveal that the child has a number of specific challenges to consider when developing

Factors to consider when developing Academic Programs

- Attention & Concentration.
- Memory.
- Organization.
- Direction Following.

programming strategies. Tyler, Blosser, and DePompei (1999) provided the following examples of common difficulties and suggestions for dealing with them:

Attention/Concentration

- Reduce distractions in student's work area (remove extra materials)
- Divide work into smaller sections. Have student complete one section at a time.
- Provide time lines for task completion.
- Ask student to orally summarize information that has just been presented.
- Establish nonverbal cueing system (e.g. eye contact, touch, etc.) to remind student to pay attention.

Memory

- Frequently repeat and summarize information.
- Teach student to use devices such as sticky notes, calendars, and assignment books as self-reminders to compensate for memory problems.

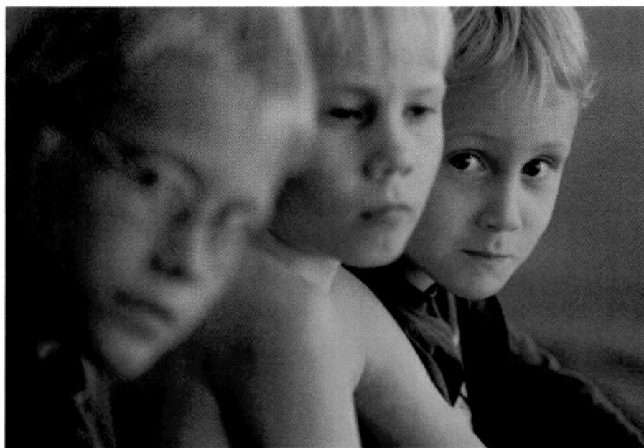

- Teach student to categorize or chunk information to aid retention.
- Demonstrate techniques such as mental rehearsal and use of special words or examples as reminders.
- Link new information to student's relevant prior knowledge.

Organization

Provide student with:

- Additional time for review.
- Written checklists of steps for complex tasks.
- Written or oral cues for organizing an activity (e.g., step one, step two...).
- Practice sequencing material.
- Color-coded materials for each class (book, notebook, and supplies).
- Assigned person to review schedule at start of school day and organize materials for each class.
- Outline coordinated to class lectures. Require student to take notes within each section.

Following Directions

- Provide oral as well as written instructions.
- Ask student to repeat instructions back to teacher or a peer.
- Underline or highlight significant part of directions on written assignments.
- Rewrite complex directions into simple steps.
- After giving directions, ask student to perform the task, check for accuracy, then give immediate feedback.

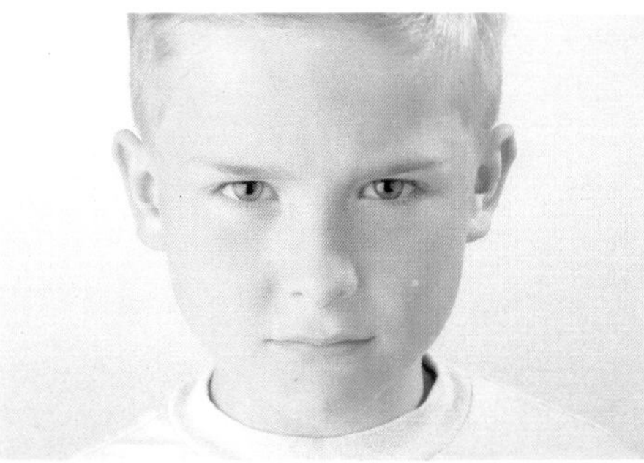

Addressing Unwanted Behaviors

Unwanted behaviors are common following brain injury. It is important for school personnel to have a clear plan for addressing behaviors when the child returns to school. Hospital/rehabilitation staff can help school personnel develop behavior intervention plans. This can be done by helping educators understand the behaviors associated with the child's brain injury, alerting them to behavioral issues during hospitalization, and sharing useful techniques for addressing the child's behavior. Tyler and Mira (1999) provided the following general guidelines to help prevent, reduce, or even eliminate unwanted behavior.

- Establish a behavioral intervention plan.

  Decrease unwanted behaviors and/or increase positive behaviors.

- Teach the child appropriate behavior.

  Clearly state what is appropriate behavior, model behavior, and reinforce appropriate behavior.

- Provide adequate supervision.

  Do not assume the child is at the same developmental level for controlling impulses and regulating behavior as peers the same age.

- Use time-out only when necessary.

  Have an established plan with a designated safe area with proper supervision if child becomes so disruptive that removal from the environment is necessary.

- Provide rest breaks.

  Unwanted behaviors often become more frequent and intensive when the child is tired.

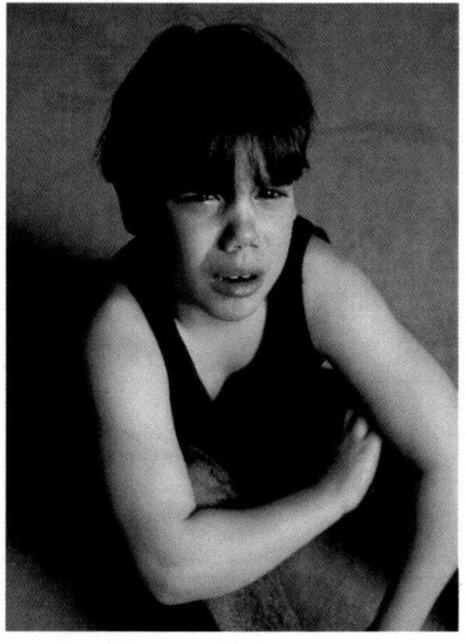

- Provide direct social skills training.

  Unwanted behaviors may occur because the child has forgotten how to interact with others.

- Arrange for positive interactions with peers.

Social isolation may cause the child to act out inappropriately to gain other children's attention. Establish a system for providing interactions with other students on a regular basis.

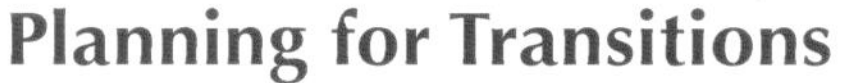

Planning for Transitions

The responsibility of hospital/rehabilitation staff does not end with the child's return to school. Rather, planning and programming for students with brain injuries is an ongoing process. It begins with planning for school re-entry the moment the student is injured and continues through transition from high school to post secondary education, employment, and community living. This planning requires the combined efforts of all those involved in the child's life, including hospital/rehabilitation staff, educators, community service providers, the child's family, and the student.

Ongoing monitoring and planning for transitions is crucial. An injury during childhood occurs to a brain that is still developing. The impact of the injury can continue to show up even years after the injury (Klonoff, Clark, & Klonoff, 1993; Eslinger et al., 1992; Price et al., 1990). New problems may arise over time, as the demands of school and life become even greater and more challenging for the student.

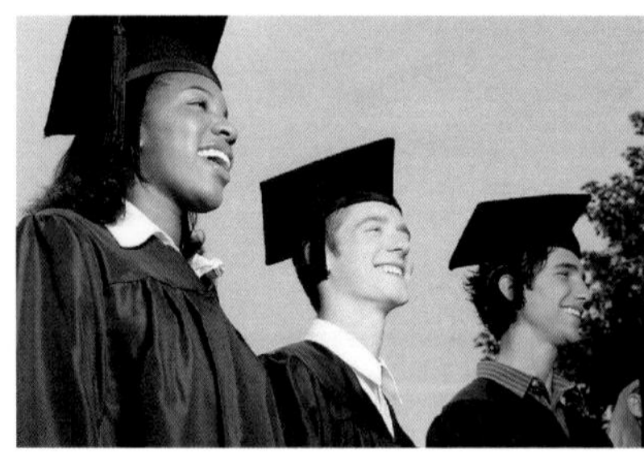

Planning not only must consider the child's current functioning, but also continual assessment of needs over the school career and on into adulthood.

The ongoing involvement of hospital and rehabilitation staff in this

School Transitions

- Recognize the need for transition planning.
- Begin transition planning early.
- Assess the new environment and determine needs.
- Prepare receiving teachers (e.g., brain injury in-service).
- Provide teachers with specific information about the student.
- Involve ancillary personnel (medical, psychological, rehabilitation).
- Continually monitor progress.

planning process is very important because of the continuing medical, rehabilitation, psychological, and cognitive needs of the child. In addition to sharing information with the school team and helping them plan for the child's return to school, hospital/rehabilitation staff must continue to provide input to help school staff and family plan throughout the years. Information from follow-up medical, rehabilitation, and neuropsychological evaluations provide valuable information to help the school determine the child's current functioning and assess progress.

Ongoing communication between school staff and the child's physicians, psychologist, and therapists allows for discussion of new concerns (e.g., late on-set seizures). It also provides important data to evaluate a current course of treatment (e.g., behavior charting of the effects of medication on behavioral performance). Because continued involvement of medical and rehabilitation staff is needed, those key persons should be listed as part of the team on the child's IEP.

Within School Transitions

Following the child's return to school, there will be many transitions over the years before finishing high school. These transitions include moving from grade level to grade level, the change from elementary to middle and then high school, and finally, graduation. While these transitions can be difficult at times for any student, they can be particularly troublesome for students with brain injuries. The student's difficulties may be partially due to cognitive and behavioral impairments that often occur following a brain injury. Such impairments may make it difficult for the student to adjust to changes in environments, routines, and expectations. As school work becomes more complex and requires higher-level thinking skills and more independent learning, new difficulties may surface as the student moves through the educational system (Tyler & Wilkerson, 1999).

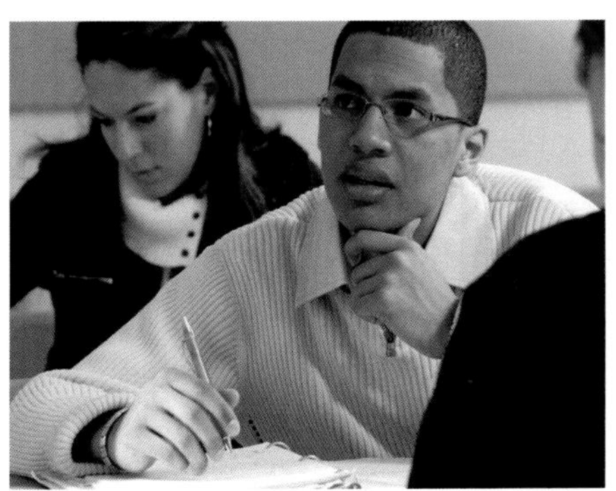

Tyler, Wilkerson, and DePompei (2001) offer the following suggestions for transitions in school:

- Recognize the need for transition planning.
- Begin transition planning early.
- Assess the new environment and determine needs.
- Prepare receiving teachers through each grade change and each school change (e.g., brain injury in-service).
- Provide teachers with specific information about the student.
- Involve ancillary personnel (medical, psychological, rehabilitation).
- Continually monitor progress.

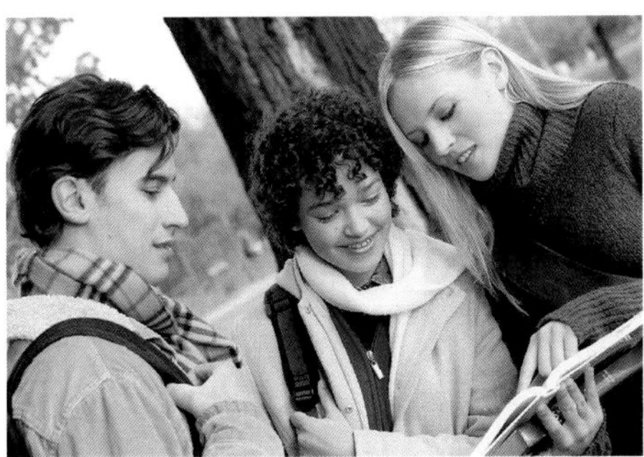

Transition to Post-Secondary Education

Available options and suitable placement must be carefully considered for students with brain injuries who pursue post secondary education (e.g., vocational school, community college, junior college, four-year university). If special education services were needed in high school, the student is likely to need special assistance or accommodations at the post secondary level.

Public Law 101-476 (IDEA), which provided funding for special education, does not apply to college. Eligibility for special education ends upon graduation from high school or age 21 years (22 in some states).

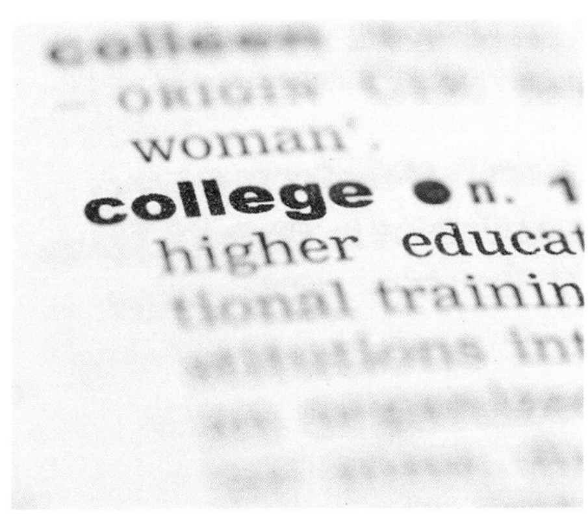

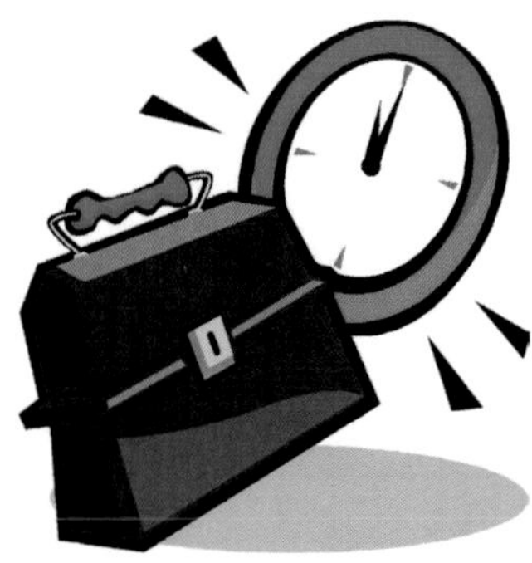

Fortunately, individuals with brain injuries can receive services under Section 504 of the Rehabilitation Act in post secondary settings. Section 504 requires all post secondary institutions that receive federal education funds to provide necessary accommodations to help students with disabilities participate. Accommodations are made on a case-by-case basis and may include such things as un-timed exams, extended time on assignments, tape-recorded textbooks, and preferential seating. The types of accommodations are determined by individual institutions and, therefore, vary widely among schools. Consequently, evaluating an institution's capacity to provide such services is critical (Goodwin & Larson, 1999; Tyler & Mira, 1999).

Some colleges offer special services, such as study skills classes, tutoring in subject areas, support groups and special counselors. These are not required, but are offered voluntarily. There may be a fee for the service. There are also a limited number of colleges with special programs designed specifically for students with brain injuries. Information about them is available from the Brain Injury Association of America or state chapters.

The high school is responsible for helping the student choose an appropriate post secondary setting if the student was injured prior to graduation. This can be done through Individual Transition Plans (ITP), a part of an IEP beginning at age 16. The high school is also responsible for preparing the student to make the transition. However, for students first entering or returning to college after a brain injury, the hospital or rehabilitation staff should provide assistance. This may come in the form of establishing linkages with campus support services to gather information and plan accommodations.

Transition to Work and Community

Schools can provide very supportive community-like environments for the student to succeed, but experiences after school can become a nightmare if not well planned. Independent living centers, community–based advocacy agencies, and other support systems need to be involved in the student's educational program before graduation to establish a coordinated transition plan from school to community.

In planning for transition to employment, coordination with community vocational resources is essential (Bergland, 1996). The transition planning team must be aware of and informed about the range of available vocational services. For example, students with brain injuries may be eligible for services from their state vocational rehabilitation agency. This may include aptitude assessment, post-high school training, and supervised trial job placement. Transition to employment planning should include vocational assessment and counseling to help identify suitable occupations.

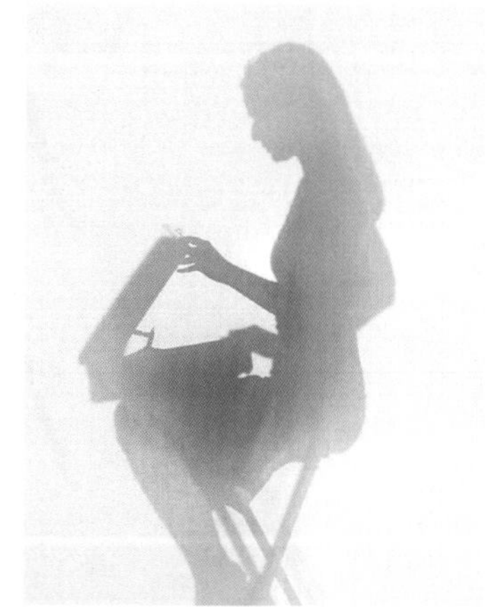

The process of determining eligibility for such services should be facilitated by the student's transition planning team. However, beware of the trap of looking for a set of jobs that are best for students with brain injuries. Rather, the focus should be on using the assessment information and the student's strengths, preferences and goals to establish vocational objectives (Tyler & Mira, 1999).

Linkages with adult service providers must be established during the high school years for the student to transition from school to community living.

Linkages include Social Security programs, independent living centers, and residential service providers. Coordination with programs that provide assistance to adults with disabilities (e.g., state head injury waiver programs) is essential. It is important for transition planners to be aware of the type and kind of services available, eligibility requirements, availability of services at the local level, and procedures for completing applications. Because some programs have waiting lists, it is important to begin planning well in advance of the need for services.

Summary

The establishment of pediatric critical care systems, new referral guidelines, and the inclusion of the category of traumatic brain injury in IDEA have given health care providers, schools, and families an opportunity to work together. By doing so, they can provide a continuum of services that will meet the special needs of the child or adolescent with a brain injury.

Early referral by health care providers and joint development of Individualized Education Plans will enable professionals to work together and provide needed services to families and children. By starting collaborative planning with schools early in the rehabilitation setting, there can be a unified, ongoing program for the child and family.

References

Bergland, M (1996). Transition from school to adult life: Key to the future. In A. Goldberg (Ed.), Acquired brain injury in childhood and adolescence (pp. 171-194). Springfield, IL: Thomas.

Blosser, J & DePompei, R (1994). Pediatric traumatic brain injury: Proactive intervention. San Diego, CA: Singular.

Centers for Disease Control (2006). "Traumatic Brain Injury in the United States: Emergency Department Visits, Hospitalizations, and Deaths."

DePompei R., Blosser, J, Savage, R, & Lash, M. (1999a). Back to school after a moderate to severe brain injury. Wake Forest, NC: Lash and Associates Publishing/Training Inc.

DePompei R, Blosser, J, Savage, R, & Lash, M (1999). Special education IEP checklist for a student with a brain injury. Wake Forest, NC: Lash and Associates Publishing/Training Inc.

DiScala, C, Osberg, JS, & Savage, RC (1997). Children hospitalized for traumatic brain injury: Transition to postacute care. Journal of Head Trauma Rehabilitation, 12(2), 1-10.

Eslinger, PJ, Grattan, LM, Damasio, H, & Damasio, AR (1992). Developmental consequences of childhood frontal lobe damage. Archives of Neurology, 49, 764-769.

Goodwin, J, & Larson, L (1999). Going to college when a student has a brain injury. Wake Forest, NC: Lash and Associates Publishing/Training.

Individuals with Disabilities Education Act of 1990, 20 U.S.C. § 1400 et seq.

Klonoff , H, Clark, C, & Klonoff, PS (1993). Long-term outcome of head injuries: A 23 year follow up study of children with head injuries. Journal of Neurology, Neurosurgery & Psychiatry, 56, 410-415.

Price, BH, Doffner, KR., Stowe, RM., & Mesulam, MM (1990). The compartmental learning disabilities of early frontal lobe damage, Brain, 113, 1383-1394.

Rehabilitation Act of 1973, 29 U.S.C. § 701 et seq.

Savage, RC (1991). Identification, classification, and placement issues for students with traumatic brain injuries. Journal of Head Trauma Rehabilitation, 6(1), 1-9.

Savage, RC (1997). Integrating rehabilitation and education services for school-age children with brain injuries. Journal of Head Trauma Rehabilitation, 12(2), 11-20.

Savage, R & Wolcott, G (Eds.) (1995). An educator's manual: What educators need to know about students with traumatic brain injury. Washington, DC: Brain Injury Association, Inc.

Tyler, J, Blosser, J, & DePompei, R (1999). Teaching strategies for students with Brain Injuries. Wake Forest, NC: Lash and Associates Publishing/Training Inc.

Tyler, JS & Mira, M (1999). Traumatic brain injury in children and adolescents: A sourcebook for teachers and other school personnel (2nd Ed.). Austin, TX: PRO-ED.

Tyler, JS & Wilkerson, LR (1999). Planning school transition for students with TBI. Brain Injury Source, 3(3), 14-16, 54.

Tyler, J, Wilkerson, L, & DePompie, R (2001). Planning In-school Transitions for Students with Brain Injury. Wake Forest, NC: Lash and Associates Publishing/Training Inc.

Ylvisaker, M, Hartwick, P & Stevens, MB (1991). School reentry following head injury: Managing the transition from hospital to school. Journal of Head Trauma Rehabilitation, 6(1), 10-22.

Ylvisaker, M,, Todis, B., Glang, A., Urbanczyk, B., Franklin, C., DePompei, R., Feeney, T., Maxwell, N.M., Pearson, S., Tyler, J.S. (2001). Educating students with TBI: Themes and Recommendations. Journal of Head Trauma Rehabilitation, 16, 76-93.

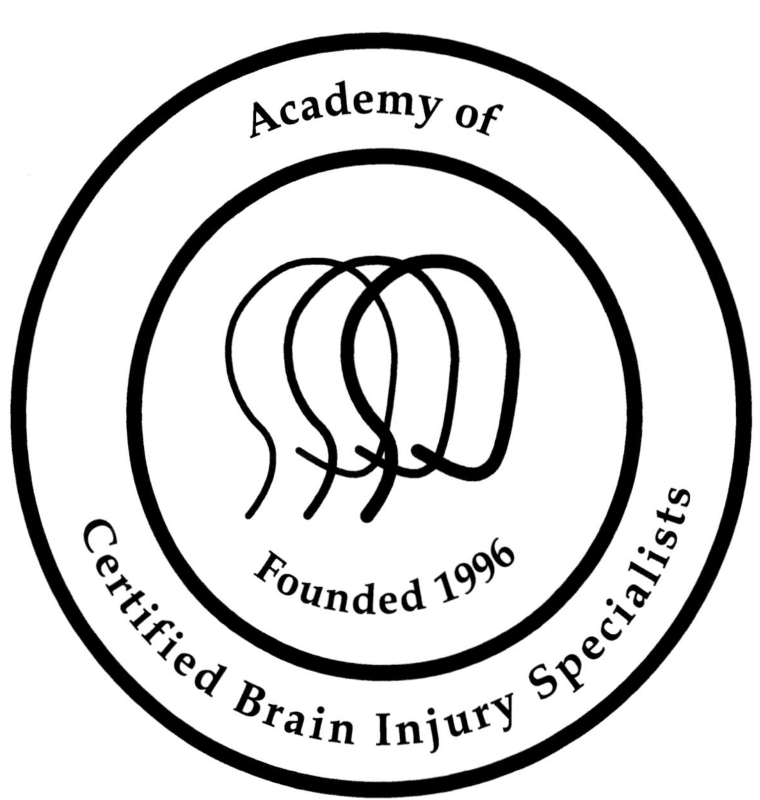
Academy of
Founded 1996
Certified Brain Injury Specialists

Chapter 7

Brain Injury: A Family Perspective

Learning Objectives

By the end of this chapter, you will be able to:

- Describe the impact of brain injury on the family.
- Understand the severity of trauma that families experience.
- Educate the family about current and future brain-related challenges.
- Identify different methods for interacting with families.

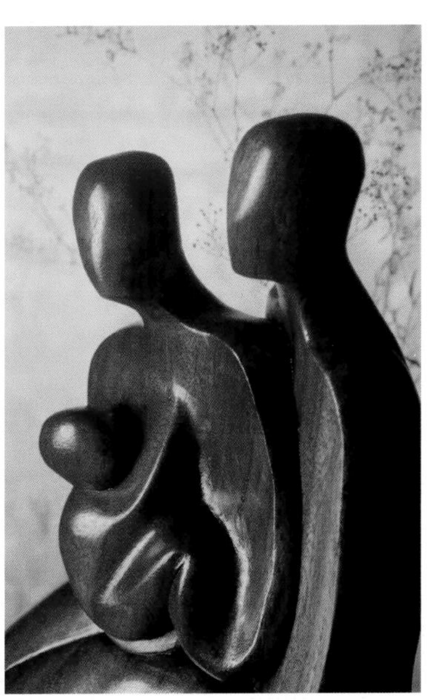

Introduction

There is a tremendous impact on families, close friends, or communities when a loved one experiences a brain injury. It is imperative that staff recognize the magnitude of challenges for the person with the brain injury, the family and other support systems in order to maximize recovery during the rehabilitation process. Education about what occurs when a loved one has a brain injury must be fused with the needs of those who are caring for the survivor. This combination of education and support is a delicate balance.

A Family's Point of View

The devastation that is associated with a brain injury is often beyond comprehension until the complexity of the injury is understood. It is not just a physical injury in which surgery or medications resolve the problems. Recovery is often dependent on many issues including access to rehabilitation services, support systems for the family, and the restoration abilities with the family system. The key often depends on pre-injury cohesiveness, family attitudes about illness and responsibilities, and economic as well as social supports. The entire support system can be strained and disrupted as a direct consequence of the individual's brain injury.

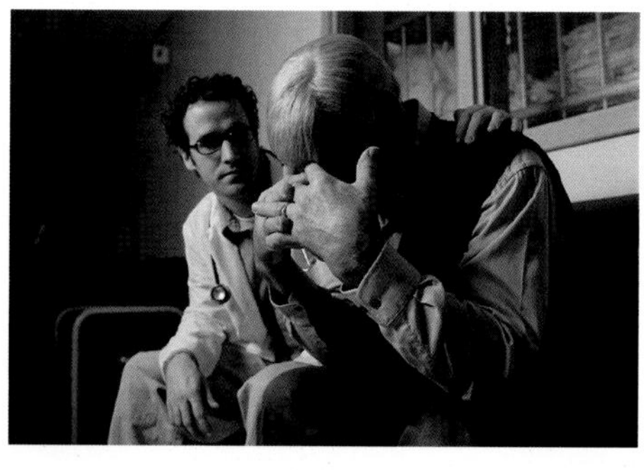

Families may experience isolation, loss of emotional support, restricted independence, and financial strain. Psychologically they may feel bewilderment, frustration, guilt, trepidation, and depression. The majority of family members typically have little or no knowledge about brain injury, rehabilitation, disabilities, or deficits. In the beginning, a family's emotions are like a roller coaster that never stops. Their feelings are constantly changing from fear to confusion to anger to pain to desolation.

A traumatic brain injury creates complex and long-term demands on the family system and often the community as well. A common denominator for all families is the awareness that they have been forcibly changed forever with no idea of what the future holds.

It is not uncommon for these demands to exhaust the most resourceful of families. It is imperative that staff who provide services of any type are aware of the multiple needs of families and understand the devastation associated with the physical injury, the emotional instability of the family, and the financial burdens associated with care.

Family Adjustments

Helping a family adjust to the impact of a brain injury requires attentive listening to their needs during the entire process of brain injury restoration. As the family struggles to achieve some sense of equilibrium, it is a difficult process of adjusting to the many problems and changes. Professionals

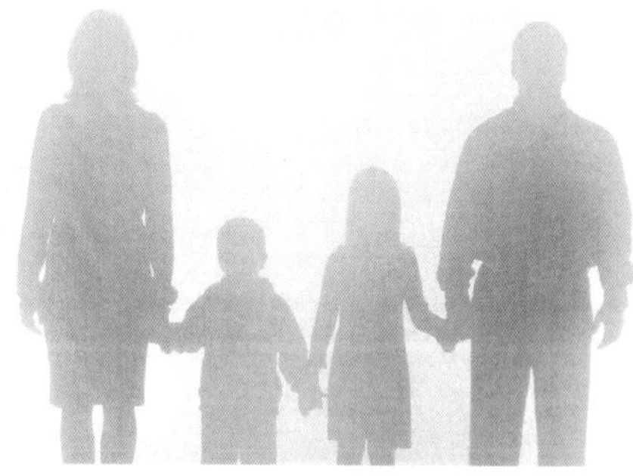

must first understand the process of recovery following a brain injury and merge this knowledge with the needs of the family. The many stages of recovery from a brain injury include the adjustments within the family unit.

Although there are different stages that are identified in the model of recovery, not all survivors progress through the systemic stages evenly. The stages of recovery for persons with brain injuries are an approximation - every survivor brings a unique recovery curve and rate of resurgence.

Stage 1 – One to Three Months

During this first stage of recovery, the shock of what has occurred dominates the minds of the family as they focus their energy on praying for

A traumatic brain injury creates complex and long-term demands on the family system and often the community as well. A common denominator for all families is the awareness that they have been forcibly changed forever with no idea of what the future holds.

recovery. They have great hopes of full recovery in a short period of time. As they adjust to the situation, they often develop denial, which is associated with the severity of the situation and with no experience about brain injury. They may assume that when their loved one wakes up, the person will be the same - maybe just a little bruised. They repress their feelings, avoid discussing the severity of the situation, and transfer their negative feelings onto others. They may revert to a child-like form of communication with the person who has been injured, even with an adult.

Stage 2 – Three to Nine Months

As the family continues to adjust to the situation, they begin to recognize the severity of the situation and their feelings of helplessness and frustration often escalate. The reality of the circumstances changes the feelings of denial to those of anxiety, anger, fear, depression, and loss. They realize that the person has a serious condition and they lack the knowledge about what will happen next or what they can do.

Stage 3 – Six to Twenty-Four Months

Family members often get a little annoyed with the survivor, thinking that the person is not trying hard enough. In reality, the person may be just starting to regain or relearn functioning in some areas. The family still expects the person to reach independence, but they may now experience feelings of depression, more guilt, and discouragement. They are starting to recognize that the person is more impaired than they first thought. Moreover, they realize that there is really nothing they can do to speed up the healing process. At this time, many family members reread the materials that are provided by the rehabilitation facilities and may start seeking additional information about the process of living with a brain injury.

Stage 4 – Ten to Twenty Four Months

This is the beginning of realism. The injured individual continues to appear different and sometimes the disability or negative behaviors bother the family immensely. The survivor may act like a child or behave rudely. Family members often have to take additional breaks to tolerate some of the un-constructive behaviors and they fear that the person may act this way permanently. At this point, some family members may reduce their time at the rehabilitation facility or change their communications from face-to-face to telephone.

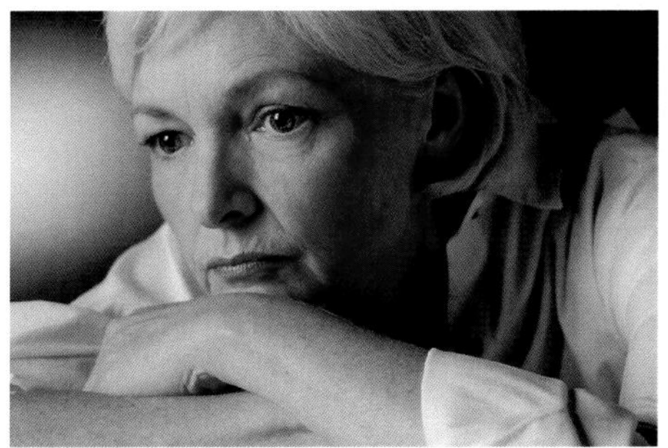

Stages of Adjustment for Families

Stage 1:	The shock of the injury dominates. Hopes for full recovery. Repressed feeling and denial of severity.
Stage 2:	Recognition of the severity of the injury. Helplessness and frustration.
Stage 3:	Start to get annoyed with survivor. Family expects full independence. Start to recognize that reality of impairments. Start information seeking about brain injury.
Stage 4:	Realism of situation sets in. Family begins to get exhausted. Reduction of time with loved one. Bereavement like emotions may occur.
Stage 5:	Profound sadness. Families begin to grieve again. Mourn the loss of loved one's personality.
Stage 6:	Greater understanding of the situation. Understand the person may never be the same. Begins to accept loved one's condition. Can now address needs of the entire family unit.

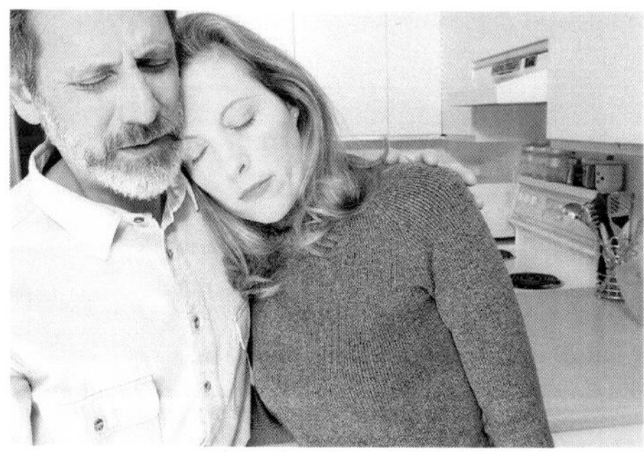

The family is also exhausted from the ordeal and lacks the stamina to continue at this pace. They feel desolated and despondent about what has occurred and they may feel trapped in the situation. Counselors are very important during this stage as the family often feels emotions similar to those of bereavement - their loved one has died and they do not know the new person in this family member's body.

Stage 5 – Twelve to Twenty Four Months

This is a time of profound sadness with few expectations. The grieving cycle often starts over again and the family requires special attention as they go through this stage. With time and support, most families pass this stage and progress toward understanding what has occurred. Family members mourn the loss of the survivor's personality characteristics, their way of responding to situations, and their shared future dreams. A part of the unique distinctiveness of the person is gone and they are aware of the void associated with the loss. They are experiencing the anguishing process of accepting the losses.

Stage 6 – Two to Three Years After the Injury

The family has now invested more time in understanding what has occurred, the severity of the injury, and the outcomes for the future. They accept that the person may never be the same as before the brain injury, but they are willing to change the roles of the family to accommodate the situation.

In healthy families, there is a dramatic change in the family as they accept their loved one's condition and the changes. Family members no longer feel guilty and become creative in helping the person who has been injured. They understand what has occurred and they now can address the needs of the entire family unit. The family has become well versed about brain injury and invests time in procuring or spending money on accommodations (e.g., ramps for wheelchairs, assistive technology for increasing self-determination, charts and devices for helping in independence, adjustments in family employment, etc). The family has transferred the anguish to something that offers family sovereignty; they have re-empowered the family unit.

As a person working with someone with a brain injury, it is important to understand the stages of recovery and the fact that not all family members go through these stages evenly. Difficulties may arise from medical conditions that complicate the process of adjusting to the stages of successful recovery. During these periods of challenges, listening to the needs of the family offers the most support that you can provide. Be creatively realistic and provide the resources for the family while understanding that the reality of the brain injury cannot be eradicated. The family can be helped to move beyond the losses to transforming the experience through healthy family relationship once again.

Working with Systems

Health care and rehabilitation systems are generally not designed to address the needs of families. The stress of working with different systems begins for families during the individual's initial treatment in the emergency department and escalates as subsequent medical procedures involve multiple transfers and introduction of new personnel both within and between hospitals. As a result, families are often separated from supports and feel abandoned early in the process. Just listening to the needs of the families provides initial support that is desperately needed to help them cope with this devastation.

The brain injury of a family member challenges the core values and resources of the family system.

Providing Information to Families

- The timing of imparting information is crucial, especially following the initial injury.
- Early and appropriate communication of information by professionals can greatly diminish a family's anxiety.
- Offering a small packet or booklet about the basics of brain injury often reduces confusion and allows the family to read the information at their own speed and in their own time.

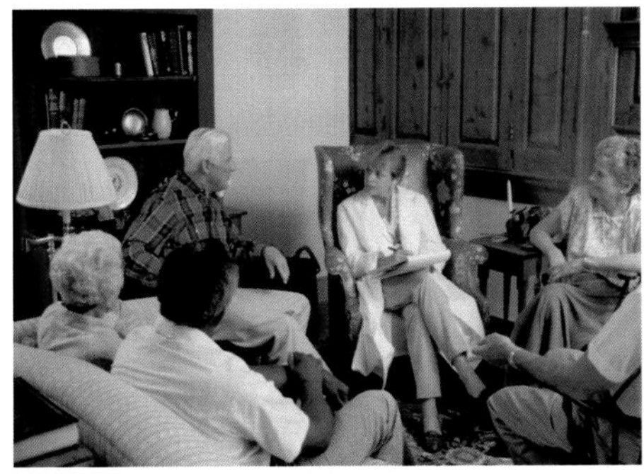

The family's understanding of brain injury depends on the kind of information provided and the ability of family members to understand and comprehend the complexities of what has occurred. The ability of staff to provide information in clear and understandable terms, to answer questions directly, and to provide diagrams to illustrate complex anatomy and procedures directly affects the family's comprehension. The interpersonal communication skills of staff during the delivery of difficult news also affect the family's understanding, as families need compassion and support as they try to absorb clinical information.

The timing of imparting information is crucial, especially following the initial injury. Health-care and rehabilitation professionals must listen to the needs of the family to determine how much information they can process at this time and to what extent. Early and appropriate communication of information by professionals can greatly diminish a family's anxiety and allow them to start working toward the inevitable change that occurs to the person with the brain injury and the family unit. Offering a small packet or booklet about the basics of brain injury often reduces confusion and allows the family to read the information at their own speed and in their own time. An organized family packet is a valuable resource because families may have difficulty assimilating and remembering information given to them, especially during these early stages (Mackay, 1997) It is also advantageous to provide information from the Brain Injury Association of

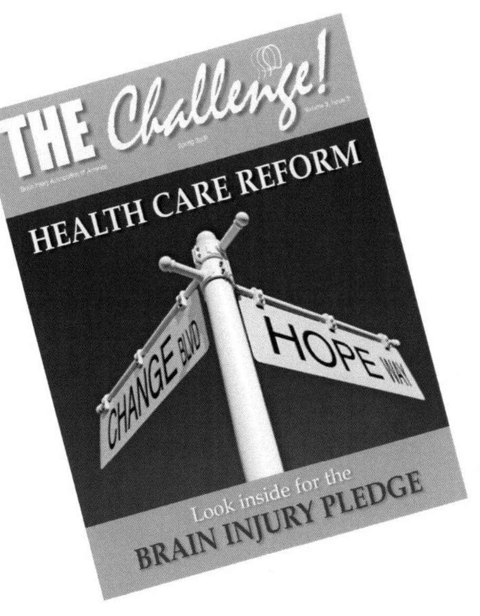

Family Strengths

1. Ability of the family to listen.
2. Shared and common perceptions of reality within the family, including the changes that often happen following a brain injury.
3. Spirituality of the family.
4. Ability of the family to realize the redemptive power of a seemingly tragic event.
5. Ability of family members to accept and assist in any disability-related problems, including education of the family about possible resolutions.
6. Ability of the family to compromise within the family unit.
7. Family members' willingness to take good care of themselves.
8. Ability to focus on the present, rather than on past events or disappointments.
9. Ability of family members to provide reinforcements for each other.
10. Ability of family members to discuss concerns.
11. Ability of family members to provide an atmosphere of belonging.
12. Use of the family's effective trans-generational coping strategies building on family strengths that have always been effective in solving problems within the family.

America, including their website, address, phone number, and family help line information. This Association has affiliations in most states that can assist families in obtaining more information.

Family's Reactions to Changes

The impact of a brain injury often alters the roles, principles or rules, and internal responsibilities of the family. All aspects of family life may be changed and major modifications in the structure and organization of the family should be anticipated. This change stresses the family unit, as routines, social status, family health, and behaviors of the individual who has been injured are altered. As a result, the family may be unable or have difficulty adjusting to the "different" person with the brain injury. Research on family functioning following a brain injury recognizes that there are standard patterns of family functioning that can place families at high risk for becoming dysfunctional. These patterns include:

- Premorbid history of family problems such as marital stress, abuse, or alcoholism.

Grief

Grief is a normal and healthy reaction to loss. However, this emotion is not a simple feeling as it is combined with the past, present, and future dreams for this loved one.

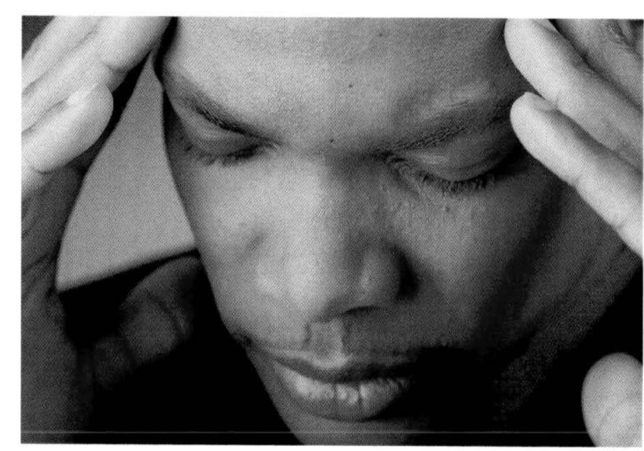

- Extended period of denial.
- Lack of basic supports.
- Persistent and severe cognitive or physical impairments of the person with the brain injury.

A recent study identified that variance in family outcome at year one follow-up was best explained by distressed family function at hospital discharge and memory/attention problems with patients with TBI (Testa, Malec, Moessner & Brown, 2006). A baseline assessment of family function is suggested to assist in the identification of families at increased risk for problems after TBI.

These difficulties must be identified by the treating professionals in the beginning of the rehabilitation process and their influences on the family unit distinctly clarified. Often these problems are identified by the direct care staff and are directed to the psychologist or social worker for family adjustments. For example, if the issue is substance abuse, the counselor may provide direct therapy or suggest support from the family's local church or AA program. This additional support may assist the family toward resolving premorbid family problems that may have been magnified by the current situation.

If some family members have not accepted what has happened to the loved one, a counselor may be able to help them start the painful mourning process together. Staff may invest additional time educating the family about the ramifications of severe impairments and differentiating between physiological versus psychological challenges. Once professionals and staff identify any dysfunction within the family, they may be able to provide additional supports to fill their current needs.

The identification of family strengths is also very important and can help pinpoint existing family resources, buttress these resources, and indicate areas where interventions may be needed. The list below may help the professional determine optimal pathways for successful interventions:

The occurrence of brain injury in a family can generate closer relationships among family members or it can fragment the family by creating a state of disorganization and dysfunction. Early and continuing intervention by health care and rehabilitation professionals, as well as other support staff (e.g., community supports), is necessary as they can be the effective catalysts for successful coping and eventual modifications. It is imperative that professionals remember that all families are uniquely complex and bring a personal history to the experience of brain injury. No two families or family situations will be exactly the same, nor will be their way of handling this event. Listening to the family is the optimum method of determining their needs and desires during this traumatic event.

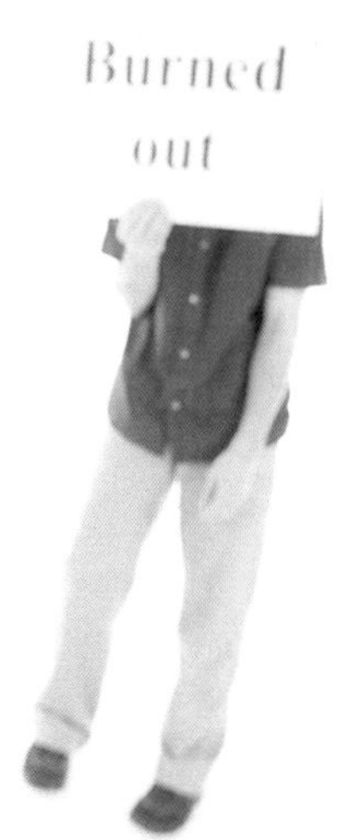

Blaming and Grieving

It is not uncommon for family members to blame or rationalize their behaviors, or the behaviors of others, for what has occurred. This response is a typical reaction to how the family views the crisis. It may indicate that they see the injury as unjust and beyond their ability to manage at this time. This is usually a method for alleviating family distress associated with the crisis.

In addition, family members often attempt to thwart intense emotional conflicts by intellectualizing what has occurred. In order to begin the healing process of this crisis, it is suggested that all significant family members discuss the dynamics of their grieving and allow each to appropriately express their emotional pain.

As a professional, you will be required to pay attention to these lost dreams while offering comfort, education, and support as you facilitate coping strategies for dealing with their losses.

Allow families to express their feelings of grief, anger, and disappointment and remember that these emotions are the natural process of grieving. In some cases, families may respond angrily to your involvement; do not personalize it, especially during the grieving process, as their pain may be more than they can bear and adds to their grief. With time and good support, family members usually return to the recovery process and redevelop a positive relationship with the professional. Opening the door for further counseling is appropriate at that time.

Family or individual counseling during the rehabilitation process can be offered on a regular basis by establishing specific times when staff, or a facility counselor can be provided. For out-patient or community programs, counseling can be obtained from local resources, such as state and city funded counseling agencies, nonprofit hospitals with out-patient programs, churches that offer professional counseling services, mental health programs provided by family insurance programs, and even schools that provide counseling. Offering assistance with any problems may increase the trust between the family and professional staff.

The behavioral, emotional, and cognitive problems are usually the most difficult for family members to manage, combined with the hidden financial and physical costs associated with caring for a person with a brain injury. These "costs" severely impair, if not destroy, many families. They always require the attention of the professional if the needs of the family are to be met.

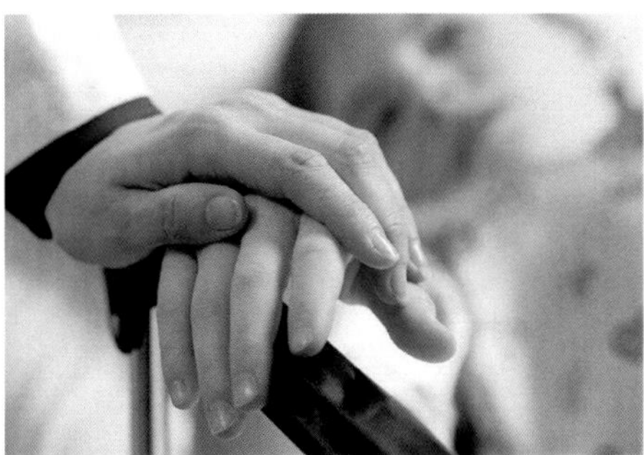

Care-Taking

The parent or spouse of the person with the brain injury is often pushed into, or takes on, the role of the primary caretaker even if the survivor is an adult. This position often places considerable strain on family resources. Problems of dependency from previous roles may develop, (e.g., an adult versus a child). It is understood that children often need assistance in some situations and adults usually accept this role without question. They may need help in basic care-taking needs, such as bathing, eating, mobility, nurturing, developing skills, etc. However, an adult who is cognitively like a child may also need these same requirements, but they are often more difficult to provide, (e.g., lifting the adult survivor into a bath, correcting inappropriate responses, teaching the basic skills again, etc.).

It is physically and emotionally exhausting and family members are thrown back into roles that they once completed during the individual's developmental stages years before. Family members, who are retired often take on the full time job as the primary caregiver. Other family members leave their current career and become the primary caregiver, which often strains the finances as well as the emotional stability of the family.

While the stresses for parents and spouses differ when the individual becomes neurologically impaired, there are some core similarities. Foremost is the need to make preparations for the lifelong care and well-being of the survivor in the future. However, problems may occur when the parents or spouse disagree over the care of the individual. In some situations, family members may experience feelings of neglect as they become overwhelmed by the demands of care-taking. Sharing family responsibilities and recognizing personal needs in relationships are as important as caring for the family member with a brain injury.

Children or Siblings

Families experience a multitude of emotions that are difficult to recognize and manage after a member has sustained a brain injury. Children may react to what has occurred with responses ranging from hysteria to shock. Physiologically, they may lack the conceptual maturity to comprehend what has happened.

A child that has been traumatized by the situation will show signs of extremes in areas of behaviors, either by under-responding or over-responding to the crisis. The signs are often found in the areas of cognitive, emotional, physical, and behavioral arenas.

The signs of traumatized children are similar to the symptoms of adults, but unfortunately children lack the abilities to process large amounts of information and to tolerate the abrupt changes in the family and situation. They do not understand the severity of the problem. They feel the void of not having the loved one available and the attention that was provided. Young children watch cartoons where people shoot each other and then get up. They see characters fly without a plane, travel in space without a spaceship, and jump off large buildings or mountains without injury (think about the cartoon of the road runner and the coyote where the road runner crashes and gets up each time). Children do not understand how permanent a disability can be for the person who has been injured nor that it has affected the entire family. If the sibling is the younger child, they may have difficulty understanding if the older role model now functions at a lower level. When assisting children who have a loved one that has sustained a significant disability, it is important to understand what they may be feeling from this crisis.

In addition, children often feel some guilt even if they were not involved or present when the injury occurred. The professional must ensure the child(ren) that they had nothing to do with the injury and remind them that, "This is why we call them accidents." They did not mean to cause such problems for the family. Families already have a great burden and their children's trauma adds to these burdens. Any individuals who are associated with these children, such as teachers, neighbors, extended family members, etc., must be in tune to the entire family's trauma which includes the children. These individuals may be able to identify the early signs of stress, notify and work with the treating professionals, and provide immediate care based on these symptoms.

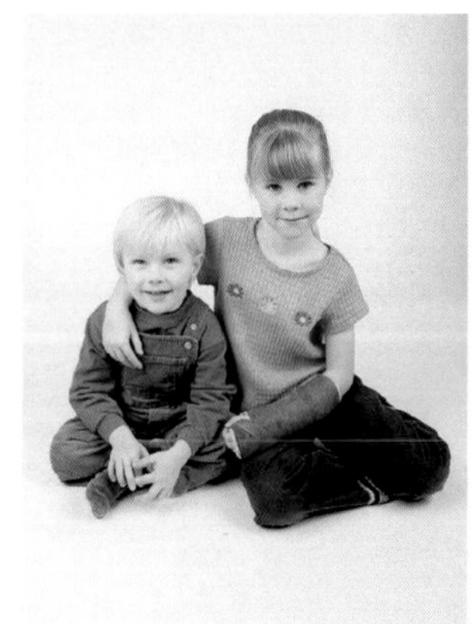

To magnify these difficulties for children, siblings often feel a major reduction in positive attention while their roles and responsibilities within the family are also changing. The person with the brain injury may be the father or mother whose young children do not understand what has occurred. The family has changed and siblings may feel cheated or angry at what has happened.

Communication about brain injury is important at this time, but information must be slowly introduced depending on age to avoid overwhelming or confusing the child. This is another part of the forced change and even children can feel this disruption in the family.

Educating the primary adult family members about how to talk with young children about the injury, the process of rehabilitation, and answering basic questions is crucial.

Children can see the disabilities and when information and explanations are not given, it often leads them to incorrect assumptions. There are many books and videos that explain a brain injury for children who have a parent with this disability. The brain injury is often a lifelong impairment and slowly educating the entire family, including the children, is imperative.

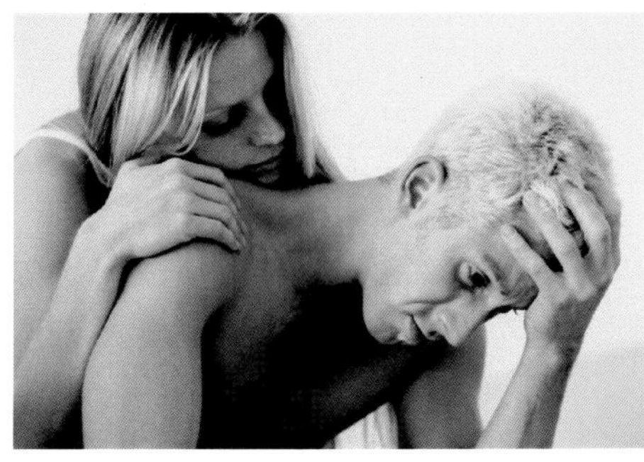

Sexual Concerns

Sexual issues for adults with brain impairments, as well as their partners, are often altered. Changes may range from impotency to aggression. For adolescents, sexual issues can result in a myriad of problems in the school setting. Depression and role changes can also affect sexual functioning. Many spouses have a difficult time changing their role from caregiver to sexual partner, especially when their spouse with the brain injury exhibits child-like behaviors.

On the other side of the spectrum, many persons with brain injuries are very vulnerable as their cognitive abilities are often immature. This leaves them at risk for harm by persons who can take advantage of the situation. Others feel that their injured spouse is very fragile and they are afraid of harming them during lovemaking.

Normal sexual interactions between adults are triggered by a large amount of physical and emotional desires. However, physiological and psychological stressors usually affect the sexual drive and often hamper the recovery of this part of the couple's relationship. In addition, damage to specific areas of the brain can alter sexual behaviors. For example, damage to the frontal lobes may result in disinhibition and the survivor may develop wanton behaviors. Memory problems and a strong desire to be touched may lead to constant demands for sexual interactions. Damage to the limbic system (in the center of the brain), medications, or hormonal imbalances may delay the person's ability to achieve orgasm or cause impotency. Alterations in the frontal neuronal connections (cingulate system) may lead to feelings of insecurity and a lack of cognitive flexibility.

A strong desire for sexual interactions may escalate to aggressive actions if these issues are not addressed. Problems occur if the person develops compulsions, negative thoughts, oppositional and argumentative behaviors, and in some cases, the person with a brain injury may have violent behaviors. The person may become very self-focused and this may result in difficulty with a reciprocal or "give and take" relationship. Medications can be suggested to help stabilize these negative behaviors and allow partners to interact in a more loving manner.

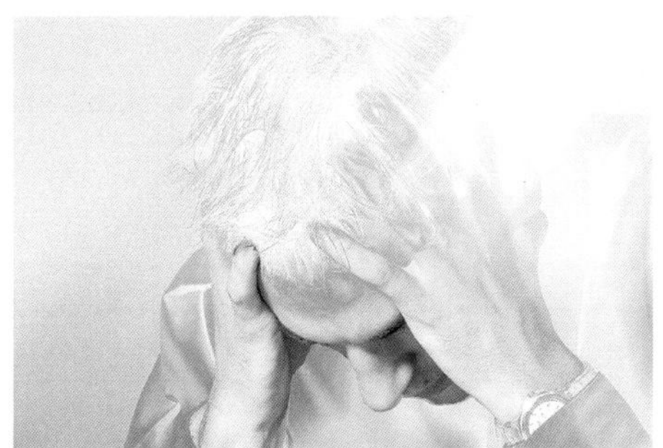

Understanding the causes of any behavioral changes, while learning about ways to communicate concerns, can maximize sexual adjustment after trauma.

Post Traumatic Stress Disorder and Families

Although most people understand the word trauma, few can actually define what an individual or a family may be experiencing following a traumatic event.

Basically trauma is defined as, "An emotional shock that creates substantial and lasting damage to the psychological development of an individual" and the main components are feelings of victimization, loss, and individual or family pathology.

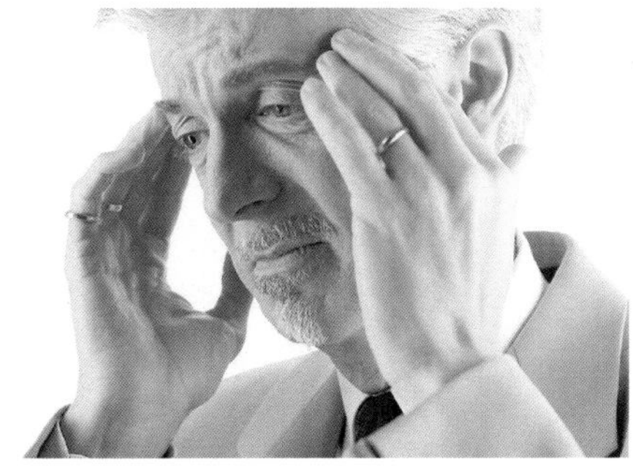

Most cases of post-traumatic stress disorder (PTSD), or acute or delayed situational stress, are healable but the experience of the trauma itself often scars the individual and the family. PTSD can also affect an entire family based on the fact that it is an anxiety reaction. For families who have a loved one with a brain injury, anxiety is usually one of the first emotions following the knowledge of the incident. As families attempt to grasp what has occurred, symptoms may appear that are often confused with simple mourning. To ensure that the

Symptoms of Post Traumatic Stress Disorder

1. **Vigilance and scanning** - Constant checking on what is going on beyond the normal questions and answers from the professionals.

2. **Elevated startle responses** - Being overly jumpy when startled and surprised.

3. **Blunted affect or psychic numbing** - There is a reduction of loss of the ability to feel. This may include a reduced ability to bond with others, especially other family members. It is usually a form of distancing in preparation for experiencing more pain.

4. **Aggressive, controlling behavior** - This form of aggression is not usually from the survivor but from family members. The person acts somewhat viciously to responses from people or situations.

5. **Interruption of memory and concentration** - Difficulty concentrating and remembering, even if just told about something.

6. **Depression** - Deep feelings of despondency, exhaustion, negative attitude, and apathy toward others.

7. **Generalized anxiety** - Tension in the body, cramps, headaches, stomachaches, etc., for no physical reason.

8. **Episodes of rage** - Not mild anger, this refers to violent eruptions to situations or people, often from a minor incident.

9. **Substance abuse** - In an attempt to reduce stress-related symptoms, the person may seek substances such as alcohol to numb feelings.

10. **Intrusive recall** - Old and negative memories suddenly appear from the past in the mind. These are the same type of responses that a person experiences during a nightmare. It makes the person feel very uncomfortable.

11. **Dissociative "flashback" experiences** - It is a form of intrusive recall where the person's mind replays a particular form of action that feels like it is happening now. It is an extremely emotionally charged memory.

12. **Insomnia** - Difficulty falling asleep or staying asleep. Sometimes the person has experienced nightmares or has reached a level of exhaustion that affects the ability to reach a restful sleep.

13. **Suicidal ideation** - There are thoughts of not wanting to live should their loved one die. The person is at a very low point in life because of what has occurred.

14. **Survivor guilt** - A common "trade off" belief where the family member prays for God to take him instead of the loved one. This is very common reaction when the survivor is a child.

professional understands PTSD, the list on page 133 can identify PTSD responses and the normal emotions of experiencing trauma.

It is important for professionals who are working with the family to pay attention to the items on the list . If a family member starts exhibiting many of these symptoms, a counselor must be contacted. It is essential to differentiate between normal mourning and PTSD, as trauma is the precursor to post-traumatic stress disorder for some individuals. Recognizing and treating these symptoms before they develop into a psychiatric disorder is one of the primary goals for the professional.

Summary

Brain injury changes and challenges the entire family system. It often confuses the present, negates the past, and distorts or destroys future dreams. To facilitate the process of learning, coping, adjusting, surviving, and living with a brain injury, the family needs timely and relevant interventions combined with authentic support.

Professionals must strive to incessantly validate what the family is experiencing, no matter how minor it may appear. Helping families cope with the emerging reality of brain injury is a process, not an event. It involves the efforts of health care and rehabilitation professionals, as well as other significant support persons who are attuned to the needs of the entire family unit including the person who has survived a brain injury.

Listen to the needs of family members as they will help you to do your job well. When their needs are met, the family's reaction to this traumatic experience comes from a position of strength, rather than by default. As professionals, we owe this to all the families and our communities.

In addition, offer extended supports such as support groups or advocacy services from the state affiliate of the Brain Injury Association of America. This provides an opportunity to get to know other families who have experienced, and continue to experience, the ramifications of brain injury. It is never easy but it is emotionally and physically survivable most of the time if they are given the right tools!

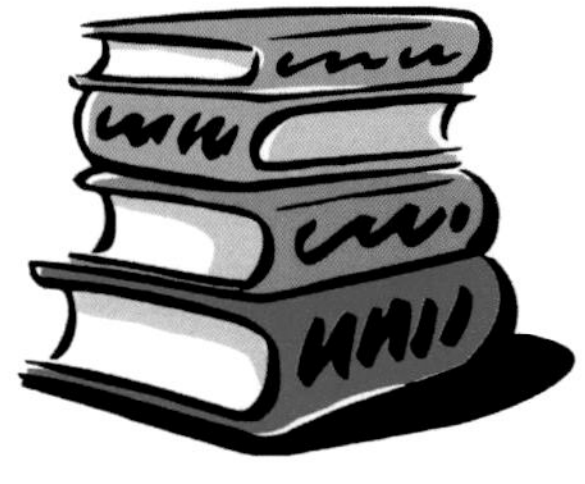

References

Amen, D (1998). Firestorms in the Brain: An Inside Look at Violent Behavior. Fairfield, CA: Mind Words Press.

Amen, D (1998). Change Your Brain, Change Your Life. New York: Random House, Inc.

American Psychiatric Association (1998). Diagnostic and Statistical Manual of Mental Disorders (4th Edition). Washington, D.C. X

Buhot, MC (1997). Serotonin receptors in cognitive behaviors. Current Opinion in Neurobiology, 7, 243-254.

Cera, RM, Vulanch, NN & Brady, WA (1995). Patients with Brain Injury: A Family Guide to Assisting in Speech, Language, and Cognitive Rehabilitation. Austin, Texas: Pro-Ed.

Colodzin, B. (1993). How to survive trauma. New York: Station Hill Press.

Curtiss, G, Klemz, S, & Vanderploeg, RD (2000). Acute Impact of Severe Traumatic brain injury on Family Structures and Coping Responses. Journal of Head Trauma Rehabilitation 15(5); 1113-1122.

Dell Orto, AE & Power, PW (1994). Head Injury and the Family: A Life and Living Perspective. Winter Park, Florida: PMD Publishers Group, Inc.

Delehanty, R. & Kieren, D. (1999). Family Perceptions of Health Professionals in Family Problem Solving After Brain Injury. The Journal of Cognitive Rehabilitation 16(3); 14-23.

Gill, DJ & Wells, DL (2000). Forever Different: Experiences of Living with a Sibling who has a Traumatic brain injury. Rehabilitation Nursing 25(3); 48-53.

Iverson, G & Osman, A (1998). Behavioral Interventions for Children and Adults with Brain Injuries: A Guide for Families. The Journal of Cognitive Rehabilitation 16(2); 14-23.

Johnson, K (1998). Trauma in the lives of children: Crisis and stress management for counselors, teachers, and other professionals. Alameda, CA: Hunter House, Inc.

Jones, C & Lorman, J (1988). Head injury: A guide for the patient and family. Stow, OH: Interactive Therapeutic.

Leventhal, JG & Shea III, LJ (2002). Families with Brain Injury: A Model for Intervention. Rusk Institute: NYU Medical Center.

Mackay, LE (1997). Crisis Intervention: Care and Involvement of the Family. In Maximizing, Brain Injury Recovery: Integrating Critical Care and Early Rehabilitation, Mackay, LE, Chapman, PA & Morgan, AS: Aspen Publishers.

Marsh, NV, Kersel, DA, Havill, JH, et. al. (1998). Caregiver Burden at 6 Months Following Severe Traumatic brain injury. Brain Injury 12(3); 225-238.

McPherson, KM, McNaughton, H, & Pentland, B (2001). Information Needs of Families when one Member has a Severe Brain Injury. International Journal of Rehabilitation Research 23(4); 295-301.

Mathewson, M (1997). Courage After Coma: A Family's Journal. Edmonton, Canada: Uneek Experience Ltd.

Osborn, CL (1998). Over my Head: A Doctor's own Story of Head Injury from the Inside Looking Out. Kansas City: Andrews McMeel Publishing.

Prigatano, GP (1991). Disordered mind, wounded soul: The emerging role of psychotherapy in rehabilitation after brain injury. Journal of Head Trauma Rehabilitation, 6(4), 1-10.

Prigatano, GP, Klonoff, PS, O'Brien, KP, Altman, IM, Amin, K, Chiapello, D, Shepherd, J, Cunningham, M, & Mora, M (1994). Productivity after neuro-psychologically oriented milieu rehabilitation. Journal of Head Trauma Rehabilitation, 9(1); 91-102.

Rosenthal, M & Muir, C (1984). Strategies for family intervention. In B. Edelsten & E. Couture (Eds), Behavioral approaches to the traumatic brain injured (pp.227-246). New York: Plenum.

Semlyen, JK, Summers, SJ, & Barnes, MP (1999). Aspects of Caregiver Distress After Severe Head Injury. Journal of Neurological Rehabilitation 12(2); 53-60.

Senelick, RC & Ryan, CE (1998). Living with Brain Injury: A Guide for Families. Birmingham, Alabama: Health South Press.

Sinnakaruppan, I & Williams, DM (2001). Family Carers and the Adult Head Injured: A Critical Review of Carer's Needs. Brain Injury 15(8); 653-672.

Stoler, DR & Hill, BA (1998). Coping with Mild Traumatic brain injury. Garden City Park, NY: Avery Publishing Group, Inc.

Tampa General Rehabilitation Center (1996). The HDI Coping Series, Number 1: Brain Injury, A Guide for Families. Houston Texas: HDI Publishers.

Testa, JA, Malec, JF, Moesser, AM & Brown, AM (2006). Predicting Family Functioning After TBI. Journal of Head Trauma Rehabilitation, 21: 236-247.

Valera, EM & Berenbaum, H (2003). Brain Injury in Battered Women. Journal of Consulting and Clinical Psychology 71(4); 797-804.

Watanabe, Y, Shiel, A, Asami, T, et al. (2000). An Evaluation of Neurobehavioral Problems as Perceived by Family Members and Levels of Family Stress 1-3 Years Following Traumatic brain injury. Clinical Rehabilitation 14(2); 172-177.

Williams, JM & Kay, T (1991). Head Injury: A Family Matter. Baltimore: Paul H. Brookes Publishing Co.

Winslade, WJ (1998). Confronting Traumatic brain injury: Devastation, Hope, and Healing. Bingham, NY: Vail-Ballou Press.

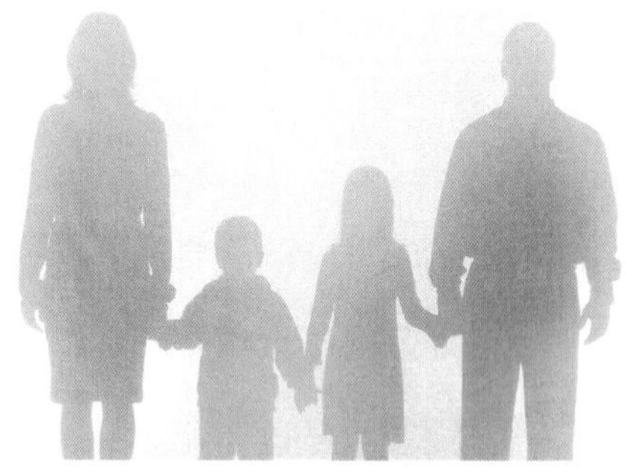

Chapter 8

Legal and Ethical Issues

Learning Objectives

By the end of this chapter, you will be able to:

1. Describe the legal rights of persons receiving rehabilitation services.
2. Explain the ethical standards of rehabilitation staff.
3. Define basic legal terms and concepts.
4. Explain the rights of an individual in rehabilitation under the Americans with Disabilities Act.

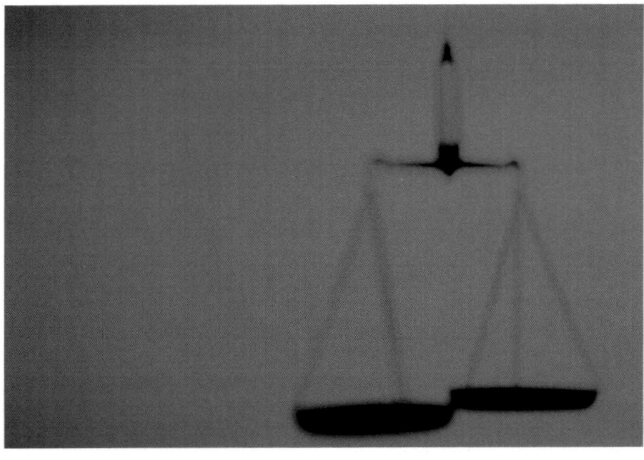

Introduction

This chapter provides an overview of the legal rights of an individual in a rehabilitation program, ethical standards for rehabilitation staff and basic legal terms and concepts pertinent to the provision of quality rehabilitation services.

Legal rights of the Individual Receiving Rehabilitation Services

Legal rights are powers or privileges that an individual has under the law. Physical or mental changes that occur after a brain injury do not alter a person's legal rights. However, if the individual is unable to exercise those rights, then a legal representative may exercise those rights for the individual as allowed by the state law.

The individual with a brain injury has the same legal rights as anyone.

Basic Sources of Law - Determining Basic Rights

There are four basic sources of law that provide individual rights at both the state and federal levels. They include:

Common law	Developed from court decisions.
Constitutional law	Based on the United States Constitution, as well as the constitution of the state where the person lives.
Statutory law	Enacted by Congress or a state legislature in the form of individual statutes, which together form a code.
Administrative Law	Created by administrative agencies, such as the Department of Health and Human Services, by statute, Congress or the state legislature. Authorizes an agency to create laws known as rules or regulations.

Resident or Individual Bill of Rights

Staff members and rehabilitation programs need to be aware of the basic rights of persons. Most states have mandated certain rights for individuals in a treatment program. Accreditation agencies may dictate how this Bill of Rights should be displayed in the common areas of the treatment program. While these rights vary from state to state, most states have statutes on the use of restrictive procedures and advocate for least restricted programming. Basically, this means that more restrictive treatments are only used when less restrictive measures have proven unsuccessful. Often these guidelines are found in the state mental health code or a similar document. Bills of Rights commonly share some of the following characteristics with which staff should be familiar.

Note

Information regarding legal definitions and principles in this chapter was obtained from multiple sources and provides only general information. Nothing in this chapter should be construed to represent legal advice regarding either general or specific issues and readers are directed to proper legal consultation for such matters.

Bill of Rights

- A bill of Rights should be posted in a prominent place in the program. This document should be written in the primary language of each resident to enhance comprehension.
- Program participants have all rights as citizens under the law.
- The Bill of Rights typically provides that each person in a program has the right to:

1. Not be physically or mentally abused or exploited.
2. Not be physically or chemically restrained unless the restraining:

   a. is necessary in an emergency to protect the person or others from injury after the individual harms or threatens to harm himself or another individual, or

b. is authorized in writing by a licensed physician for a limited and specified period of time.

3. Participate in restrictive interventions only in accordance with least restrictive treatment guidelines.

4. Be treated with the respect, consideration, and recognition of the individual's dignity and individuality. In a residential program, a person shall receive personal care and private treatment in a safe and decent living environment.

5. Not be denied appropriate care on the basis of the individual's race, religious practice, color, national origin, sex, age, disability, marital status, or source of payment.

6. Not be prohibited from communicating in the individual's native language with other individuals or employees for the purpose of acquiring or providing any type of treatment, care or services.

7. Be encouraged and assisted in the exercise of the individual's rights. A person may present grievances on his/her own or another's behalf to the director, manager, state agencies, or other persons without threat of reprisal in any manner. The person providing services shall develop procedures for submitting complaints and recommendations and for assuring a response by the person providing services.

8. Receive and send unopened mail.

9. Engage in unrestricted communication, including personal visitation with any person of the individual's choice, including family members and representatives of advocacy groups and community service organizations at any reasonable hour.

10. Make contacts with the community and achieve the highest level of independence, autonomy, and interaction with the community of which the person is capable.

11. Manage financial affairs, or shall be given at least a quarterly accounting of financial transactions made on the individual's behalf by the program should the program accept the individual's written delegation of this responsibility for any period of time in conformance with state law.

12. Have confidential records that cannot be released without the individual's written permission. A person may inspect his or her personal records maintained by service providers.

13. Have the person providing services answer questions concerning health, treatment, and condition unless a physician determines that the knowledge would harm the individual. The physician must record that determination in the individual's record.

14. Choose a personal physician.

15. Participate in planning the individual's service plan.

16. Be given the opportunity to refuse treatment, including medications after the possible consequences of refusing treatment are fully explained.

17. Be provided unaccompanied access to a telephone at a reasonable hour in case of an emergency or personal crisis.

18. Privacy (not a single bedroom).

19. Retain personal clothing and possessions as space permits. The number of personal possessions may be limited for health and safety reasons which are documented in the individual's record.

20. Determine the individual's dress, hairstyle, or other personal effects according to individual preference, except the resident has the responsibility of maintaining personal hygiene.

21. Retain and use personal property in the immediate living quarters and to have a private locked area (cabinet, closet, drawer, footlocker, etc.) in which to keep personal property.

Examples of Basic Rights Under the Bill of Rights

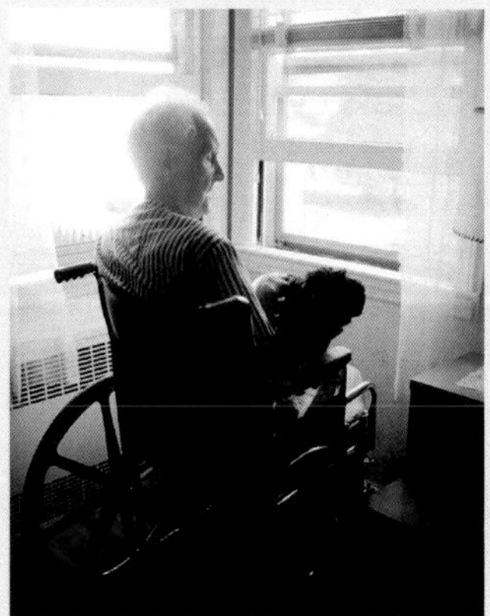

Be treated with respect, consideration and dignity.

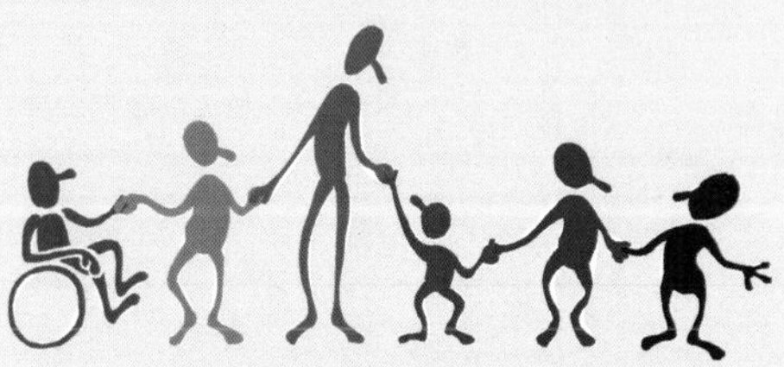

Not be denied appropriate care on the basis of one's race, religion, national origin, sex, age, disability, marital status or funding.

Receive and send unopened mail.

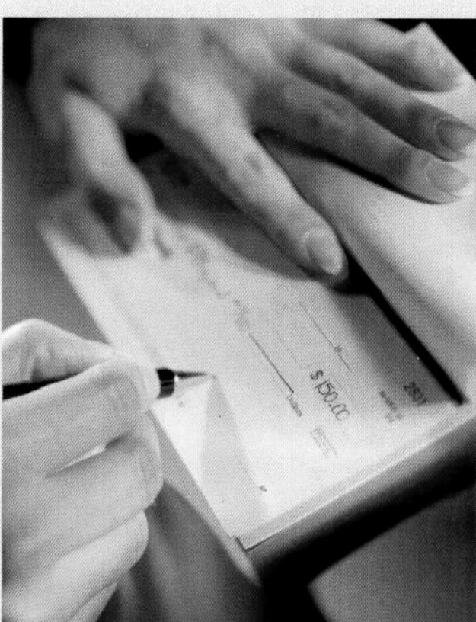

Manage financial affairs or be given an accounting of transactions.

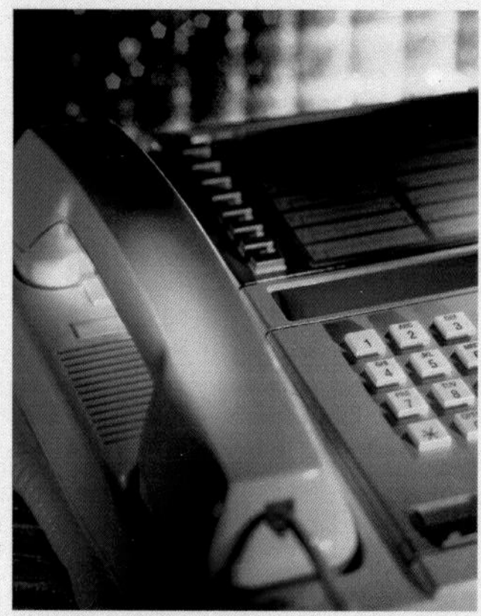

Be provided unaccompanied access to a telephone for emergency or personal crisis.

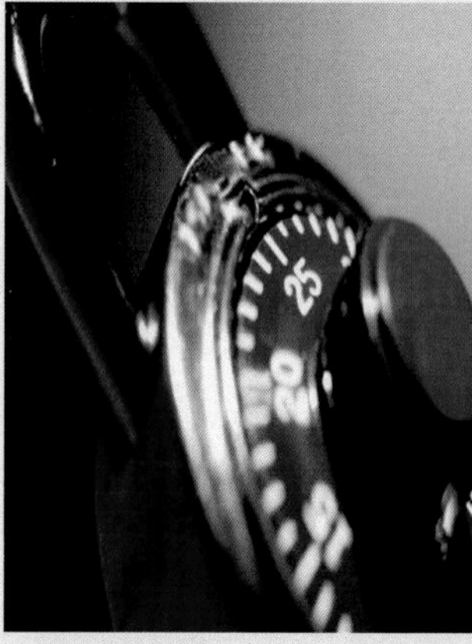

Retain & use personal property in the immediate living quarters and have a private locked area.

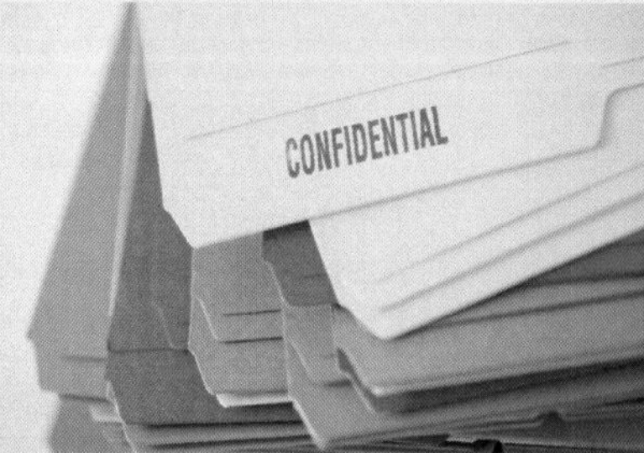

Have confidential records released only with written permission.

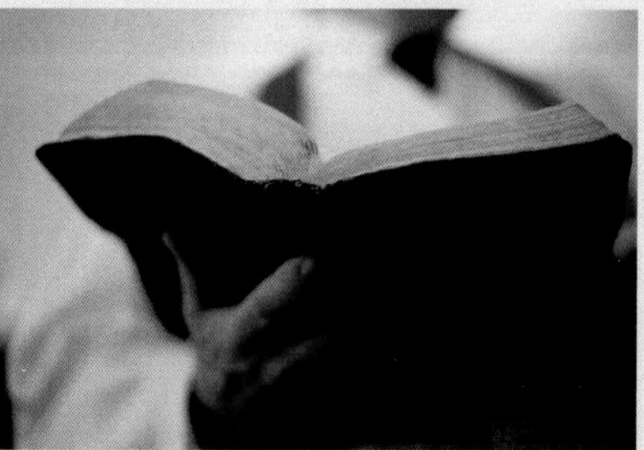

Make contacts in the community and achieve the highest level of independence possible.

22. Refuse to perform services for the program, except as contracted for by the individual and facility.

23. Be informed, in writing, by the person providing services of available services and the applicable charges if the services are not covered by Medicare, Medicaid, or other form of health insurance.

24. Unless previously arranged, not be transferred or discharged, except in an emergency situation. The individual, the guardian (if applicable) and other responsible persons shall be notified immediately.

25. Leave the program temporarily or permanently, subject to contractual or financial obligations.

26. Not be deprived of a constitutional, civil, or legal right solely by reason of residence in a program for persons with brain injury.

27. Have access to the services of a representative of the state agency or program charged with regulating licensing, or monitoring the program.

The client Bill of Rights is a written guarantee of basic rights for persons in treatment programs. Staff members are accountable to adhere to these rights in their treatment activities. A violation of any of these rights could be an unlawful act or potential grounds for a lawsuit.

Use of Seclusion and Restraint

Overview

The inappropriate use of seclusion or restraint violates the Constitutional rights of an individual. It is important to remember that every United States citizen is guaranteed constitutional rights regardless of ability or disability. In Youngberg v. Romeo, the United States Supreme Court held that a basic liberty under the Constitution is to be free from undue bodily restraint. Congress and state legislatures have also recognized this right and enacted laws on allowable and prohibitive uses of seclusion and restraint.

Medical professional standards also respect this basic human right. The American Medical Association advocates that people "have a fundamental right to be free from unreasonable bodily restraint" and that restraints should only be imposed when "in the best interest of the patient." [American Medical Association, Use of Restraints, Code of Medical Ethics, Section E-8.17]

State and federal law, as well as accrediting organizations such as JCAHO and CARF, mandate that seclusion and restraint can only be used as a measure of last resort. This means that these measures should only be used when other less restrictive procedures have been documented as being unsuccessfully attempted and the patient or others are in imminent danger. In many states, the use of seclusion and restraint is viewed as crisis intervention rather than effective treatment and is only to be used when other treatment has failed. Furthermore, in these states, each episode of seclusion or restraint requires review by the patient's treatment team to reassess current treatment protocols and determine how programming can be changed to reduce or prevent the subsequent need for these restrictive procedures.

Restraint

Restraint is generally defined as any manual, mechanical, chemical or other means of restricting movement or access to one's body, against one's will. This may include other people holding a person; restricting movement through straps, belts, helmets, placement in wheel chairs or geri-chairs that the person cannot get out of, or other mechanical means; or using medications or other chemical compounds to subdue a person's actions.

Seclusion

Seclusion is generally defined as isolating a person from others and physically preventing him or her from leaving a confined area. Different states have different definitions of seclusion, but this may include placing a person in a locked time out room, placing a person in solitary confinement, or physically preventing a person from leaving his or her room by stopping the person in the doorway.

Seclusion and restraint procedures are never allowed for retribution, staff convenience, or to make up for inadequacies of the treatment program such as an unsafe environment, inadequate staffing, inadequate training of staff, poor professional oversight, lack of treatment planning, or other such factors. These factors contribute in a vicious cycle to the dangerous behaviors on the part of patients that inappropriately "justify" the use of these restrictive procedures. The application of such procedures validates the "dangerousness" of the patient, which in turn validates the presumed need for these interventions. Substantial research has documented that programs that successfully address the above factors have a much lower incidence of seclusion and restraint usage, than programs that do not.

Seclusion and restraint procedures can also be very dangerous to patients and staff. Each year a small, but significant number of patients die as a result of these procedures, especially because of positional asphyxia due to improper restraint techniques that impair breathing, resulting in suffocation. Other people die because of medical complications when they are inadequately monitored during seclusion procedures. Finally, a substantial number of staff injuries and worker compensation claims are related to episodes of patient seclusion and restraint.

Seclusion & Restraint

Seclusion and restraint procedures are never allowed for retribution, staff convenience, or to make up for inadequacies of the treatment program such as an unsafe environment, inadequate staffing, inadequate training of staff, poor professional oversight, lack of treatment planning, or other such factors.

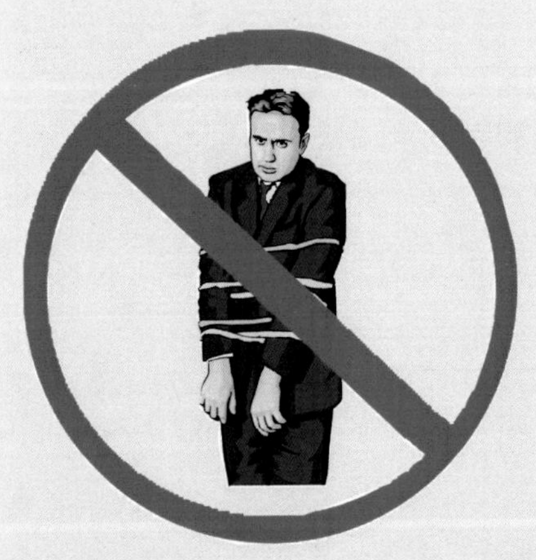

Guidelines for the Use of Seclusion and Restraint

Despite these concerns there may be situations in which seclusion or restraint is necessary. As previously noted, this includes when a person truly is an imminent danger to him/herself or others and other less restrictive procedures have not been effective. Most states require an order for seclusion or restraint from an independent licensed professional and that the procedure only be used as long as necessary to reduce the danger of the situation. These procedures should never be used to enforce compliance.

It is critical to constantly monitor the physical and psychological status of the individual who is being restrained and secluded. Most states require that the individual be evaluated by a qualified health professional during and after the procedure to assure the person's physical and emotional safety and lack of enduring negative effect. The professional literature reports that the safest and most effective way to do this is through constant, in person, staff supervision of a person in seclusion or restraint. Additionally, most states require a debriefing with the patient and staff involved in the procedure to review the factors that lead to seclusion or restraint as well as steps that all parties can take the next time to prevent the need for such procedures.

Use of Restraint & Seclusion

- Used only if less restrictive means have failed
- May require an order from a licensed professional
- There is imminent danger to oneself or others
- Ongoing monitoring of the person must occur while in seclusion or restraint
- Follow up after restraint or seclusion should occur with staff and patient

Medications or other chemical compounds that are used to subdue a person's actions are considered restraints.

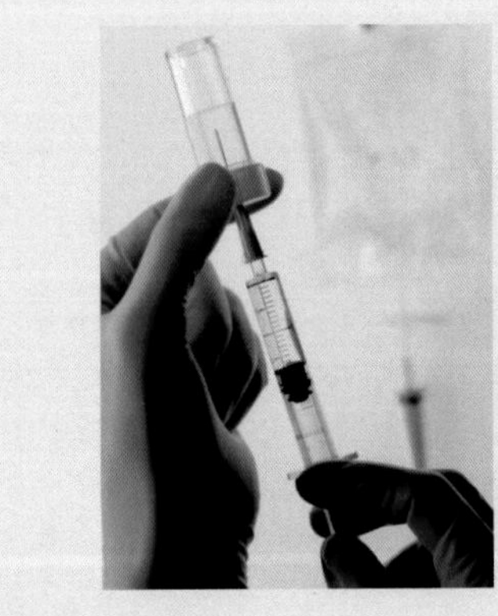

Medically prescribed restraints are often considered as a different class from restraints used to address behavioral challenges. Medically prescribed restraints may include vests to help prevent people from falling out of beds, helmets for people prone to falling due to seizures, lap belts on wheel chairs, lap trays on wheel chairs, and other devices that promote the safety and function of the individual. In most cases, these devices can be managed by the individual or are applied and removed under the patient's direction. They also have to be prescribed by a physician and must be carefully monitored for safety. However, these types of restraints generally do not carry the same level of monitoring and oversight as behavioral restraints. Laws on seclusion or restraint vary among settings and patient populations. For example, laws on the use of seclusion or restraint in psychiatric treatment facilities may not be applicable in brain injury rehabilitation. Federal or state law may also set different standards for children than for adults. It is important that staff be aware of laws and policy applicable to their treatment setting and for patients under their care.

Finally, staff members may be held personally responsible and accountable for their role in the use of seclusion or restraint in some states. For both the safety of the patient and the protection of staff, it is essential that staff be trained on the proper and safe administration of seclusion and restraint.

Critical Questions for Staff About Seclusion and Restraints

- What interventions are considered seclusion or restraint in your state?
- Who may order seclusion or restraint and should the order be in writing?
- When are seclusion or restraints allowable?
- What types of seclusion or restraints are allowable in the brain injury rehabilitation setting?
- What types of seclusion or restraints are allowable for adults and what types for children?
- How do you properly implement a seclusion or restraint?
- Who is responsible or accountable when a seclusion or restraint is imposed?

Accreditation Standards and the Law

Accreditation primarily addresses the safety and quality of care provided by a facility. It may be a voluntary effort or it may be required for state licensing requirements or federal certification. An accreditation is essentially a seal of approval that indicates a high performance standard. Major accreditation organizations include the Joint Commission on Accreditation of Health care Organizations (JCAHO) and the Commission for the Accreditation of Rehabilitation Facilities (CARF).

Accreditation standards often vary with the setting. A standard for a hospital may be different from one for a rehabilitation facility; one may be more restrictive than the other. All the standards for accreditation may not be required under the law. However, an accredited facility requires staff to follow them, as they are standards of care for the facility.

Ethical standards

Rehabilitation staff must follow both the law and a broader standard of ethics. Ethical standards are standards of professional conduct rooted in the moral principles and values of society and the profession. Regulatory boards, such as the state board of nursing, often establish ethical standards in professional codes of

conduct in state regulations. Employers and professional organizations may also set ethical standards.

> Legal rights are anchored in ethical standards, yet ethical standards exceed legal rights.

The ethical standards of health care professions usually reflect the principles listed in the box below.

Legal Terms and Concepts

There are legal terms and concepts that staff often come across in brain injury rehabilitation. A basic understanding of these terms and concepts protects the patient as well as staff. Each concept explained in this section is far more complex than this overview. These terms and concepts are governed largely by state law, which may vary greatly from state to state.

Competency or Capacity

> Competency or Capacity is a legal term that describes a person's mental ability to understand *the nature and effect of one's decisions and acts.*

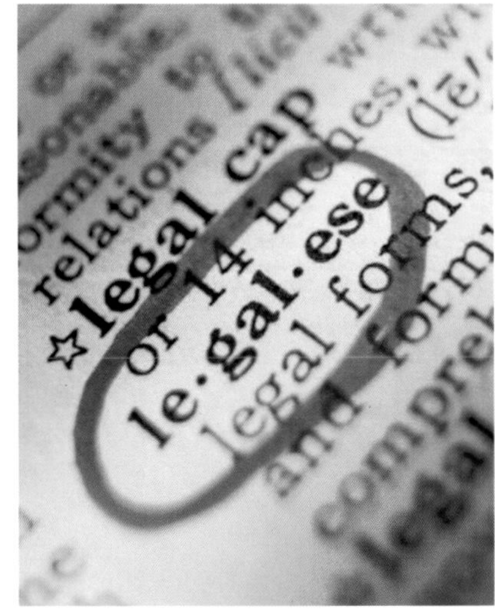

Generally, the law presumes that an adult individual is competent unless proven otherwise. State law provides the process to determine competency. Only a court may determine that an individual is legally incompetent. If a court determines that an individual is legally incompetent, the court may appoint a representative who will make the decisions that the individual is incapable of making.

In the health care setting, competency may be described as the ability of an individual to make an informed decision about health care. If staff believes that a legally competent patient is not, in fact, competent, then this concern should be presented to a supervisor as soon as possible. The same is true if staff believe that a legally incompetent patient may be, in fact, competent.

What Staff Members Should Know About Competency

- Legal competency status of the patient
- When and how to contact a patient representative
- Who is responsible for notify-

Principles of Ethical Standards

Respect	Esteem for the human dignity of each patient
Beneficence	Doing good for each patient
Autonomy	Recognition of the right of each patient to make choices (self-determination)
Non-discrimination	Fairness and equity in the provision of services
Loyalty	Faithfulness to the patient
Truthfulness	Honesty with the patient and others
Competence	Delivery of patient care by personnel with sufficient skills and knowledge for safe and quality care
Compliance	Adherence to laws and employer rules and policies
Confidentiality	Safeguarding of patient confidences and information

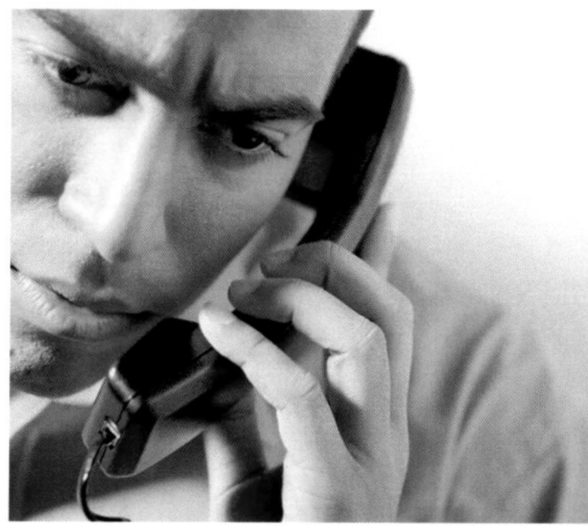

ing supervisor if competency or incompetency is in question.

Guardianship

A Guardianship is a legally enforceable arrangement under which one person, the guardian, has the legal right and duty to care for another, the ward.

A Guardian of the Person manages and makes decisions about the personal affairs of the ward, ensures that the ward has food, shelter and clothing as well as medical care, education and rehabilitation. By contrast, a Guardian of the Estate manages the financial affairs and property of the ward.

Parents are the natural guardians of minors or children. Once a child reaches the age of adulthood, the "natural" guardianship of the parent automatically dissolves unless legal action is taken. This is true even for the individual with a disability, such as a brain injury.

To establish Guardianship for an adult, a court must appoint a guardian and do so through the process and by the standards required by state law. Guardianship restricts the right of the individual/ward to make certain decisions. Often a court appoints a guardian, only if it is the least restrictive alternative for assistance. Many states restrict the powers and duties of the guardian to only those necessary to address the unique limitations of the ward. Guardianship does not necessarily extinguish the legal rights of the ward, such as the right to vote or to marry. A court may remove an inappropriate guardian by standards described in state law.

Guardianship

Guardian of the Person - Cares for the personal needs of the ward

Guardian of the Estate - Cares for the property of the ward

Plenary Guardianship - Cares for personal needs and the property of the ward.

What Staff Members Should Know about Guardianship

- Extent of powers and duties of the Guardian
- Who the Guardian is
- How to reach the Guardian
- Who is responsible for notifying supervisor if the Guardian is not performing as expected.

Limits of Guardianship

A Guardian may misunderstand the scope of duty. A person with a guardian does not lose basic legal rights. The limitations of Guardianship must always be carefully explained and understood.

Examples

A Guardian who is also a parent may want to limit or restrict access of the ward (a son or daughter) to an ex-husband or wife if there have been conflicts in the past. If the ward chooses to have contact with this person, the ward can do so unless there is a court order restricting such access.

A Guardian may request that a staff member open all mail to be kept informed of all communications with the ward. However, the ward has the right to personal privacy, including written and telephone communications. Therefore the guardian's request cannot be met.

Power of Attorney

A Power of Attorney is a document in which a competent person, the principal, appoints another, the agent, to act for him in legal and financial matters. The agent may have broad or limited powers. The appointment of the agent can be immediate or it may become active if and when something happens, such as the physical incapacity of the principal. The appointment may also be durable. This means it is not changed when the principal becomes disabled or incompetent. A guardian may be appointed after Power of Attorney has been granted should circumstances change. Under state law, a guardian can override or revoke the Power of Attorney.

Living Will and Durable Power of Attorney for Health Care

A Living Will is a document, often called an Advance Directive. It provides written instructions by a competent adult to a physician on providing, withholding or withdrawing life-sustaining procedures when the individual is in a terminal or permanently unconscious condition. The right to refuse medical treatment is protected by the Constitution. The federal Self-Determination Act requires that health care facilities receiving Medicare and Medicaid funds inform patients of their right to execute a Living Will or Advance Directive. Most, if not all states recognize the Living Will, although the specifics of the law vary.

A durable Power of Attorney for health care is also known as a medical Power of Attorney or a health care proxy. It is a document in which a competent adult, the principal, appoints an agent to make decisions about medical care in the event that the principal is unable to make those decisions. This decision-making power is not limited to end-of-life decisions, although they may be included. Through the document, the principal expresses wishes regarding a variety of health care decisions.

Power of Attorney

A document in which a competent person, the principal, appoints another, the agent, to act for him in legal and financial matters.

What Staff Members Should Know About Power of Attorney

- Extent of powers and duties of agent
- Who the agent is
- How to reach the agent
- Who is responsible for notifying supervisor if agent not performing as expected.

Living Will and Durable Power of Attorney for Health Care

It provides written instructions by a competent adult to a physician on providing, withholding or withdrawing life-sustaining procedures when the individual is in a terminal or permanently unconscious condition.

What Staff Members Should Know About a Living Will or a Durable Power of Attorney for Health Care

- How to access the document
- Contents of the document related to staff care
- Who the agent is
- How to reach the agent
- Who is responsible for notifying supervisor if the agent is not performing as expected.

Confidentiality and Privilege

Health care providers have a duty to maintain patient Confidentiality. A basic tenet in health care is that patient trust is essential for quality care. A patient should feel free to fully disclose information to a health care provider. The patient must also believe that the health care provider will respect the confidential nature of information and only disclose information when required by law or when given written consent to do so by the individual or the guardian.

The importance of medical confidentiality is rooted deeply in history. It is in the Hippocratic Oath taken by

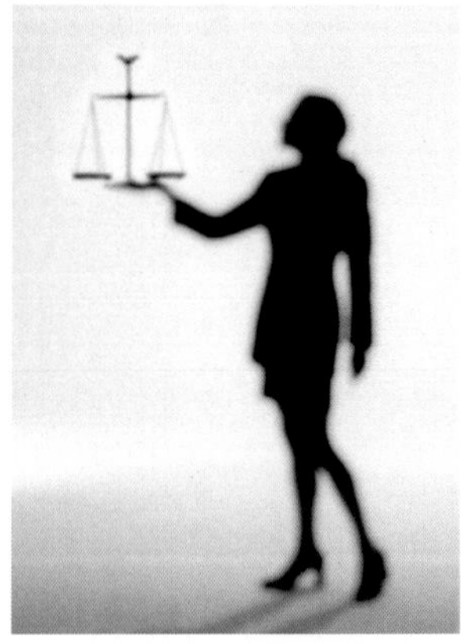

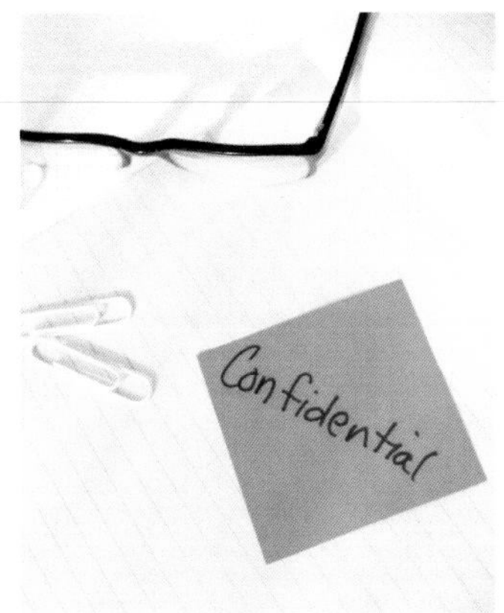

physicians and emphasized repeatedly in the Ethical Standards of many health care professions. The law, in turn, imposes a duty on health care professions to maintain patient confidentiality.

In 1996 the federal Health Insurance Portability and Accountability Act (HIPAA) was enacted and required that regulations be developed to protect individually identifiable health information. These regulations came into effect in April 2003 and created national standards to protect medical records and other protected health information.

HIPAA

Overall, Protected Health Information (PHI), identifying health information which can be linked to a person individually, may not be used or disclosed for reasons other than treatment, payment, or service operations without specific authorization from the individual or a guardian.

The HIPAA Privacy Standards:

- Limit the non-consensual use and release of private health information.
- Give individuals new rights to access their medical records and to know who else has accessed them.
- Restrict most disclosure of health information to the minimum needed for the intended purpose of providing health care.
- Establish new criminal and civil standards for improper use or disclosure.
- Establish new requirements for access to records by researchers and others.

Failure to protect health information can result in the staff member being held liable. The following examples illustrate breaches in protecting health information.

Well intended family members may call a facility and ask for updates on their niece, neighbor, church member or friend. While well intended, it is important to ensure that the individual's confidentiality is upheld. Information cannot be given out without the person's or guardian's written consent.

This issue of confidentiality comes up sometimes when a family member is visiting and asks staff about another person in the program whom their family member has befriended. "How is Jack doing? He told me he was going home in 2 weeks, is he?" Again, while well intended, Jack's confidentiality needs to be maintained. The best response may be to say something like, "I am sorry but I cannot provide that information about Jack. However, he is going to be around later, maybe you could talk to him then."

Confidentiality & Privilege

What staff members should know about confidentiality and privilege

- Pertinent requirements on confidentiality under the law and under facility policy
- When patient privilege may be over-ridden
- With whom patient information may be discussed.

Another common example is when a staff member may be in the community with an individual as part of the out patient rehabilitation program. The staff member may meet someone and be expected to make introductions. The best introduction may be to simply say, "This is Jack." It is important to not disclose that the person is a participant in rehabilitation as in, "This is Jack. He is a client at the rehabilitation program where I work."

However, in a case of emergency, staff members need to identify themselves if in contact with the police, ambulance, etc.

Privilege is a right of the patient to prevent disclosure of health care information by a health care provider. In most states, a physician may assert the patient's privilege when asked for information in court or legal proceeding. The patient may waive privilege by consenting to release information. Many states require that the consent be in writing.

State law may also override patient privilege and allow particular types of information to be disclosed without a release, when the state deems it is in the public interest. Common

Informed Consent

Informed Consent refers to a patient's right to consent to care only after the health care provider fully discloses risks and facts necessary to make an informed decision about health care.

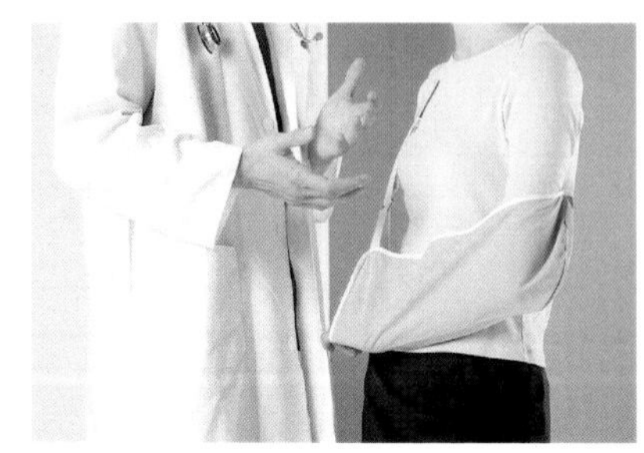

examples include reporting communicable diseases, gunshot wounds, child abuse, and abuse of the elderly. A health care provider may also have a Common Law or statutory Duty to Warn third parties of a risk of violence, a contagious disease or other risk. A staff member who is uncertain about these duties can get advice from a supervisor overseeing the patient's care or from the agency's legal counsel.

Informed Consent

Informed Consent refers to a patient's right to consent to care only after the health care provider fully discloses risks and facts necessary to make an informed decision about health care. The Informed Consent doctrine is a principle of law that recognizes patient autonomy or freedom of will.

An individual must have information to make an informed decision on whether or not to consent to care or to decide on the type of care. The individual must be given accurate and timely information in a format and language that the individual can understand.

The information should include:

- Nature and purpose of the care.
- Benefits of care.
- Risks of care.
- Options available, if any, and their respective risks.
- Experience of professional giving the care.
- Prognosis with and without the care.

Staff should notify the health care professional who will give the care if the patient has questions, so there can be further discussion with the patient.

Each patient has a right to an informed decision, whether the patient is legally competent or incompetent. When a patient is deemed incompetent, a legal representative may make the informed decision within the limits of state law.

Abuse, Neglect and Exploitation

All states have protective laws against the maltreatment of dependent, incapacitated or institutionalized adults. State protective laws are often found in adult protective services laws, mental health laws, institutional abuse laws, the laws of the long-term care ombudsman's program and criminal laws.

Typically, the types of maltreatment addressed by the laws are abuse, neglect and exploitation.

The laws on abuse, neglect and exploitation vary significantly among the states, but they usually:

- Define the maltreatment.
- Require reporting and investi-

Abuse

The willful infliction of injury, unreasonable confinement, intimidation, or punishment with resulting physical harm, pain or mental anguish. This also includes the deprivation by an individual, including a caretaker, of goods or services that are necessary to attain or maintain physical, mental, and psychosocial well-being.

Neglect

Neglect is usually a failure to provide for the basic needs of a dependent individual.

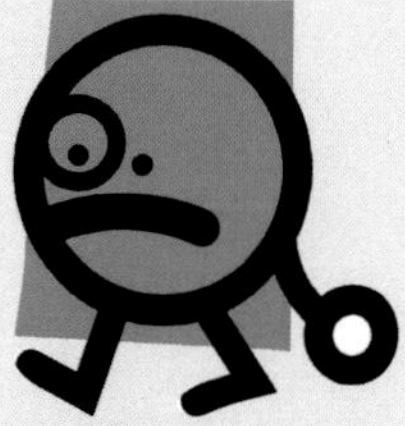

Exploitation

The use of a dependent individual's property illegally or without the consent of the individual, or the expenditure of funds. Usually, the act is considered exploitation if done for profit or other advantage.

gation of the maltreatment.

- Penalize the perpetrator.
- Include social services to help the victim's recovery.

The Center for Medicare and Medicaid Services, 42 CFR 488.301, defines abuse as, "the willful infliction of injury, unreasonable confinement, intimidation, or punishment *with resulting physical harm, pain or mental anguish. This also includes the deprivation by an individual, including a caretaker, of goods or services that are necessary to attain or maintain physical, mental, and psychosocial well-being.*

Abuse also may be verbal or emotional. It can be the result of intentionally inflicting emotional or mental anguish through ridicule, derogatory remarks or threats. Emotional abuse may also include unreasonable use of restraints or seclusion for punishment or as a substitute for treatment. The term abuse may also include sexual abuse or sexual exploitation.

Neglect is usually a failure to provide for the basic needs of a dependent individual.

Basic needs include food, shelter, clothing or health care. They may also include toileting, bathing and safety measures. Neglect may also include abandonment of an individual without a reasonable effort to provide necessary services.

Exploitation is the use of a dependent individual's property illegally or without the consent of the individual.

Exploitation includes the expenditure of funds. Usually, the act is considered exploitation if done for profit or other advantage.

State laws provide for civil or criminal remedies (or both) of abuse, neglect and exploitation. Civil remedy is in the form of a lawsuit. Criminal penalties range from misdemeanor to felony penalties, the latter of which may include substantial prison time and fines.

Persons (i.e. staff) with reasonable cause to believe that abuse, neglect and exploitation has occurred, or is occurring, are required by law to report the activity immediately to the appropriate government authority or to be subject to penalty themselves. Most states provide immunity from punishment for the person reporting, unless the person reporting is the actual perpetrator.

What staff members should know about abuse, neglect and exploitation:

- How the state law defines *abuse, neglect and exploitation*
- *How and to whom to report*

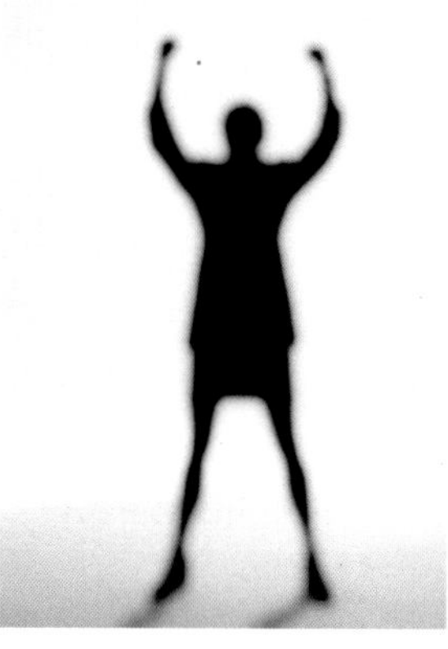

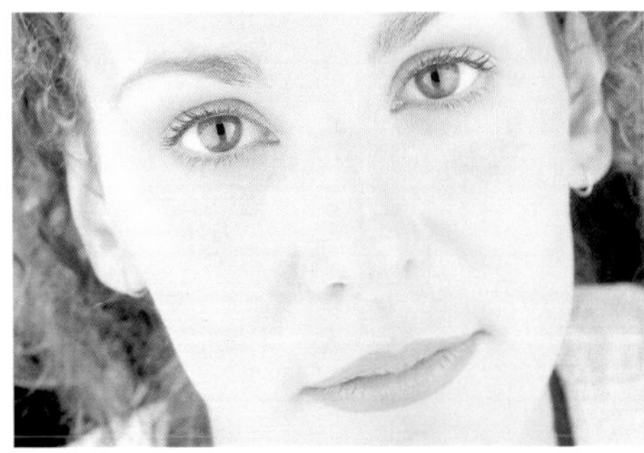

incidents of abuse, neglect and exploitation.

Advocacy

An advocate is an individual or organization who serves on behalf of an individual. An advocate may be obtained to act on behalf of an individual with a brain injury who is in a rehabilitation program. The advocate may serve the individual through a formal legal arrangement, as does a lawyer or guardian. Or the advocate may assist through an informal arrangement with the individual. An advocate may help the individual in legal or ethical issues, to pursue funding or services, or many other ways. Each individual has the right to seek the assistance of an advocate without reprisal.

The Brain Injury Association of America (BIAA) is a national organization with state affiliates that advocate for the needs of individuals with brain injury. In addition, many state advocacy groups exist to address issues of individuals with disabilities.

The federal government has created specialized advocacy and legal advocacy centers to represent the needs of individuals with a variety of disabilities. These Protection and Advocacy (P&A) Systems exist in every state. In 2000, the federal government created a specialized program within the P&As dedicated to individuals with traumatic brain injury. The P&A staff have authority to investigate allegations of abuse in public facilities, to represent individuals or groups of individuals with disabilities in advocacy matters, including complaints and litigation.

Americans with Disabilities Act

In 1990, Congress enacted the Americans with Disabilities Act (ADA), a landmark Civil Rights Act, to prohibit discrimination against individuals with disabilities. The ADA defines an "individual with a disability" as:

- A person who has a physical or mental impairment that substantially limits one or more major life activities (A major life activity includes any activity that an average person can perform with little or no difficulty such as: walking, breathing, seeing, hearing, speaking, learning and working); or

- A person who has a history or record of such an impairment; or

- A person who is perceived by others as having such impairment.

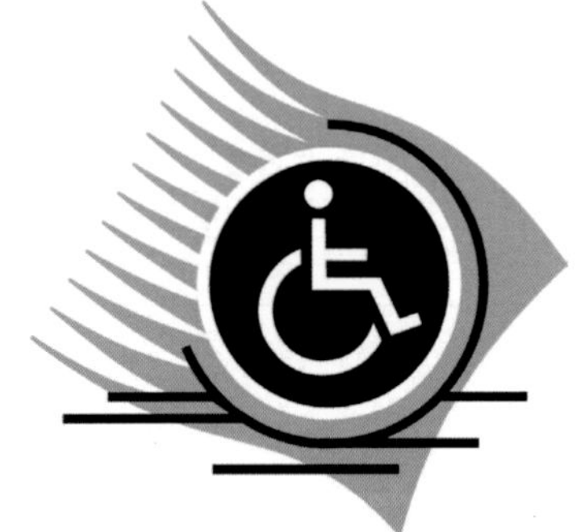

The act protects individuals with disabilities against discrimination in the following areas: employment, state and local government services, transportation, public accommodations, and telecommunications.

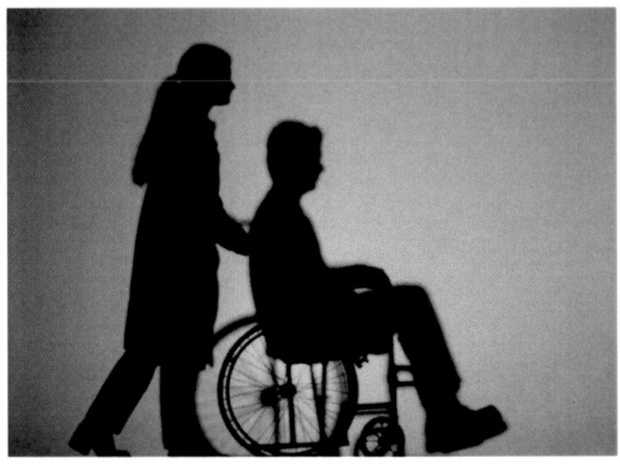

Title I: Employment

Title I of the ADA prohibits discrimination against individuals with disabilities in recruitment, hiring, promotions, training, pay, social activities and other privileges of employment. In order to be protected under the ADA, an individual with a disability must be qualified to perform the essential functions or duties of the job with or without reasonable accommodation. Reasonable accommodations may include, but are not limited to, making existing facilities used by employees readily accessible to and usable by people with disabilities, job restructuring, modifying work schedules, reassignment to vacant positions, acquiring or modifying devices, adjusting/modifying examinations, training materials, or policies and providing qualified readers or interpreters. A reasonable accommodation is required as long as it does not constitute an "undue hardship" on the employer's business.

Complaints of possible employment discrimination are filed with:

United States Equal Employment Opportunity Commission
1801 L Street, NW, room 8023
Washington, DC 20501

State and local government services, and instrumentalities thereof Title II of the ADA prohibits discrimination against qualified individuals with disabilities in all programs, activities and services of public entities. Title II covers all activities of state and local governments, including their departments, agencies and contractors. Title II requires state and local governments to give individuals with disabilities an equal opportunity to benefit from all of their programs, services and activities, such as public education, employment, transportation, recreation, health care, social services, courts, voting and town meetings.

As a result of the Olmstead Supreme Court decision in 1999, state and local governments are required to provide services in the most integrated setting appropriate to the needs of the individual with a disability.

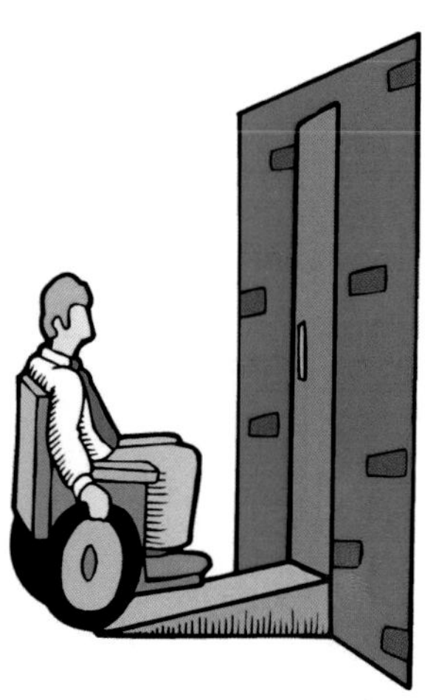

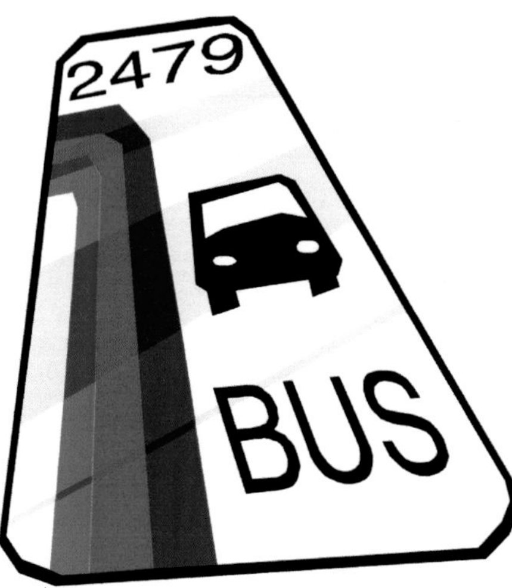

Under Title II of the ADA, state and local governments are required to follow specific architectural standards in the new construction and alteration of buildings. They must also relocate programs or make modifications to provide access in older inaccessible buildings. However, public entities are not required to take actions that would result in undue financial burden or hardship. Rather, they are required to make reasonable modifications to policies, practices and procedures where necessary to avoid discrimination, unless they can demonstrate that doing so would alter fundamentally the nature of the service, program or activity provided.

Responsibility for oversight of Title II rests with the US Department of Justice although it may also involve other federal agencies such as the Departments of Education, Health and Human Services, and Housing and Urban Development.

Title II: Transportation

The transportation provisions of Title II of the ADA cover public transportation services such as city buses and public rail transit (e.g., subways, commuter rails, Amtrak). Public transportation authorities may not discriminate against individuals with disabilities in the provision of their services. They must comply with the requirements for accessibility in newly purchased vehicles, make good faith efforts to purchase or lease accessible buses, remanufacture buses in an accessible manner and, unless it would result in undue burden, provide para-transit where they operate fixed-route bus or rail systems.

Para-transit is a service provided to individuals who are not able to use the regular transit system independently (because of a physical or mental impairment). Para-transit picks up and drops off passengers at their destinations.

Responsibility for oversight of transportation issues rests with the US Department of Transportation.

Title III: Public Accommodations

Title III of the ADA covers all businesses and nonprofit entities that provide a service to the public. A public accommodation is a private entity that owns, operates, leases from or leases to public facilities such as restaurants, retail

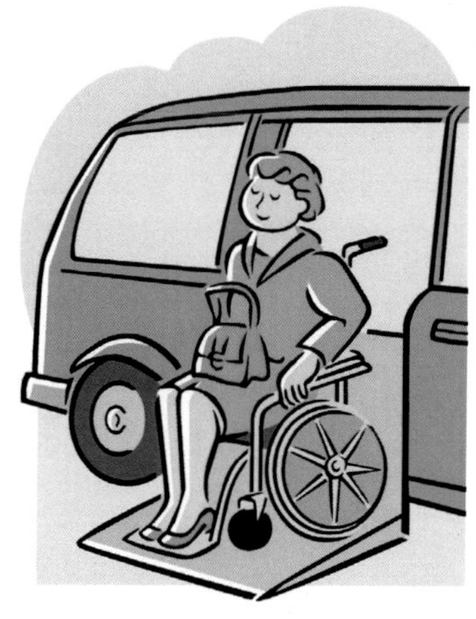

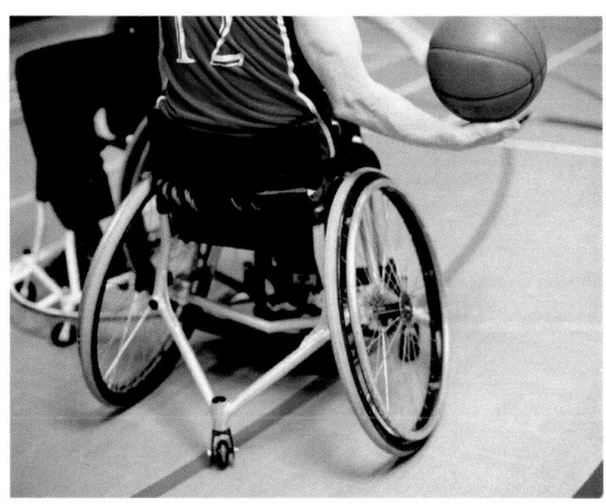

stores, hotels, movie theaters, private schools, convention centers, doctors' offices, homeless shelters, transportation depots, zoos, funeral homes, day care centers and recreation facilities, including sports stadiums and fitness clubs. Public accommodations must comply with basic nondiscrimination requirements that prohibit exclusion, segregation and unequal treatment. They also must comply with specific requirements related to architectural standards for new and altered buildings, reasonable modifications to policies, practices and procedures and provide effective communication for people with hearing, vision or speech disabilities. Public accommodations also must remove barriers in existing buildings where it is easy to do so or not unduly expensive.

Courses and examinations related to professional, educational or trade-related applications, licensing, certifications or credentialing must be provided in a place and manner accessible to persons with disabilities or alternative accessible arrangements must be offered.

Private clubs and religious organizations are exempt from Title III requirements for public accommodations. Further, the ADA generally does not cover private residences. If a public accommodation, such as a doctor's office or day care center is located in a private residence, however, the business portions of the residence are subject to the ADA's requirements.

Oversight of Title III rests with the US Department of Justice.

Title IV: Telecommunications

Title IV of the ADA addresses telephone and television access for people with hearing and speech disabilities. It requires common carriers (telephone companies) to establish interstate and intrastate telecommunications relay services (TRS) 24 hours a day, seven days a week. TRS enables callers with hearing or speech disabilities who use telecommunication devices for the deaf (TDDs) or teletypewriters (TTYs) and callers who use voice telephones to communicate with each other through a third party communications assistant. The Federal Communications Commission (FCC) has set minimum standards for TRS services. Title IV also requires closed captioning of federally funded public service announcements.

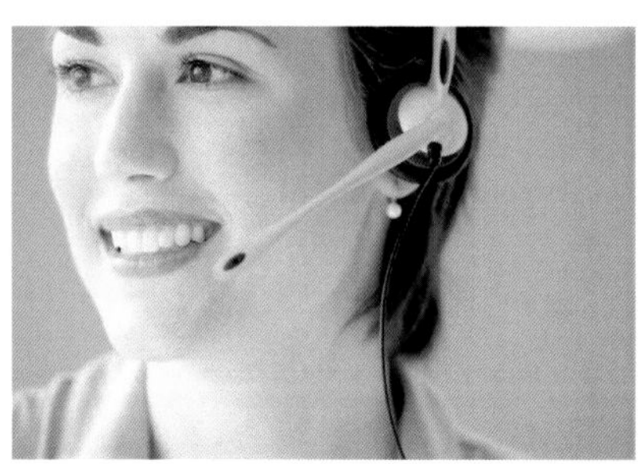

Oversight of Title IV rests with the Federal Communications Commission.

If you observe or experience discrimination that you think violates the ADA, contact your local government agency to file a complaint.

For more information about the ADA, contact:

Disability Rights Section
Civil Rights Division
US Department of Justice
P.O. Box 66738
Washington, DC
20035-6738

1-800-514-0301 (voice)
1-800-51400383 (TTY)

www.usdoj.gov/crt/ada/adahom1.htm

Summary

It is important to understand the legal rights of the individual in brain injury rehabilitation as well as the ethical standards required of staff. An understanding of the basic legal concepts encountered in the day-to-day world of brain injury rehabilitation helps protect the patient, as well as the rehabilitation facility and its staff.

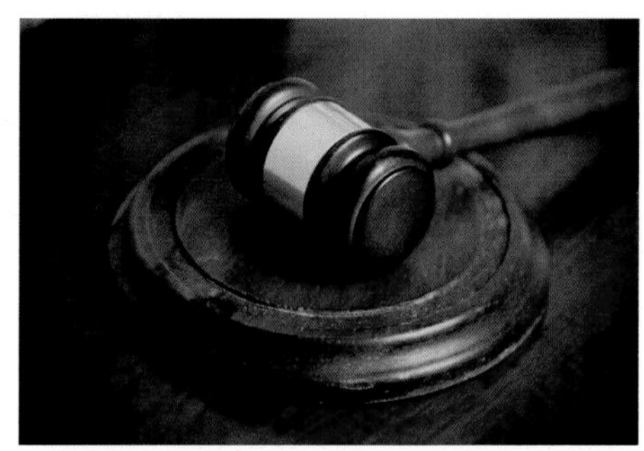

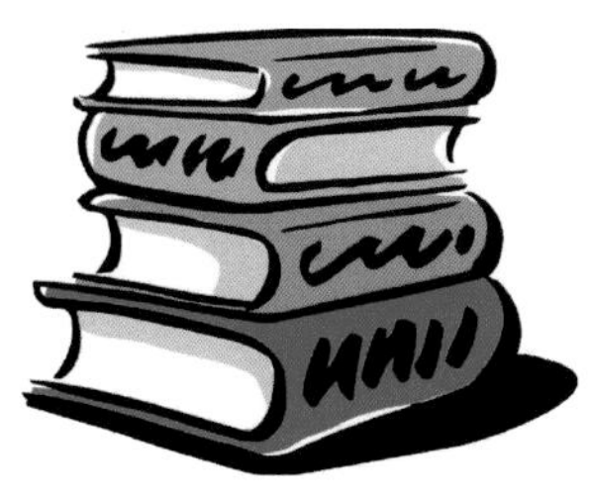

References

Braun JA, Capezuti EA (2000). The legal and medical aspects of physical restraints and bed side rails and their relationship to falls and fall-related injuries in nursing homes.

DePaul Journal of Health Care Law 4:1-72.

Capezuti EA, Lawson WT (1999). Falls and restraints-liability issues. In: Nursing Home Litigation: Investigation and Case Preparation (ed) P Iyer. Lawyers and Judges Publishing Co. Tucson, Arizona.

Capezuti E, Strumpf N, Evans L et al (1998). The relationship between physical restraint removal and falls and injuries among nursing home residents. J Gerontol 53A:M47-M53.

Capezuti E, Talerico KA, Cochran I et al (1999). Individualized interventions to prevent bed-related falls and reduce side rail use. J Geron Nursing 25:26-34.

CARF Standards Manual & Interpretive Guidelines for Medical Rehabilitation, CARF (1997). Tucson, AZ: The Commission for the Accreditation of Rehabilitation Facilities.

The Joint Commission Accreditation Manual for Hospitals 1992. Chicago, IL: Joint Commission on the Accreditation of Health care Organizations.

LaVigna, G. (1998). Alternatives to Punishment. New York: Irvington Publishers, Inc.

U.S. Department of Health &Human Services, Health Care Financing Administration, Guidance to Surveyors-Long-Term Care Facilities transmittal 274:44, June 1995.

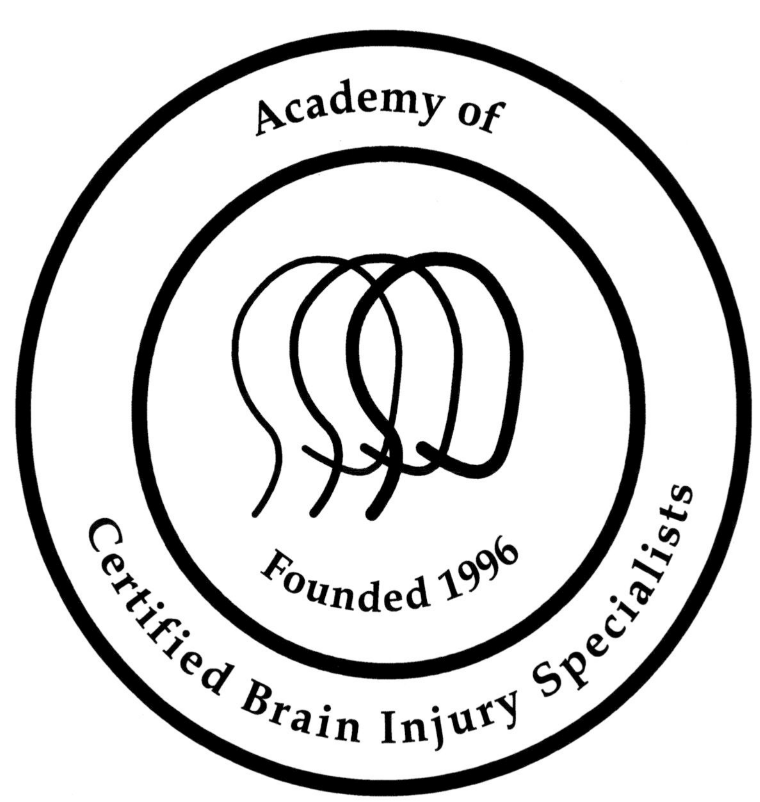
Academy of
Founded 1996
Certified Brain Injury Specialists

Glossary

A-B-C data	"A" stands for antecedents to the behavior. "B" is for the behavior. "C" is for consequences to the behavior. A-B-C data collects information, not only on the unwanted behavior, but also on what immediately precedes and follows the behavior.
Absence seizures	Formerly known as petit mal, there is transient loss of consciousness. Person may cease physical movement, have loss of attention or stare vacantly, neither speaking nor apparently hearing what is said. There may be excessive eye blinking, staring or chewing movements. Seizures so brief that may not be recognized.
Acquired brain injury	An injury to the brain occurring after birth that is not hereditary, congenital or degenerative; does not refer to brain injuries induced by birth trauma.
Active treatment interaction	Very broad concept that avoids caring for a person in a custodial sense or behaving in ways that are likely to increase dependency within the relationship. The term implies directed action, teaching, and a certain degree of risk taking.
ADA	Americans with Disabilities Act.
Administrative Law	Law that is created by administrative agencies, such as the Department of Health and Human Services by statute, Congress or the state legislature. Administrative law authorizes an agency to create laws known as rules or regulations.
Advance Directive	Term used for a living will.
Advocate	An individual or organization chosen to serve on behalf of another individual. May be a formal legal arrangement or an informal arrangement with an individual.
Akathisia	Inability to sit or stand still; motor restlessness.
Akinesia	Slowness and loss of movement.
Americans with Disabilities Act	Known as the ADA, its purpose is to eliminate discrimination on the basis of disability in the full and equal enjoyment of the goods, services, facilities, privileges, advantages, or accommodations of any place of public accommodation by any person who owns, leases (or leases to), or operates a place of public accommodation.
Amygdala	Close to the hippocampus, the amygdala is a "fight or flight" structure closely tied with emotional memories and reactions.
Anosognosia	Lack of awareness of deficits.
Anoxia	Stop in oxygen getting to the brain.
Anoxic	Lack of oxygen.
Anxiolytics	Anti-anxiety medications.
Aphasia	Difficulty understanding speech and/or difficulty expressing thoughts.
Apraxia	Inability to conduct purposeful movement.

Glossary

Arachnoid	Like a spiderweb that bridges the brain's many wrinkles and folds.
Arousal	General state of readiness of an individual to process sensory information and/ or organize a response.
Aspiration	Inhalation of foods, liquids or vomitus into the lungs.
Ataxia	Impaired ability to coordinate movement.
Atrophy	Wasting of size or functional activity.
Axon	A long, slim "wire" in the neuron that transmits signals from one cell body to another via junctions known as synapses.
Basal ganglia	Four nerve cell clusters of the basal ganglia or "nerve knots" help handle physical movements by relaying information from the cerebral cortex to the brainstem and cerebellum.
Brain stem	Located at the top of the spinal column, the brain stem relays information in and out of the brain. It is like the "point person" for all incoming and outgoing information and basic life functions. It is a major trunk at the top of the central nervous system, made up of the medulla, the pons, and the midbrain. The brainstem contains many of the centers for the senses of hearing, touch, taste, and balance. It does not affect sight and smell.
Brocca's area	Located in the lower portion of the motor cortex in the left frontal–temporal lobe; controls muscles of the face and mouth and enables the production of speech.
CARF	Commission for the Accreditation Rehabilitation Facilities is a national accreditation agency with standards for rehabilitation programs.
CDC	Centers for Disease Control and Prevention.
Cellulitis	Inflammation of the skin.
Cerebellum	Located in the lower back section of the brain, the cerebellum is the "movement" part of the brain that coordinates, modulates, and stores all body movement.
Cerebral cortex	This is divided into two hemispheres dedicated to the highest levels of thinking, moving, and acting. The right and left hemispheres are further divided into four lobes – frontal, parietal, temporal and occipital.
Cerebrospinal fluid (CSF)	Special fluid that bathes the brain inside the skull.
Clonic	Alternating contraction and relaxation of muscles.
Closed head injury	Skull is intact after an injury to the head.
Cognition	Conscious process of knowing or being aware of thoughts or perceptions, including understanding and reasoning.

Glossary

Cognitive impairment — Difficulty with perception, memory, attention and reasoning skills. Activities of daily living, such as hygiene, eating, household management, community re-integration, and many other aspects of day-to-day living are affected by cognitive changes.

Cogwheel rigidity — Rigidity with little jerks when the muscles in the arms and legs are stretched by the examiner.

COMBI — The Center on Outcome Measurement in Brain Injury is an online resource for detailed information and support on outcome measures for persons with brain injuries.

Common law — Law that is developed from court decisions.

Community skills — Abilities that enable someone to live and function safely in the community.

Competency or ***capacity*** — A legal term that basically reflects a mental ability to understand the nature and effect of one's acts.

Complex partial seizures — Formerly known as psycho-motor or temporal lobe seizures, consciousness is impaired. May be a warning or aura seizures usually last one to three minutes and may be followed by some confusion.

Confidentiality — Basic tenet in health care respecting confidential nature of patient information.

Constitutional law — Law based on the United States Constitution, as well as the constitution of the state where an individual lives.

Contractures — Abnormal, usually permanent condition of a joint characterized by flexion and fixation due to wasting away and abnormal shortening of muscle fibers and loss of skin elasticity.

Corpus callosum — Complex band of nerve fibers that exchanges information between the two hemispheres.

Cortex — "Thinking" part of the brain.

Corti — Organ where transmitted sound waves vibrate thousands of tiny sensitive hairs. Each hair is connected to thousands of nerve fibers which send signals through the eighth cranial (acoustic) nerve to the brainstem. There, many of the nerve fibers cross over before taking signals up to the tops of the temporal lobes for analysis.

Coup-contracoup — Effect when the back of the head is struck and the front of the brain is injured by the brain bouncing back and forth.

Deep venous thrombosis (***DVT***) — Blood clot in one of the deep veins of the body.

Dendrites — Networks of short "wires" in the neuron that branch out from a cell body and synapse with the ends of axons from other neurons.

Diencephalon — Located centimeters above the midbrain, the diencephalon is made up of the thalamus, hypothalamus, and other structures. It is a master relay center for forwarding information, sensations, and movement.

Glossary

Diffuse axonal injuries	Injuries caused by individual nerve cells stretching and breaking throughout the brain.
Dilatation	Widening.
Disability	Under the Americans with Disabilities Act, disability means "a physical or mental impairment that substantially limits one or more of the major life activities" of an individual (Source: 42 U.S.C. § 12102).
Dura mater	Outer hard matter of the brain, which is like a heavy plastic covering.
Duration	Length of time that a behavior occurs.
Duty to warn	Obligation of health care provider under common law or statutory third parties to inform when there is a risk of violence, contagious disease or other risk.
Dysphagia	Difficulty swallowing.
Electroencephalogram (EEG)	An electrical study of the brain's activity.
Empathy	Ability to identify with and understand another person's feelings or difficulties.
Escape and avoidance	Behavior that gets someone out of an unpleasant situation, or removes the threat of one.
Ethical standards	Standards of conduct rooted in the moral principles and values of society.
Executive functioning	The ability to plan, initiate, direct, and monitor one's activities. Involves organizing, planning, creating, evaluating, and initiating projects and activities.
Exploitation	Use of a dependent individual's property illegally or without the consent of the individual.
Expressive communication	Ability to express oneself to others through speech and language.
External physical force	Cause of traumatic brain injury, including motor vehicle crash, sports/recreation injury, falls, or assault.
Extinction	Weakening of a behavior by absence of a positive consequence.
Fading	Use of gradual change from artificial to more natural cueing stimuli.
Frequency	Number of times that a skill or behavior is observed to occur.
Frontal lobes	Include everything in front of the central fissure. When injured or damaged, an individual's ability to synthesize signals from the environment, assign priorities, make decisions, initiate actions, control emotions, behave and interact socially, make plans, and other executive like functions are severely compromised.
GAO	Government Accounting Office.
Gastrostomy tube	Tube placed through a surgical opening into the stomach to administer liquid feedings.

Glossary

Generalized seizures	Sudden burst of abnormal, generalized discharges that usually affect both hemispheres; subclassified as tonic-clonic and absence seizures.
Glial cells	Non-communicating ("glue") cells that support and nourish the neurons.
Guardian of the estate	Person who cares for the property of the ward.
Guardian of the person	Person who cares for the personal needs of the ward.
Guardianship	A legally enforceable arrangement under which one person, the guardian, has the legal right and duty to care for another, the ward.
HCBS	Home and Community-Based Services Waivers.
Health issues	Any factor that affects a person's physical well-being.
Health maintenance organization	An organizational structure of managed care that oversees the individual's care, usually with a gate-keeping mechanism that includes incentives for enrollees to use network providers. Includes elective contracting with providers, quality controls and risk-sharing arrangements.
Hematomas	Accumulation of blood or a collection of blood trapped in the tissues of the skin or in an organ
Hemiparesis	Weakness of one side of body.
Hemiplegia	Paralysis of one side of body.
Heterotopic ossification (HO)	Creation of abnormal growth of bone in soft tissues or around joints.
Hippocampus	A paired–organ, one on each side of the brain sitting within the temporal lobes, "between your ears" so to speak. Most commonly associated with memory functioning.
HMO	Health maintenance organization.
Household management	Meal preparation, housekeeping, money management, and other activities related to managing where one lives.
Hydrocephalus	Excess cerebrospinal fluid.
Hyperreflexive bladder	Bladder in which the need to empty is triggered easily.
Hypertension	Elevated blood pressure exceeding 140/90 mm Hg.
Hypotension	Low blood pressure (below 90/50).
Hypothalamus	Control center for hunger, thirst, sexual rhythms, endocrine levels, and temperature regulation. Also involved in many complex responses like anger, fatigue, memory, and calmness. Serves as the "conductor" of a person's emotional orchestra.
Hypoxia	Decreased amount of oxygen getting to the brain.

Glossary

IEP	An individualized education plan for a student found eligible for special education and/or related services that designates the kinds and extent of services that the student needs.
In school transitions	Change in school, including moving from grade level to grade level, elementary to middle and then high school, and finally, graduation.
Incidental teaching	Interactions between staff and individuals with brain injuries that occur outside the structured program.
Inclusion	Incorporation and welcome of the individual into the community, regardless of a disability.
Indemnity policy	The insurer assumes the responsibility of paying medical benefits for services performed and covered under a policy in return for premium payments.
Indwelling catheter	Foley catheter that remains in the bladder and drains urine continuously.
Informed consent	A patient's consent to health care based on a full disclosure of facts necessary to make an intelligent decision.
Initiation problems	Difficulty engaging in activities unless prompted.
Integration	Based on the expectation that people fit in, be alike and reach for similar standards.
Integumentary system	Skin, hair, nails, sweat, sebaceous glands.
Interdependence	An interconnection or an interrelationship between two or more entities that suggests a partnership between entities that maximizes potential for both groups.
Interdependent paradigm	Refers to a blended framework where people are seen to have gifts and capacities to build supports to engage community. Interdependence focuses on finding the points of connection between people.
Internal occurrence	Cause of injury to the brain by stroke, infectious disease, tumor, or loss of oxygen.
Intracranial pressure	Pressure inside the skull that builds as the brain swells; relieved by inserting special devices into the skull to monitor it.
Ischium	Back lower portions of the hip bones.
JCAHO	Joint Commission on the Accreditation of Health care Organizations, a national accreditation agency with standards for rehabilitation programs.
Larynx	Voice box.
Latency	Length of time that it takes a person to initiate (or complete) a behavior.
Legal rights	Powers or privileges that an individual has under the law.
Leisure skills	Ability to use free time in ways that are not harmful (i.e., substance abuse, or other dangerous activities).

Glossary

Limbic system	Located in the middle section of the brain, the limbic system sits on top of the brain stem and is involved in emotions and basic elemental feelings.
Living will	A document in which a competent adult provides written instructions to a physician on the provision, withholding or withdrawing of life-sustaining procedures when the individual is in a terminal or permanently unconscious condition.
Magnitude	Measurement of intensity, which is especially important for unwanted behaviors; seldom used because of difficulty in objectively measuring the intensity of an aggressive or self-injurious response.
Medicaid HCBS	A state can waive one or more of the requirements of eligibility for funding and provision of services providing the average per capita cost of providing these services does not exceed the cost of institutional care.
Medical model	Framework for delivering services that views a disability as a form of illness or sickness; most effective as a treatment model when the goal is to address sickness or establish medical stability.
Medical paradigm	Refers to the scientific framework that reduces the focus of attention to the deficits or dysfunction of the person. The medical paradigm is very narrow and looks to fix people's major problems.
Medulla	First area in the lower part of the brain stem which is involved in many basic living functions. It contains reflex centers which control many involuntary functions such as breathing, heart rate, blood pressure, swallowing, vomiting, and sneezing.
Memory problems	Considered the most disabling consequence of brain injury, impaired memory affects a person's ability to learn, retain, and use new information and may significantly affect a person's ability to live independently.
Meninges	Three membranes that cover the brain, containing the Dura mater, Arachnoid and Pia mater layers.
Midbrain	Smallest part of the brainstem and responsible for alertness and arousal.
Mild brain injury	Characteristics include: loss of consciousness for less than 30 minutes (or no loss); Glasgow Coma Scale of 13-15; post-traumatic amnesia for less than 24 hours; temporary or permanently altered mental or neurological state; post concussion symptoms.
Mobility	Ability to move about, either by walking, or with the aid of an assistive device; also includes the ability to transfer from one position to another.
Moderate brain injury	Characteristics include: coma more than 20-30 min., but less than 24 hours; Glasgow Coma Scale of 9-12; possible skull fractures with bruising & bleeding; signs on EEG, CAT or MRI scans; some long term problems in one or more areas.
Modified barium swallows	Specialized x-ray study that provides serial images of barium mixed with food of different consistencies.
Mutual reinforcement	Exchange of reinforcers or desired events between two or more people.

Glossary

Myoclonic seizure	Sudden brief contraction of muscle groups, producing rapid jerky movements in one or more extremities of the entire body.
Negative reciprocal relationship	Also called negative reciprocity, this refers to relationships that involve ongoing exchange of unwanted events between people.
Negative reinforcement	The removal of something unpleasant following a behavior that makes the behavior more likely to occur again.
Neglect	Failure to provide for the basic needs of a dependent individual.
Neurochemical transmitters	Leap the synaptic gaps between each neuron's axon and the other neurons with which an axon makes contact.
Neurogenic bladder	A neurologic impairment that affects bladder function.
Neurons	Billions and billions of tiny brain cells making up the nervous system which are the "communicators". Each neuron has a cell body, axon and dendrite.
NIDRR	The National Institute on Disability and Rehabilitation Research, under the US Department of Education, provides funding for a research and demonstration projects on various aspects of disability and rehabilitation.
No blame	Concept that proposes that if people are predisposed to behave in certain ways in certain situations, then holding them at fault or blame for unwanted actions does not make good sense.
Occipital lobes	The primary visual center which is located as far away from the eyes as possible in the back of the skull.
Olmstead decision	Interpreted Title II of the Americans with Disabilities Act to require states to administer services, programs, and activities "in the most integrated setting appropriate to the needs of qualified individuals with disabilities".
Open head injury	Skull is broken and the brain is exposed after an injury to the head.
Optic chiasm	Located near the back of the eyes, the optic nerves carrying these signals meet at this "crossing" where optic fibers from the inner half of each retina cross to the opposite hemisphere of the brain.
Outcome criteria	Evaluation of results based on therapeutic goals directly related to functional improvements in the individual.
Outcome oriented model	Identifies areas of agreement between people that are related to the goals of their assistance. This model stresses the accomplishments and successes of the person in question.
Outcome-driven treatment planning	Discharge site or the next placement is a primary focus for treatment planning, although the individual is the constant element in the treatment plan.
Parietal lobe	Caps the top of the brain behind the central fissure and merges into the occipital lobe. Responds to touch, heat, cold, pain, and body awareness; injury to the parietal lobe can cause a loss of these sensing abilities.

Glossary

Partial seizures — Arise from disturbances in specific, localized areas of one hemisphere of the brain; subclassified as simple partial or complex partial.

Patient's rights — Rights that an individual may exercise in addition to basic citizenship rights provided under the Constitution and other laws. Federal law provides patient's rights under the Medicare and Medicaid law. Patient's rights are also often a statutory set of rights in state law.

Percent of opportunities — Useful measure for knowing whether or not a behavior occurred when the opportunity was available.

Peristalsis — Coordinated, rhythmic contractions of smooth muscle that forces food through the digestive tract.

Person-centered treatment planning — Inclusion of the individual, whenever possible, in the development and design of the treatment plan as well as discussion of expected discharge site, outcome criteria, goals, objectives, and treatment methods.

Phlebitis — Inflammation of a vein.

Pia mater — Tender matter which molds around every tiny crook and crevice on the brain's surface.

Plenary guardianship — Person who cares for personal needs and the property of the ward.

Polydipsia — Excessive thirst.

Pons — Bridge of nerve fibers just above the medulla that connect the cerebral cortex and the cerebellum.

Positive reinforcement — The addition of something enjoyable that follows a behavior and makes it more likely to occur again.

Post-concussion symptoms — May or may not persist and include: headache, dizziness, vomiting, sleep disturbance, memory problems, changes in personality, irritability, depression, changes in personality, difficulty in problem solving, diminished attention span.

Postictal state — Person awakens after seizure to a state of confusion, extreme fatigue and no memory of the seizure.

Power of attorney — A document in which a competent person, the principal, appoints another, the agent, to act for him in legal and financial matters.

Preferred provider organization — A model of managed care with a specific organizational structure, elective contracting, quality controls and risk sharing arrangement.

Pre-frontal cortex — Located at the very front part of the frontal lobes (right over one's eyebrows), the prefrontal cortex is responsible for various emotional responses to circumstances.

Privilege — Right of the patient to withhold information that is communicated between the patient and health care provider.

Prolonged coma — Also known as minimally conscious state. Individuals still can breathe and their hearts beat, even without life supporting equipment. For individuals with

Glossary

minimal levels of consciousness, there may also be some minimal level of awareness to basic stimulations, (e.g., touch, light, temperature).

Punishment — A negative consequence of behavior that makes it less likely to happen again.

Rate — Number of times that a behavior occurs in a specified time period.

Receptive communication — Ability to understand others through speech and language.

Regurgitation — Return of swallowed food into the mouth which increases risk of aspiration.

Restraint — Any physical, mechanical, chemical or other means of restricting movement or access to one's body, against one's will.

Reticular activating system (RAS) — Collection of nerve fibers and nuclei within the brainstem that modulates or changes arousal, alertness, concentration, and basic biological rhythms.

Rewards — Good things that happen after a behavior and make it more likely to be repeated in the future. A reward strengthens or reinforces a behavior.

Seclusion — Isolating a person from others and physically preventing the individual from leaving a confined area.

Section 504 — Part of the Rehabilitation act of 1973 that requires schools receiving federal funding to provide reasonable accommodations to allow an individual with a disability to participate.

Seizures — Hyperexcitation, and abnormal, disorderly discharge of electrical activity in the nerve cells of the brain.

Selective Seratonin Reuptake Inhibitors — Antidepressant medications.

Self-help skills — Bathing, dressing, eating, grooming, and toileting; often referred to as activities of daily living (ADL skills).

Sensorimotor impairments — Changes affecting muscles groups and sensory modalities. Depending on the location and extent of injury to the brain, sensori-motor impairments can be localized to one extremity or side of the body or generalized.

Severe brain injury — Characteristics include: coma longer than 24 hours, often lasting days or weeks; Glasgow Coma Scale of 8 or less; bruising, bleeding in brain; signs on EEG, CAT or MRI scans; long term impairments.

Shaping — Reinforcement is provided only when a person gets progressively closer to the ultimate target behavior.

Simple partial seizures — Formerly known as focal motor or jacksonian seizures, person does not lose consciousness. Abnormal, localized electrical activity in the motor area of the brain may result in motor symptoms such as stiffening or jerking of muscles, eye movements, and unusual tongue movement, blinking and facial twitching.

Spasticity — Involuntary increase in muscle tone (tension) which causes the muscle to resist being stretched.

Glossary

Standard precautions	Approach to infection control that helps prevent transmission of bloodborne pathogens.
State demonstration projects	The Health Resources and Services Administration administers the TBI State Grant Program and funds demonstration projects by states to integrate services, establish policy, and procure financial support to bring about systems change by expanding and improving state and local capacity to care for individuals with TBI and their families.
Status epilepticus	Seizure that lasts longer than 5 minutes, or two or more seizures without time between for the person to recover consciousness.
Statutory law	Law that is enacted by Congress or a state legislature; statutory law is in the form of individual statutes which together form a code.
Sub-dural hematomas	Bleeding into the space between the dura mater and the Arachnoid layers of the meninges.
Surveillance	Ongoing and systematic collection, analysis and interpretation of data used to describe and monitor a health event.
Tardive dyskinesia	Side effect of antipsychotic medications resulting in involuntary movement disorder characterized by lip smacking, rhythmic darting of the tongue, chewing movements, aimless movements of the arms and legs and in severe cases, difficulty breathing and swallowing.
TBI Model Systems	Research centers involved in prospective, longitudinal multi-center efforts to examine the course of recovery and outcomes following TBI.
Temporal lobes	Rest on both sides of the brain and are the centers for language, hearing, and may be where memories are permanently stored.
Thalamus	Sits on the very top of the brain stem just beneath the cortex. Acts as a major relay station for incoming and outgoing sensory information. Each sense (except smell) relays its impulses through the thalamus.
Tonic	Excessive muscle tension/contraction.
Tonic-clonic seizures	Formerly known as grand mal, there is abrupt loss of consciousness. Body stiffens in tonic contraction at onset. Person may cry out, drop unconscious to the ground, roll up eyes or turn to the side, and bite tongue.
Torticollis	Twisted position of the neck.
Trachea	Wind pipe.
Tracheostomy	Surgical opening made through the neck with a tube inserted into the trachea to help with breathing.
Traumatic brain injury	An insult to the brain, not of a degenerative or congenital nature but caused by an external physical force, that may produce a diminished or altered state of consciousness, which results in an impairment of cognitive abilities or physical functioning. Defined under the Individuals with Disabilties Education Act as: "...an acquired injury to the brain caused by an external physical force, resulting in total or

Glossary

partial functional disability or psychosocial impairment, or both, that adversely affects a child's educational performance. The term applies to open or closed head injuries resulting in impairments in one or more areas, such as cognition; language; memory; attention; reasoning; abstract thinking; problem–solving; sensory, perceptual and motor abilities; psychosocial behavior; physical functions; information processing; and speech. The term does not apply to brain injuries that are congenital or degenerative, or brain injuries induced by birth trauma" (Section 300.7b[12] 1999).

Traumatic Brain Injury Act — Passed in 1996, this federal legislation expanded efforts for effective prevention, biomedical research and the improvement of services through state demonstration projects.

Urinary urgency — Sudden urge to urinate.

Vocational skills — Behaviors needed to get and keep a job.

Void — Urinate.

Wernicke's area — Located in the left temporal parietal lobe; governs a person's understanding of speech and the ability to make sense of the thoughts that are spoken.